Corneal Emergencies

Bhavana Sharma • Jeewan S. Titiyal
Editors

Corneal Emergencies

Springer

Editors
Bhavana Sharma
Department of Ophthalmology
All India Institute of Medical Sciences
Bhopal, India

Jeewan S. Titiyal
Cornea, Cataract and Refractive Surgery Services
Dr Rajendra Prasad Centre for Ophthalmic Sciences
All India Institute of Medical Sciences
New Delhi, India

ISBN 978-981-16-5878-5 ISBN 978-981-16-5876-1 (eBook)
https://doi.org/10.1007/978-981-16-5876-1

This Springer imprint is published by the registered company Springer Nature Singapore Pte Ltd.
The registered company address is: 152 Beach Road, #21-01/04 Gateway East, Singapore 189721, Singapore

Foreword

The contemporary medical literature affirms that the most common ophthalmic diagnoses addressed in emergency departments are problems related to the anterior structures of the eye, including the lids, cornea and conjunctiva. For this reason, both the ophthalmologist and the emergency medicine physician must be able to recognize, triage and manage these disorders effectively. In this volume, Profs Sharma and Titiyal and their colleagues have compiled a truly comprehensive treatise on urgent and emergent disorders of the cornea and external eye.

Beginning with the basic pathophysiology of corneal injuries and the requisites for diagnosis and treatment, this book progresses from minor corneal injuries to severe trauma, corneal infections, management of perforations, chemical injuries, postsurgical complications, contact lens-associated emergencies, peripheral ulcerative keratitis, complications of ectatic diseases, systemic inflammatory diseases affecting the ocular surface, keratomalacia and the medicolegal aspects of corneal emergencies.

In the setting of a busy emergency department, ocular emergencies are often deemed less urgent, even when permanent vision loss may be the result. The reason for this, in part, is the press of potentially life-threatening emergencies that may preempt attention to other 'less immediate' issues. However, the downgrading of urgency may also be the result of lack of familiarity with the nature of corneal emergencies. For this reason, it is even more important that the emergency medicine physician understand the degree of urgency that accompanies corneal disease and trauma in the emergency department.

Enlisting a group of experienced clinicians as contributors, the editors provide us with a book that is a truly comprehensive resource for the corneal specialist, the general ophthalmologist and the emergency medicine physician. Both a scholarly text and a useful 'manual', this volume will be an important clinical opus in our field.

Mark J. Mannis, MD, FACS
Fosse Endowed Chair in Vision Science Research
Professor and Chair
Department of Ophthalmology and Vision Science
University of California Davis Eye Center
Davis, Sacramento, CA, USA

Preface

Corneal emergencies are one of the most common ocular emergencies. They may be accidental or iatrogenic in nature and encompass a plethora of conditions including trauma, infections, chemical injuries and postsurgical complications. Together, they constitute a significant burden of avoidable corneal blindness and warrant immediate intervention to prevent sight-threatening sequelae.

This book is a comprehensive compilation of the various corneal emergencies encountered by ophthalmologists in their day-to-day practice. The chapters systematically cover the basic pathophysiology, clinical examination, essential investigations and treatment algorithms for the different corneal emergencies. Special attention has been paid to incorporate the recent advances in the diagnosis and treatment of emergencies associated with ocular surface disorders, corneal ectasia and microbial keratitis. The written material is structured in a lucid fashion with numerous tables, flowcharts and colour illustrations to help the readers understand and assimilate the information easily. The highlights of each chapter are summarized at the end as key points in order to provide the important information at a glance.

The myriad corneal emergencies may manifest in different forms requiring a good diagnostic acumen and meticulous management approach. The immediate treatment received at the point of first contact is a significant determinant of final visual and anatomical outcomes in any ocular emergency. Ophthalmology, like all of medicine, is increasingly becoming specialized with surgeons mastering specific skill sets; however, a knowledge of corneal emergencies is imperative for all ophthalmologists regardless of their field of interest. This book provides a comprehensive overview of the presentation of various corneal emergencies and details a step-by-step management to enable optimal outcomes. I believe this book would serve as a useful guide and valuable resource not just for the residents and fellows who often handle the emergency department but also for the senior corneal specialists.

I would like to express my sincere gratitude to all the authors for their valuable contributions to this book. I would also like to thank Springer publications and their staff for facilitating the publication and distribution of this book.

New Delhi, India Jeewan S. Titiyal

Preface

Corneal emergencies are visually debilitating ocular conditions of fairly common occurrence necessitating emergency intervention. Its management has undergone significant transformation with new diagnostic and therapeutic options that have changed the treatment paradigm over the last several decades. The editors and authors have endeavoured to provide the most recent resource for residents, fellows, clinicians and researchers in the management of corneal emergencies. One of the great strengths of this book is the vast experience and clinical expertise of contributors of this book. It gives the distilled experience of the world's leaders in this field and outlines their approach and justification for the same

This book was conceptualized while observing residents as they managed various emergencies during their training period. I felt that there was a need for a concise, informative and practical book on corneal emergencies. Subsequently, I conversed with residents and fellows and also reached out to those who had completed their residency, regarding the need and utility for such a book. The feedback on the need for an authoritative resource in the field of corneal emergencies was unanimous rendering confidence that comprehensive knowledge of corneal emergencies can be unravelled through this book.

The book deals with an important and yet uncovered subtopic of the cornea through thoughtfully curated chapters, clinical photographs and key points incorporated in the chapters. It intends to provide comprehensive knowledge of corneal emergencies, their risk factors, causative agents, diagnostic pearls, treatment challenges and management options through explanatory flow diagrams and diagnostic and treatment algorithms accompanied by numerous illustrative photographs, diagrams and sketches. The figures and illustrations have been designed to provide an informative and vivid representation of referenced conditions. Much emphasis is on practical management, supplemented with preferred practice patterns, guidelines and other authoritative sources.

Corneal emergencies are an integral part of postgraduate curriculum. This book shall serve as essential reading for postgraduate students, trainees, fellows and ophthalmic practitioners in addition to supplementary/recommended reading for undergraduate students. Ophthalmic practitioners would immensely benefit from this book by way of its comprehensive approach to the diagnosis and management of corneal emergencies which would further their understanding to better manage such cases and to avoid potential consumer litigations.

I am extremely grateful for input, advice and support received from colleagues, staff and students, in particular Dr Deepak Soni who was instrumental in meticulous data curation and overall editing. Dr Sajith Haridas and Dr Ananyan Sampath for their contribution towards skilful sketches and drawings without which many of the images in the book would not have been possible. We thank colleagues From Dr RP Centre AIIMS New Delhi for graciously allowing the use of clinical photographs from their collection. Finally, I would like to acknowledge the support and commitment of the staff at Springer Nature in completing the book to perfection.

Bringing out a book on a subject like corneal emergencies was enormous and complex and was made possible by the concerted efforts of the contributing authors of this book. I am obliged to all the contributing authors for sharing their knowledge and expertise and the time and effort they have put into the writing of this book. I am extremely grateful to Prof Mark J Mannis for being a source of great inspiration in the field of academics, research and clinical care. He has been kind enough for taking the time to contribute a brilliant foreword for this book. I am indebted to my co-editor Padmashree Prof Jeewan Singh Titiyal for his invaluable help and guidance at every step. I would also like to acknowledge my family for their patience and constant support to accomplish this work.

We hope this book will benefit students, practising ophthalmologists and thereby the patients for years to come.

Happy reading!

Bhopal, India Bhavana Sharma

About the Editors

Bhavana Sharma is currently the Head of Department of Ophthalmology and Dean Examinations at All India Institute of Medical Sciences, Bhopal, India. She completed her graduation and postgraduation from the Regional Institute of Ophthalmology, Bhopal, and was conferred with gold medal for the best outgoing postgraduate student. She further completed her training in cornea and cataract from Dr RP Centre AIIMS, New Delhi. She specializes in Cornea, Cataract and Ocular Surface Diseases. She is presently deliberating her academic, clinical and administrative duties at AIIMS Bhopal in addition to being in charge of cornea clinic and eye bank services. She has numerous publications in international and national journals to her credit, in addition to chapters in various books. She serves as a reviewer for major international and national journals and text books, in addition to being an editorial board member of prestigious international ophthalmology journals. She has been conferred with achievement award of All India Ophthalmological Society for significant contribution towards academics. She has presented more than 150 papers in various conferences and has been awarded best paper awards of cornea, cataract and trauma sessions and the most coveted Best of Best Paper Award. She is frequently invited as guest faculty by various organizations to deliver guest lectures and chair scientific sessions in addition to conducting instruction courses. She has served as vice president, treasurer and general secretary of divisional ophthalmic societies in addition to chair of various institutional and government committees.

Jeewan S. Titiyal completed his graduation, postgraduation and training from All India Institute of Medical Sciences (AIIMS), New Delhi, and is presently the chief at Dr Rajendra Prasad Centre For Ophthalmic Sciences, AIIMS New Delhi. His areas of expertise include cataract surgery keratoplasty, refractive surgery, stem cell transplantation, contact lens and low vision aids. He has dedicated his academic career to the pursuit of excellence in the field of Ophthalmology, and this book is a part of his endeavours to transmit knowledge and skills to the generation of Ophthalmologists. He has been invited by various organizations to deliver keynote addresses, orations and guest lectures and chair scientific sessions. Dr Titiyal is the first Indian to perform live surgery at the American Society of Cataract and Refractive Surgery (ASCRS), USA. He has to his credit numerous publications in peer-reviewed journals and various books and chapters as well. He has been awarded the 'Senior Achievement Award' by the American Academy of Ophthalmology (2016), the 'Achievement award' by the Asia Pacific Academy of Ophthalmology (2015), the APACRS Educator Award (2015), the prestigious RP Dhandha Award and P. Siva Reddy Award by the All India Ophthalmological Society and numerous gold medals. The 'Padma Shri', one of the highest civilian awards in 2014, was conferred on him in recognition of his exemplary contributions in the field of medicine by the Government of India.

Contents

1 Anatomical, Pathophysiological, and Wound Healing Aspects in Corneal Emergencies

Harsha Saxena, Samendra Karkhur, Arvind Maurya, and Bhavana Sharma

1.1 Introduction

Cornea is the predominant refractive component of the eye. It forms the outermost layer of the eye along with sclera, accounting for nearly 70% of the refractive power of human optical system [1]. The optical clarity and corneal dimensions serve as essential integrals for focusing the light, un-deviated over the retinal surface. Additionally, it serves as a structural barrier protecting the eye against physical, biological, and chemical threats. Loss of cellular integrity of cornea can be a cause of impaired visual acuity. However, the unique cellular anatomy of cornea enables rapid restoration of afflicted tissue, in order to maintain anatomical and functional integrity. Consequent to the disruption of corneal function, as a result of infectious, inflammatory, or traumatic insult, there is a simultaneous ingress of inflammatory cells, differentiation of fibroblasts, collagen and extracellular matrix synthesis, and subsequent scar formation with or without fibrovascular proliferation.

This chapter would focus on anatomical and pathophysiological aspects of corneal emergencies, the main events in corneal wound healing and maintenance of corneal transparency.

1.2 Anatomical Considerations

Cornea is a biconvex, aspheric, and avascular structure with an anterior and posterior curvature of 7.8 mm and 6.5 mm, respectively. With a refractive index of 1.376, cornea contributes nearly 2/3rd of the total refractive power of about 48 D [1, 2].

H. Saxena · S. Karkhur · B. Sharma (✉)
All India Institute of Medical Sciences, Bhopal, Madhya Pradesh, India
e-mail: head.ophtho@aiimsbhopal.edu.in

A. Maurya
All India Institute of Medical Sciences, Bibinagar, Andhra Pradesh, India

B. Sharma, J. S. Titiyal (eds.), *Corneal Emergencies*,
https://doi.org/10.1007/978-981-16-5876-1_1

The central corneal thickness ranges from 551 to 565 μm and the peripheral corneal thickness from 612 to 640 μm [1, 2]. Corneal thickness gradually increases from center to the periphery, due to increase in the amount of collagen in the peripheral stroma.

The corneal layers from superficial to deep are epithelium, Bowman's layer, stroma, Descemet's membrane, and endothelium. A well-defined, acellular layer in pre-Descemet's region known as Dua's membrane has gained attention recently (Table 1.1) [2].

Corneal layers serve specific functions in maintaining the physiology, thereby combating the pathology. Epithelium, being the outermost layer, plays a critical role in preserving the integrity and transparency of cornea, while stroma provides mechanical strength. Endothelium maintains relative dehydration besides being a resistant structure for infectious or inflammatory insult and limbal stem cells play a vital role in the maintenance of outermost epithelial layer of the cornea (Table 1.2).

Descemet's membrane is tightly adherent to the posterior surface of the corneal stroma and reflects any alteration in the stromal contour. Certain factors could result in the rupture of Descemet's membrane such as compression birth injury, mechanical trauma, etc., subsequently resulting in the ingress of aqueous into the corneal stroma, leading to stromal edema.

1.3 Physiological Considerations

1.3.1 Epithelium

Tissue transparency is the structural and functional requisite for refractive property. The corneal epithelium along with the tear film maintains an optically smooth surface and protects the underlying layers from infection and impairment. The epithelium possesses remarkable regenerative power to restore any breach in surface epithelium, through mitotic activity and cellular migration. The tight desmosome connections between the epithelial cells, comprising of "zonula occludens" with surface glycocalyx prevent the binding of pathogens and provide a selective barrier for penetration of unwanted substances, besides maintaining the corneal deturgescence [3].

1.3.2 Stroma

Corneal stroma is sandwiched between two layers which possess distinct structural and functional properties. A stratified layer of epithelial cells protects the cornea from external environment and tear-borne pathogens while providing the first physical barrier. The endothelium lines the inner surface of the stroma toward anterior chamber and is constituted by a fragile single layer of cells with limited regenerative capacity.

Table 1.1 Anatomy of cornea

Corneal layer	Thickness (μm)	Embryonic origin	Composition and function
Epithelium	50–90	Surface ectoderm	Uniform layer composed of nonkeratinized stratified squamous epithelium, with five or six layers of three different types of cells: superficial cells, wing cells, and columnar basal cells. It provides a smooth regular surface for hydrophilic spread of the tear film with each eyelid blink. The intercellular tight junction complexes prohibit tears from entering the intercellular spaces and maintain relative dehydration of cornea
Bowman's membrane	8–14	Mesodermal	This smooth layer is not a true membrane and is acellular condensation of Type I and V collagen with proteoglycans and helps the cornea maintains its shape. It is relatively resistant to infection and injury. It has no regenerative ability
Stroma	500	Neural crest	Stroma is made up of keratocytes and ECM, which is composed of regularly arranged collagens (Type I, III, V, VI) and glycosaminoglycans like keratan sulfate, chondroitin sulfate, and dermatan sulfate. This attributes to the physical strength, stability of shape, and transparency of cornea. The uniform arrangement and continuous slow turnover of collagen fibers in the stroma are essential for corneal transparency
Dua's membrane (pre-Descemet's membrane)	15		It is a well-defined, acellular layer, which is impervious to air and provides strength
Descemet's membrane	6–10	Neural crest	Descemet's membrane is elastic and made up of Type IV collagen and laminin. It curls on getting severed. Endothelial cells continuously secrete Descemet's membrane
Endothelium	5	Neural crest	The endothelium is a single layer structure. The cells are orderly arranged cuboidal metabolically active cells. The endothelial cells contain high density of pumps, which maintain relative corneal dehydration. Endothelial cells do not regenerate.

The mechanical strength and optical characteristics of the corneal stroma are owing to a unique structure and spatial arrangement of collagen fibers. Corneal stromal fibers exhibit a uniform spacing that is maintained by virtue of intramolecular forces in extracellular matrix (ECM), as well as by a tightly controlled movement of water molecules. Additionally, membrane-active ion transport works to

Table 1.2 Wound healing response of corneal layers in various emergencies

S. No	Corneal emergency	Epithelial response	Stromal response	Endothelial response	Limbal response	Outcome
1.	Microbial keratitis	1. Expression of IL-1 and IL-6 2. Increase in the number of cells attaching to fibronectin matrix 3. Expression of integrin in corneal epithelial cells 4. Corneal epithelial cell migration through modulation of the fibronectin–integrin system	1. Direct degradation by collagenase produced by pathogen 2. Degradation by MMPs released from bacterial elastase activated keratocytes 3. Keratocytes and infiltrated cells secrete cytokines/growth Factors to modulate cells in the healing of corneal stroma	Endothelial–mesenchymal transformation with change in size and shape followed by migration to the affected area	Limbal Stem Cells divide by terminal differentiation to replace damaged cells	1. Tissue necrosis 2. Corneal perforation 3. Scarring
2.	Corneal Perforation	1. Release of growth factors and cytokines 2. Secretion of mediators like KGF, HGF, IL-1, PDGF, EGF, IGF, and TGF-β 3. These mediators regulate transformation of keratocytes to myofibroblasts	1. Infiltration of PMNs from the limbal vessels 2. Myofibroblastic transformation of keratocytes 3. Deposition of ECM, resulting in stromal remodeling with or without fibrotic changes	ECM proteins, fibronectin, and TSP-1 stimulate migration of corneal endothelial cells	Proliferation of cells increases many folds in both central and peripheral limbus	Hypertrophic scar

3.	Corneal Sloughing	Releases IL-1α and TGF-β2 into the stroma	1. IL-1α induces some of the stromal keratocytes to undergo cell death, others to proliferate, which secrete MMPs, and transform into an activated phenotype 2. TGF-β2 induces keratocytes to transform into myofibroblasts that secrete ECM	Growth factors like EGF, FGF-2, IL-1β, PDGF-BB, TGF-β2, and VEGF, promote endothelial migration and wound healing	Deficient equilibrium between the centripetal movement of epithelial cells, differentiation of basal cells, and the desquamation of epithelial cells	Pseudo-cornea/Anterior staphyloma
4.	Corneal Laceration	1. Epithelial cell differentiation, proliferation, and migration 2. Up-regulation of fibronectin–integrin system interactions, hyaluronan, and modulation of the ECM by newly expressed proteolytic enzymes	Keratocytes transdifferentiate into myofibroblasts and actively produce matrix components	Endothelium closes the wound gap mainly by migration and increased cell spreading	Limbal fibroblasts markedly upregulate KGF expression and limbal epithelial cells show elevated expression of its receptor	Complete healing with scar formation of variable depth

(continued)

Table 1.2 (continued)

S. No	Corneal emergency	Epithelial response	Stromal response	Endothelial response	Limbal response	Outcome
5.	Peripheral Ulcerative Keratitis	1. Inflammatory stimulus in the peripheral cornea results in neutrophil recruitment and complements activation 2. Release of cytokines and proteases	1. Infiltration of mononuclear cells, granulocytes secreting MMPs and other proteolytic enzymes 2. Imbalance between MMPs and their tissue inhibitors (TIMPs)	Provoke endothelial cell apoptosis and ensuing healing	T-cell mediated antibody production and formation of immune complexes deposition in marginal cornea	1. Thinning 2. Tissue necrosis of stroma 3. Variable scarring
6.	SJS / TEN [10–12]	1. Recurrent erosion due to mechanical degradation and dry eye 2. Release of cytokines like TNF-α, IL1, and MMP 3. Impaired integrity of corneal epithelial junctional complexes	1. Keratocyte apoptosis 2. VEGF and TGF-β contribute to neovascularization, with ECM components supporting the growth of new vessels	Disruption of pump mechanism in severe cases, results in variable healing.	1. Deficiency of limbal stem cells results in impairment of corneal epithelial homeostasis	1. Persistent epithelial defects 2. Recurrent ulcers and perforation 3. Dry eyes 4. Conjunctivalization

7.	Alkali Injury [10, 13]	1. Direct tissue damage such as protein hydrolysis, and saponification 2. Neutrophil chemo attraction by expression of inflammatory cytokines and MMPs 3. PMN release collagenase and superoxide free radicals that damage the tissue further	1. Tear neutrophils adhere to the surface of the denuded stroma and release tissue-degrading MMPs 2. The proinflammatory cytokine TNF-α is up-regulated in response to injury 3. VEGF and TGF contribute to injury-induced neovas-cularization, with ECM components supporting the growth of new vessels	1. Interfere with the pump mechanism 2. Reversible corneal edema 3. Simultaneous loss of glycosaminoglycans	1. Severe inflammation leads to limbal stem cell damage 2. Remaining stem cell population heals first by propagation of pluripotential epithelial stem cells around the corneal periphery and then by centripetal growth of phenotypic cells	1. Delayed healing 2. Persistent epithelial defects/perforation 3. Conjunctivalization 4. Scarring
8.	Contact Lens Related Hypoxia [14, 15]	1. Disrupts renewal mechanisms, producing a thinned, stagnant epithelium 2. LDH enzyme released by damaged or dying cells 3. IL-1 release in response to microtrauma	1. Low oxygen transmissibility results in a shift to anaerobic metabolism 2. Increase in stromal lactic acid and CO_2 3. Drop in stromal pH 4. Stromal swelling	1. Inhibit endothelial Na/K ATPase. 2. Pleomorphism and polymegathism	Limbal epithelium exhibits a higher proliferative activity and a lower differentiation capability	1. Corneal edema 2. Epithelial Haze 3. Variable scarring

(continued)

Table 1.2 (continued)

S. No	Corneal emergency	Epithelial response	Stromal response	Endothelial response	Limbal response	Outcome
9.	Advanced Corneal Ectasia [5, 16, 17]	1. Release IL-1 in response to microtrauma occurring after eye rubbing 2. Early degeneration of the basal epithelial cells 3. Disruption of the basement membrane 4. Breaks in the epithelial layer with epithelium growing posteriorly into Bowman's layer and collagen growing anteriorly into the epithelium	1. Increased sensitivity of keratocytes to IL-1 by increased binding sites 2. Up-regulation of proteolytic enzymes result in degradation of the extracellular matrix of the stroma and subsequent thinning 3. IL-1 induces apoptosis of stromal keratocytes	1. Pleomorphism and polymegathism	Limbal Stem Cells divide by terminal differentiation to replace damaged cells	1. Thinning 2. Perforation 3. Scarring
10.	Refractive Surgeries [18–20]	1. Damage to epithelial cells and corneal nerves result in increased production of cytokines like TGF-β, IGF, etc., which goes to stroma 2. Up-regulation of migration of precursor cells from limbal stem cells 3. Resurfacing of damaged epithelium	1. Keratocytes death leads to activation of stromal cells 2. Immune cell infiltration, 3. Myofibroblast transformation 4. Accumulation of fibrotic ECM 5. Variable scarring/haze depending on the amount of fibrotic remodeling	1. Endothelial–mesenchymal transformation 2. Cell apoptosis and ensuing healing	Limbal Stem Cells divide to replace lost cells	1. Epithelial/stromal haze 2. Variable Scarring

prevent the development of edema and supply the substrates for ongoing metabolic activity of its outer stratified epithelium and inner monocellular endothelium.

The corneal stroma is normally maintained in a relatively dehydrated state by balancing out of the forces between, inter-fibrillary imbibition of fluid and the fixed negatively charged keratan and chondroitin sulfate repelling each other. The swelling tendency is termed as the swelling pressure (SP). Imbibition pressure (IP) is a negative force that draws fluid into the stroma. The equation that describes the relationship between these parameters is: IP = IOP – SP [2].

The corneal stroma swells if the efficiency of the endothelium pump is diminished or lost, leading to an alteration in the regular interval between collagen fibrils. The disturbance in regular arrangement of the inter-fiber distance scatters the light passing through cornea and results in haziness.

1.3.3 Endothelium

The corneal endothelium is critical toward preventing stromal edema and maintaining normal corneal thickness, via a membrane-active ion-transport mechanism, essential for corneal homeostasis.

A minimum number of functioning endothelial cells is critical to prevent corneal swelling and subsequent opacification. This limit has been reported to be 500–800 cells/mm^3 [4]. Endothelial cells contain Na^+-K^+-ATP-ase on the side-walls, which ensures a relatively dehydrated state of the cornea. However, the endothelial layer possesses weak mitotic activity and poor regenerative capacity [2].

1.4 Corneal Wound Healing

Status-quo in the corneal anatomical structure is vital toward efficient functioning of the physiological, immunological, and optical roles of corneal tissue. The cornea being vulnerable to external insults is equipped with an active biodefense system and possesses a robust immune system, responsible for wound healing. Being an avascular structure, cornea differs from rest of the body in wound healing. Wound healing mechanism varies significantly in different layers of cornea, which themselves vary mutually, in their anatomical and physiological attributes.

The epithelium healing is consequent to migration and differentiation of limbal stem cells without undergoing transformation to morphologically distinct cell types. In contrast, during stromal wound healing, the stromal keratocytes differentiate into fibroblasts and myofibroblasts; this requires significant recruitment of resident and circulating immune cells. Corneal endothelium, unlike any other cellular components of cornea, heals by cellular migration and spreading. It may also additionally include endothelial–mesenchymal transformation; however, cell proliferation only contributes secondarily to this phenomenon [5].

1.4.1 Epithelial Healing

1.4.1.1 Cellular Events

The epithelium plays an integral role in maintaining corneal transparency and clear vision. Besides, it secretes the epithelial basement membrane which, along with a stable and smooth tear film is a prerequisite for a healthy corneal healing. Corneal epithelium has a turn-over time of 7–10 days, during which the outermost cells are shed into the tear film. Any breach in corneal epithelium accelerates this process leading to quicker healing of purely epithelial injuries [2].

Corneal epithelial wound healing entails:

- Cellular migration
- Proliferation
- Adhesion to basement membrane
- Differentiation with cell-layer stratification.

Corneal epithelium is constantly replaced by fresh cells from limbal epithelial stem cells (LESC) that exclusively reside in limbus. These cells migrate centripetally to the injured part of the cornea, multiply rapidly, and differentiate into mature epithelial cells. As these cells move from the limbus to the central cornea, they also differentiate and migrate from the deeper layers to the more superficial ones (Fig. 1.1). This process occurs in normal homeostasis as well as wound healing. The limbus stem cells participate in the regeneration and maintenance of cornea through centripetal cell migration [6]. Deficiencies or damage to LESC, as in cases of chemical burns, lead to alteration in corneal wound healing, stromal neovascularization and conjunctivalization of cornea, resulting in corneal opacification [5, 7].

1.4.1.2 Molecular Events

Corneal epithelial healing involves complex interplay of growth factors, cytokine, and extra cellular matrix (ECM) and their signal-mediated interactions at the site of injury, to restore integrity and homeostasis. Corneal cells express various growth factors and cytokines, which have specific effects on epithelial cells. Noteworthy among them are epidermal growth factor (EGF), platelet-derived growth factor (PDGF), transforming growth factors(TGF) α and β, fibroblast growth factors (FGF), acidic fibroblast growth factors (FGF-1) and basic fibroblast growth factors (FGF-2), insulin-like growth factor (IGF-I), keratinocyte growth factor (KGF),

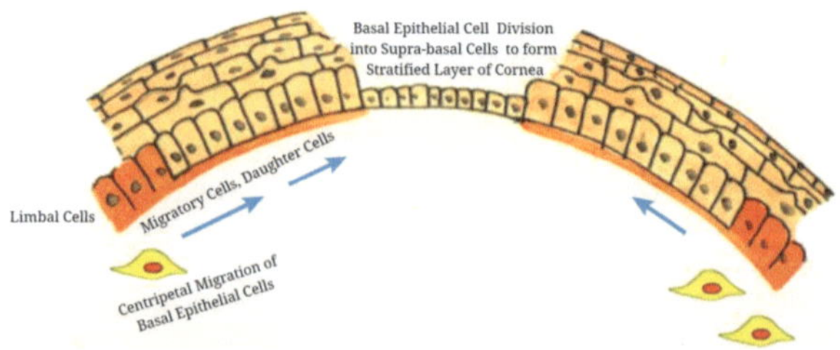

Fig. 1.1 Limbal cell migration and epithelial healing

hepatocyte growth factor (HGF), thymosin-β_4,(Tβ_4), interleukins (IL)-1, -6, and -10, and tumor necrosis factor (TNF)-α [5–8]. These factors are up-regulated in corneal wound healing, and triggering a cascade of events resulting in migration of epithelial cells [5].

EGF is a polypeptide and a potent stimulator of corneal epithelial cells' proliferation. It also promotes cellular adhesion to fibronectin matrix [5, 8]. The stimulatory effects of EGF are modulated by TGF. It also promotes migration of corneal epithelial cells. FGF-2 is a polypeptide growth factor which stimulates the proliferation of several other cells. Matrix metalloproteinases (MMPs) are released early during wound healing and initiate the mechanisms to disengage cell–cell and cell–matrix adhesion. Interleukins regulate the responses of the immune system, evoke inflammation, and vary tissue responses to environmental stimuli. They modulate the immune or inflammatory cell activity, both locally and systemically [5].

Cellular migration depends on the controlled interaction of cells, in coherence with underlying ECM. The migratory cells attach to the ECM proteins such as fibronectin, tenascin, and laminin, which act as their scaffold [5]. The control is governed by timely cessation of the cell to cell and cell to matrix attachment. The disengagement is done by degradation of matrix proteins. This controlled process of attachment and termination of attachment results in cell migration. The epithelial basement membrane also has important function in regulating cellular motility. On the one hand, the damaged basement membrane (BM) undergoes rearrangement and reintegration, along with various chemotactic factors to regulate migration of epithelial cells into the wound. On the other hand, discontinuity of the BM results in bidirectional passage of the cytokines like TGF-β and PDGF between epithelium and the stroma [5, 9].

1.4.2 Epithelial Wound Healing Response

Epithelial wound healing includes a complex cascade of cellular phenomena, depending on the severity of affliction. The response of epithelial cells to varied grades, types, and duration of insult determines the outcome with reference to visual and structural integrity. Any breach in the corneal epithelium can activate a series of growth factors (GFs) and cytokines, which are responsible for cellular interactions that heal and renew the affected area. The complex dynamic process is mediated by fibronectin–integrin interaction and ECM modulation by newly expressed enzymes, under control of various cytokines and growth factors [5, 10–20]. Epithelial wound healing response in common corneal emergencies is described below.

1.4.2.1 Corneal Abrasion

An abrasion in cornea is a defect in the continuity of the superficial layers of the cornea, not involving the Bowman membrane. The epithelial response to corneal abrasion is initiated by retraction of basal and squamous epithelial cells at the margin of the defect with chemotaxis of polymorphonuclear cells (PMN's) and limbal stem cells.

Migration from the basal to superficial layers is quite rapid, as compared to the centripetal movement from the limbus to the corneal center. The normal physiologic process of corneal homeostasis is exaggerated in the event of a corneal injury. While healing, the corneal epithelial cells flatten, spread, and migrate across the defect until it is fully covered. Cellular proliferation begins, approximately 24-h after injury and is independent of cellular migration. Limbal stem cells respond by proliferation, giving rise to transient amplifying cells. These cells migrate to fill the tissue defect and proliferate to restore the normal corneal integrity [21]. Healing of the epithelium is considered to be complete when the regenerated epithelial cells anchor themselves to the underlying Bowman membrane. It is only when the basement membrane is secreted and organized during the cellular migration that the epithelial cells develop strong, permanent adhesions.

The magnitude and extent of corneal regenerative response to a corneal abrasion is directly proportional to the size of the wound. Large epithelial defects bring about enhanced amplification in the rate of epithelial cell migration and limbal stem cell mitosis. Stevens–Johnson syndrome (SJS), chemical injuries, and contact lens-induced keratopathy could result in irreversible limbal damage and hence cause delayed corneal wound healing, recurrent corneal epithelial erosions and vascularization, and conjunctival epithelial in-growth [5, 22].

1.4.2.2 Corneal Ulcer

Cornea acts as a physical barrier in protecting intraocular milieu, owing to the tight intercellular junctions in the epithelial layer. Discontinuation of normal corneal epithelium associated with necrosis of ulcer base and surrounding tissue leads to formation of corneal ulcer (Fig. 1.2). As the ulcer develops, cellular reorganization and proteinase synthesis occur. This causes the loosening of cell adhesion, like desmosomes, hemidesmosomes and changes in collagen type VII fibers arrangement [23]. The cells assume a flattened morphology and move to fill the defect. Subsequently, the distal cells proliferate and migrate to replenish the wound, followed by cellular differentiation and stratification. Finally, the cell adhesion structures are remodeled, and ECM is synthesized. During the process of epithelial renewal and repair, the secretion of ECM components is altered, influencing the expression of MMP. MMPs are responsible for catalyzing ECM molecules, such as collagen, proteoglycans, and fibronectin, helping to maintain the corneal structure and functions. The expression and performance of MMPs are regulated by GF and cytokines, such as IL-1 and TGF-b, enabling cell migration and tissue repair (Fig. 1.2) [5, 22].

1.4.2.3 Thermal Burns

Thermal injury results in corneal abrasions. Direct thermal injury to the cornea induces collagen shrinkage, with prominent stress lines radiating centrifugally from the injury. Epithelial healing response resembles that of abrasion.

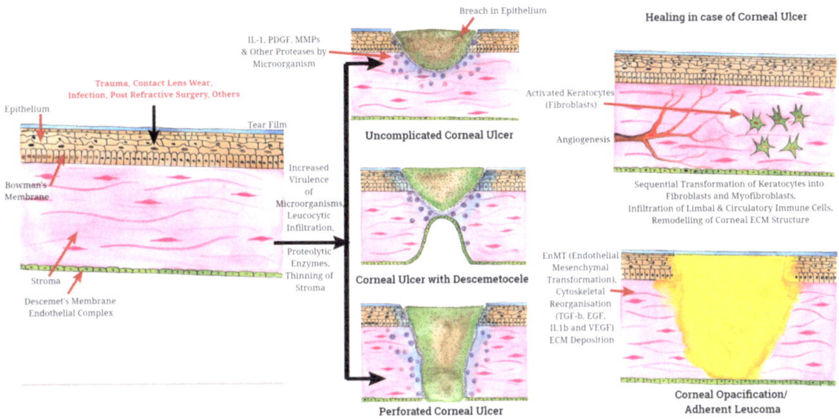

Fig. 1.2 Wound healing response in corneal ulcer

1.4.2.4 Stevens–Johnson Syndrome

SJS is a severe cutaneous adverse reaction (SCAR), a subcategory of adverse drug reactions (ADR). The epithelium is damaged both clinically and histologically, at an initial stage. It is associated with loose hemidesmosome adhesions. The integrity of corneal epithelial tight junctions is based on the interaction between—epithelial cells' derived cytokines, immune cells stromal keratocytes, and tear fluid. The damage to the junctional integrity disrupts existing intercellular equilibrium and results in epithelial erosions.

Severe inflammation and dry eye could also lead to damage to the ocular surface integrity, mediated by the interaction of keratocytes with cytokines. TNF-α, IL-1, and MMP are the key cytokines that are involved in surface damage and repair. IL-1 is a key inducer of other inflammatory cytokines, including TNF-α and MMP and is also up-regulated in dry eye disease [24]. There is late infiltration with lymphocytes in the epithelium. TNF-α is secreted by keratocytes or monocyte and macrophage cells, which play a vital role in corneal wound healing. SJS is also associated with poor limbal stem cells reserve, which promotes conjunctivalization and episodes of recurrent erosions [25].

1.4.2.5 Chemical Injuries

An ocular chemical injury results when a corrosive substance comes in contact with the eye and/or peri-ocular tissues. The pathophysiological event starts with an abnormally rapid change of tissue pH (Fig. 1.3). Alkaline agents contain the "hydroxyl ion," which brings about saponification of fatty-acids in the cell membranes and results in cellular disruption; the alkalis, in general, penetrate the tissue deeper than acids. Once the epithelium is compromised, alkaline solutions penetrate more rapidly into the underlying tissues, destroying proteoglycan

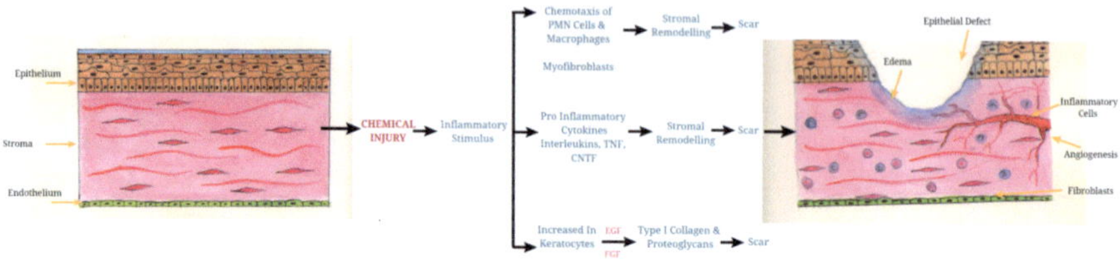

Fig. 1.3 Wound healing response in acute chemical injury

ground substance and the collagen matrix. Acidic agents denature tissue proteins, resulting in a coagulation necrosis and resulting in the formation of a barrier that prevents further tissue penetration [26]. Alkalis, on the other hand, continue unabated tissue destruction, due to the lack of formation of a similar chemically-induced tissue-barrier.

The lysis of cell membrane results in release of chemotactic and inflammatory mediators, such as interleukins, leukotrienes, and prostaglandins initiating a rapid immunological response. Within the first few hours after corneal epithelial injury, the margin of intact epithelium propagates fine extensions toward the site of injury [27]. Fibronectin and other proteins from the tear film are laid on the corneal stroma or intact Bowman's membrane. Marginal, basal epithelial cells attain motility by losing hemi-desmosomal attachments. They migrate centripetally into the denuded zone, carrying layers of cells. When the entire epithelium has been denuded and the LSCs have been wiped out—it is the conjunctival epithelium that acts as the source to replenish corneal epithelial layer. Once re-epithelization of the cornea is completed by conjunctival epithelium, a phenotypic change in the cellular structure takes place by the process of trans-differentiation. Gradually pseudostratified columnar conjunctival epithelium becomes pseudostratified squamous, and there is an attrition of goblet cells. After this, vascularization of the healing tissue occurs, with return of goblet cells and conjunctivalization of the corneal surface. This is initiated and catalyzed by the damage of limbal stem cells due to chemical injury (Flow Diagram 1.1).

Direct chemical injury to the conjunctiva would result in scarring, symblepharon, and cicatrix formation. Destruction of conjunctival goblet cells and limbal stem cells results in dry eyes, corneal opacification, and neovascularization due to loss of progenitor epithelial cells. The wound healing response depends on the severity of chemical burns. The determining factor is the extent and severity of damage to conjunctiva, limbus, and corneal tissue—epithelial and stromal. Factors like degree of limbal ischemia and corneal haze, depth of corneal involvement, presence of endothelial injury are prognostic indicators. As the severity of the burn increases, the healing response also increases [28].

1.4.2.6 Contact Lens Wear

Prolonged use of contact lenses causes limited oxygenation from the atmosphere and results in switching of aerobic to anaerobic metabolism with consequent accumulation of lactic acid in corneal tissue. Corneal edema results because of epithelial

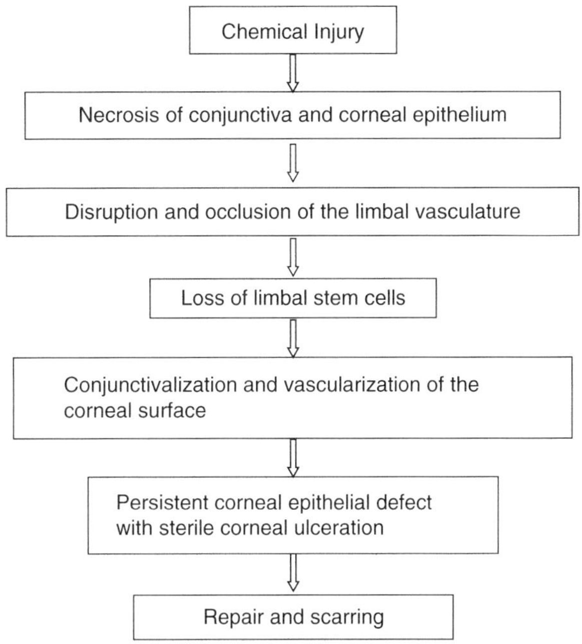

Flow Diagram 1.1 Cascade of events in acute chemical burn

hypoxia, hypercapnia, and recurrent trauma due to improper fitting or over-wear, or a combination of these factors. Chronic use can stimulate angiogenesis and related complications [14].

1.4.3 Stromal Wound Healing

1.4.3.1 Cellular Events

Corneal stroma is unique in structural integrity by virtue of regular array of collagen fibers interspersed in extracellular matrix. The collagen secretes a procollagen triple helix into the extracellular space, synthesizes glycosaminoglycans (GAGs), as well as maintains the transparency. Keratocytes, upon transformation secrete MMP, which along with various growth factors, like EGFs and TGFs, participate in ECM remodeling and eventually in corneal wound healing. Continuous interactions (cross-talk) between the epithelium and stroma play a vital role in the repair of stromal injury. This complex and orchestrated process comprises:

1. Keratocyte death and repopulation
2. Sequential transformation of keratocytes into fibroblasts and myofibroblasts
3. Immigration of limbal and circulating immune cells
4. Remodeling of the corneal ECM structure.

1.4.3.2 Molecular Events

Corneal stromal wounds are common outcome of trauma, infection, and surgeries. Healing of stroma is synonymous to remodeling. Stromal remodeling is initiated by direct damage to the stromal cells or/and indirectly by release of mediators due to damage to the corneal epithelium. Injury to epithelium activates release of inflammatory and profibrotic cytokines and growth factors like IL-1, TNF-α, PDGF, TGF-β, and IGF-1. On the one hand, these mediators cause apoptosis of keratocytes and induce chemotaxis of PMNs and macrophages. While, on the other hand, they facilitate activation of cell cycle of keratocytes with acquirement of contractile properties, resulting in trans-differentiation to myofibroblasts. Additionally, they assist in production of ECM-degrading enzymes which promote stromal remodeling. Stromal remodeling involves neighboring cells to fill void thereby to close the wound and ECM changes for rearrangement of collagen lamellae. These sequences of events are reflected in fibrotic response of stroma [2, 5].

1.4.4 Stromal Wound Healing Response

Similar to epithelial wound healing response, physiological response in stromal wound healing largely depends on extent and severity of affliction. Thus, the final outcome with regard to optical clarity is dependent on restoration of regular collagen organization, which is disturbed at the site of injury. The stromal wound healing response in different corneal emergencies is described in detail.

1.4.4.1 Corneal Ulcer

Three different pathways [2, 5] which bring about the degradation of collagen fibers of stroma during infectious ulceration are:

1. Direct degradation of the corneal stroma, by collagenase enzyme produced by various microorganisms causing infectious keratitis.
2. Degradation of stroma by MMPs released from keratocytes, which are transdifferentiated into myofibroblasts. This trans-differentiation is activated by various factors such as elastase, produced by bacteria or other pathogens causing ulcers.
3. Infiltration of inflammatory cells in corneal stroma, which leads to activation of various pathways. Both keratocytes and infiltrated cells secrete cytokines and growth factors that modulate the response of cells in the healing of corneal stroma.

Keratocytes trans-differentiate into myofibroblasts in response to corneal stromal injury and actively secrete matrix components. A fibrotic response involves rapid contraction of the wound and closure of the defect by activated keratocytes (fibroblasts) followed by tissue scarring. Corneal scarring thus heals the tissue, but fails to restore optical clarity. Based on the depth of cornea involved in the ulceration, various types of corneal opacities may occur, namely, nebular (50% stromal involvement), or leukomatous (>75% stromal involvement) [29].

Some corneal ulcers extend to the deeper tissues rapidly and involve full thickness of the corneal stroma, sparing the Descemet's membrane. The Descemet's membrane resists the inflammatory process, but yields to the intraocular pressure in the absence of adjoining support and subsequently bulges through the corneal ulcer in the form of a transparent membrane, known as descemetocele. This may eventually perforate, if there is a spike in the intraocular pressure, even transiently because of any strenuous activity.

1.4.4.2 Peripheral Ulcerative Keratitis (PUK)

It is a progressive peripheral necrosis of the corneal stroma, through immune complex mediated activation of the complement pathway resulting in chemotactic recruitment of inflammatory cells, i.e., neutrophils, lymphocytes, and macrophages (Flow Diagram 1.2). Collagenase and protease released by the neutrophils and macrophages destroy corneal stroma. Stromal keratocytes produce matrix metalloproteases under influence of proinflammatory cytokines and induce breakdown of tissue. The peripheral cornea, unlike the avascular central cornea, is in close proximity to the limbal conjunctiva and hence a source of immune competent cells. Any external stimulus inducing inflammation in the peripheral cornea may initiate local and systemic immune responses, resulting in neutrophil chemotaxis and complement pathway activation. This is the major pathophysiologic mechanism of PUK, which results in tissue degradation and corneal stromal necrosis brought about by the by proteolytic enzymes, secreted predominantly by neutrophils [30, 31].

Histopathology of the conjunctiva adjacent to a PUK lesion reveals numerous lymphocytes, plasma cells, and mast cells in various stages of degranulation and phagocytic vacuole formation. Leukocyte infiltrations are observed in the advancing edge of the lesion. Bowman's membrane and the epithelium overlying the lesion are lysed, and infrequently, all that eventually remains is Descemet's membrane. Once

Flow Diagram 1.2 Pathophysiological mechanisms in PUK

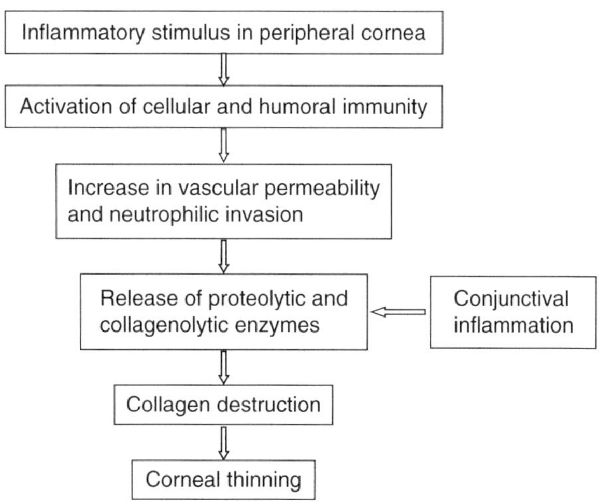

healing is completed, conjunctival epithelium and vessels grow over the residual thinned corneal stromal lamellae [32].

1.4.4.3 Corneal Lacerations

Mechanical corneal trauma involving the deeper stromal layer constitutes corneal laceration. Apoptosis and epithelial injury of the corneal cells lead to the disruption of their attachment to the basement membrane. Subsequently, cells from the wound margin in their response to this insult flatten and begin centripetal migration (Fig. 1.4). The sliding of cells is accompanied by restoration of cellular adhesions, which covers the wound. These cells then undergo proliferation and differentiation to restore the integrity [33]. Laying down of a temporary ECM during wound healing facilitates epithelial migration and covers the wound with fibronectin, fibrin, and hyaluronic acid. During the final phase, the cells induce new hemidesmosomes' formation, for anchorage and integrity [21].

After epithelial injury keratocyte apoptosis, beneath the wound, is the first response seen in corneal stroma, initiated by cytokines, such as IL-1, from damaged epithelial cells [33]. Activation of surrounding keratocytes results in their differentiation into fibroblasts. These then begin to migrate toward the site of injury and subsequently proliferate and repopulate. Various growth factors mediate corneal wound healing, including TGF-β, PDGF, FGF-2, and EGF. As soon as the stromal wound closure, mediated by myofibroblast/fibroblast is completed, the density of myofibroblasts reduces in the stroma. Stromal remodeling occurs in an attempt to restore transparency [7]. As a result, the disorganized scar-tissue matrix is gradually replaced by regular and optically clear corneal ECM.

1.4.4.4 Refractive Surgeries

The usual cascade of events in photorefractive keratectomy (PRK) initiates with death of keratocytes, activation of inflammatory pathway, stromal cell activation beyond the ablation zone, infiltration by immune cells, and myofibroblast formation. Although the cornea is flattened out, thus changing its refractive properties; the epithelium regrows, with the absence of Bowman's layer and increased thickness of stroma. Initial epithelial coverage is fairly rapid, but the epithelial basement membrane restoration, nerve regeneration, and stromal remodeling are time-consuming processes [5]. Haze occurs in all patients initially, due to complex biological events,

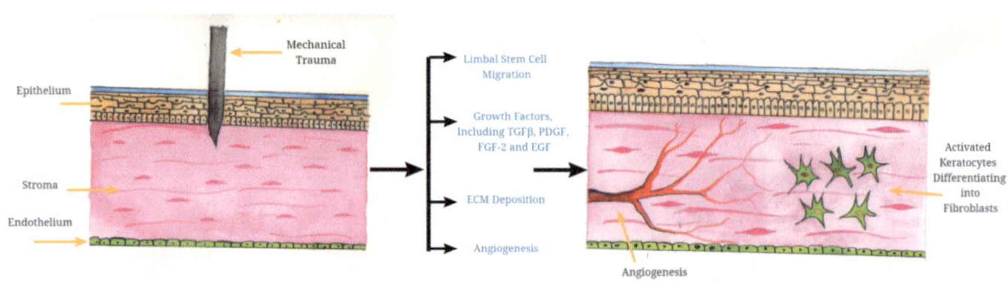

Fig. 1.4 Wound healing response in corneal laceration

which involve TGF-β induced myofibroblasts and excessive ECM production, during remodeling of stroma [34]. Most patients of corneal refractive surgeries have an uneventful postoperative period. However, persistent stromal haze occurs, when previously accumulated excessive stromal matrix and residual wound healing cells fail to regress (Flow Diagram 1.3).

In Laser assisted in-situ keratomileusis (LASIK), stromal remodeling occurs at the flap margin, and haze is usually absent, except in complicated cases [5]. Myofibroblasts appear transiently mainly at the flap margin, with increased production of MMP and fibrotic ECM accumulation. Collagen, basement membrane components, and tenascin-C are laid down to further reinforce flap-adhesion [5]. Flap margin displays fibrotic changes whereas interface of the flap displays a hypocellular scar, with scant fibrotic ECM deposition [5, 18]. Contrary to PRK, LASIK is associated with minimal corneal haze in uncomplicated cases. In Flap procedures, proliferation and apoptosis of keratocytes occur within the stroma, both above and beneath the flap interface as opposed to PRK, where keratocyte apoptosis occurs in the anterior stroma and its proliferation occurring in the peripheral and posterior stroma [19].

1.4.4.5 Acute Chemical Injuries

The basic pathophysiological cascade of events in acute chemical injuries is an outcome of change in tissue pH and subsequent tissue damage. After a chemical burn, number of keratocytes increase by mitosis, and newer ones migrate toward the area of injury, under an intact epithelium. EGF and FGFs both contribute in the production of new collagen and proteoglycans by the keratocytes. The newly formed collagen is type I, which is not same as that of the intrinsic collagen, which results in formation of scar and decreases the transmission of light [13]. In chemical burns of lesser severity, the complex mechanisms by which the stroma responds lead to minimal scarring. However, in severe chemical injuries, with long chemical contact

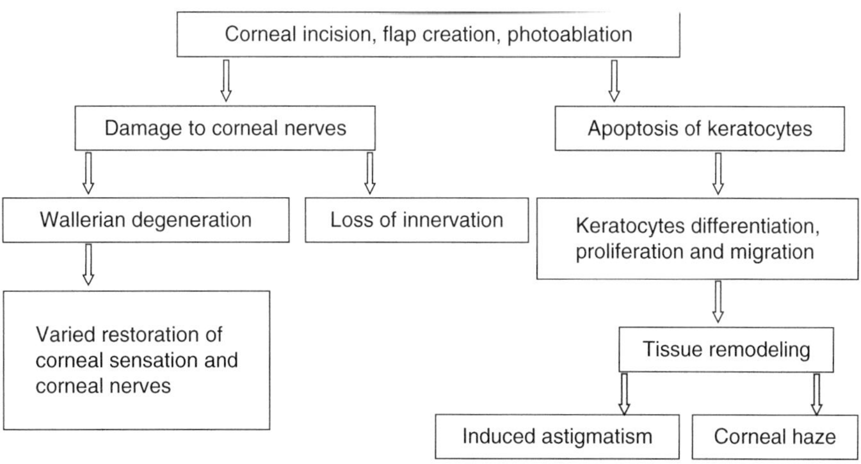

Flow Diagram 1.3 Cascade of events after corneal refractive surgeries

time and maximal variances from physiological pH, the overwhelming stromal response is that of degradation or melting (Fig. 1.3).

1.4.4.6 Advanced Corneal Ectasia

Fragmentation of the epithelial basement membrane, axial stromal thinning, and breaks in Bowman's membrane, with consequent scarring—are the primary structural changes, involved in advanced corneal ectasia [16]. There is marked reduction in number of collagen fibers and loss of normal quiescent phenotype of keratocytes with ongoing depletion. The cellular involvement is through disruption of collagen fibers, lamellae, and proteoglycans. Stretching of Descemet's membrane can lead to breaks and subsequent acute hydrops [16, 35]. Endothelial cells demonstrate considerable pleomorphism and polymegathism which can be correlated with severity and duration of disease. Pathophysiological processes are mediated through activated caspase pathways and mitochondrial deoxyribonucleic acid (DNA) damage. Oxidative stress could activate degradative enzymes and that of tissue inhibitors like MMP. Additionally, there is over-expression of inflammatory cytokine mediators mainly IL-6 and TNF-α [16, 17].

1.4.4.7 Corneal Transplantation

Surgical corneal wounds trigger a complex healing process, involving inflammation, cell-signaling activation, production and release of various cytokines, apoptosis, proliferation, and migration. This is followed by adhesion, differentiation, and remodeling of the ECM. Corneal transplantation results in a long-term reduction of central endothelial cells. This is due to a depletion of the peripheral storage zone with relatively higher endothelial cell densities. Human corneal wound does not heal simply by re-anastomosis of the severed ends of collagen lamellae. Rather, it takes place by the deposition of a provisional matrix, intercalating with the existing lamellae, within the wound site. Hence, the wound architecture does play a role in the healing process, involved in penetrating keratoplasty. After keratoplasty, the levels of type III collagen and large proteoglycans in the regenerating area are increased and gradually decrease as the reconstruction process proceeds [19, 36].

Following persistent epithelial defects or wound dehiscence after penetrating keratoplasty, the corneal epithelial cells rapidly migrate to fill the incisional gap. Keratocytes synthesize new ECM, following their migration into the wound where they transform into myofibroblast-like cells. The epithelial plug is gradually replaced by this newly synthesized ECM. The sensory nerve function does not recover fully after penetrating keratoplasty (PKP) until 1 year [37], which could account for the delayed epithelial healing [18, 36].

1.4.4.8 Corneal Graft Rejection

Cornea is considered an "immune privileged," tissue; a feature that is critical for a successful corneal transplantation. Following are the important factors which form the basis of relative success of corneal transplantation and the reason for which it is considered as "immune privileged" [38–40].

1. Bone-marrow derived group of specialized macrophages, known as Dendritic Langerhans cells, are absent in the central cornea. These cells are implicated in antigen processing and result in graft rejection.
2. The cornea expresses lesser extent of major histocompatibility complex (MHC) antigens, as compared to other body parts.
3. The cornea is an avascular structure, which limits access of lymphocytes and other immune responsive cells.
4. The immunomodulatory factors and neuropeptides; mainly TGF-β2 and α-melanocyte stimulating hormone (α-MSH), produced by stromal keratocytes function by inhibiting T-cell and complement pathway activation.
5. The expression of CD95 (Fas) ligand induces apoptosis of activated T cells, adding to immune privilege.
6. Anterior chamber-associated immune deviation (ACAID) is a specialized mechanism for suppression of systemic immune response to the antigens present in anterior chamber.

In spite of all the immune privileges corneal graft rejection is not uncommon in clinical practice. The aforementioned factors can be compromised by prolonged inflammation, secondary glaucoma, extensive vascularization, and other local and systemic risk factors. This results in establishment of lymphatic drainage channels to cervical lymph nodes, Langerhans cells' (LCs) migration into the cornea, resident epithelial LCs and stromal dendritic cells' (DCs) maturation, which may then function as antigen presenting cells (APCs) to initiate immune surveillance. Consequently, there is up-regulation of proinflammatory cytokines, like IL-1 and TNF-α, which later accentuate MHC expression and maturation of DCs, thereby upregulating the expression of adhesion and chemotactic factors [38, 39, 40]. This unique physiological response is the cause of graft rejection in high-risk corneal transplantation.

1.4.5 Endothelial Wound Healing

1.4.5.1 Cellular Events

Corneal endothelium is integral to maintenance of deturgescence and corneal transparency. Consequent to an acute or chronic tissue insult, the reconstitution of an intact and functional, monolayer of endothelium, is paramount for the sustenance of corneal transparency. Cell migration and enlargement (pleomorphism and polymegathism) chiefly cause endothelial wound healing, rather than by cellular proliferation [41].

Healing occurs in three stages [5, 7, 25]:

1. Stage I (0–3 days) is characterized by an initial covering of the wound by cells. These cells are pleomorphic spindle-shaped cells, but with incomplete barrier function and less pump density.

2. Stage II (4–7 days) is characterized by cells assuming a flattened configuration, an irregular polygonal shape, and eventually establishing a normal pump-, site density and barrier function.
3. Stage III (8–30 days): Remodeling and rearrangement of the endothelial cell monolayer occur in the final stages of healing, followed by an exchange of adjacent cells by sliding past one another.

1.4.5.2 Molecular Events

Endothelial wound healing mainly occurs by enlargement in the cell size and change in shape of the cell along with migration of these cells to the injured site. In the presence of endothelial cell injury, adjacent cells initiate repair by extending their membranes toward the wound area. This process continues until cells migrate and the affected area is covered requiring cells to attain a temporary contractile and migratory properties subsequently achieved by endothelial–mesenchymal transformation (EnMT) [5]. EnMT is characterized by cytoskeleton reorganization, increased cell motility and cell junction destabilization, and is mediated by TGF-β, EGF, FGF-2, IL-1β, TGF-β2, PDGF-BB, and VEGF [5, 25].

1.4.6 Endothelial Wound Healing Response

Endothelium as opposed to other corneal layers has the lowest regenerative capacity. Therefore, for repair of damaged endothelial cells, the remaining cells migrate and enlarge, to remodel the cellular monolayer. Consequently, barrier function of the cells is re-established and their pumping activity is resumed. It is important to study the endothelial would healing response in the background of the following clinical situations.

1.4.6.1 Corneal Perforation

Corneal ulcer often perforates when the patient suddenly exerts, such as during coughing, sneezing, or straining. Due to rapid increase in intraocular pressure, an already compromised corneal tissue gives way through the ulcer bed. Smaller perforations result in the iris plugging the same, which may later organize into an adherent scar tissue resulting in formation of "pseudocornea." If the perforation is large, the iris prolapses out and healing in such cases results in formation of adherent leukoma. The cicatricial tissue is not strong enough to withstand raised intraocular pressure and the scar tissue becomes ectatic and gradually bulges forward, resulting in the formation of anterior staphyloma.

In view of negligible mitotic activity, the endothelial wounds heal by reorganization and enlargement of the surrounding remaining cells. As soon as the defect is covered, the endothelial cells resume their pumping activity and a fresh basement membrane is deposited underneath.

Following corneal injury, the phenomenon of EnMT ensues, wherein the usually quiescent endothelial cells attain fibroblast-like characteristics and begin to proliferate. This is characterized by loss of apical-basal polarity, loss of cell-junctions, and actin-skeleton reorganization [2, 33]. The process relies on TGF-β, IL-1β, and FGF-2. EnMT leads to the deposition of fibrous ECM (retrocorneal fibrous membrane), posterior to Descemet's membrane leading to endothelial cells loss and corneal opacification secondary to ECM deposition [25, 33].

1.4.6.2 Refractive Surgery

Laser-based keratorefractive surgery usually results in none or minimal endothelial changes. But if it is performed on a thin cornea, it induces acute, temporary endothelial cell stress (increased polymegathism and decreased pleomorphism) as a response to healing. Besides, it results in the loss of barrier function, resulting from the shockwave produced by laser ablation. However, long-term endothelial cell effects have not been linked to refractive laser surgery [18, 19].

1.4.6.3 Contact Lens Associated Corneal Edema

Secondary to extended contact lens wear, acute reversible corneal edema could occur and if continued, would potentially result in signs of endothelial cell stress, namely increased polymegathism and decreased pleomorphism. The corneal endothelium employs the same carbohydrate metabolic pathway for energy generation, as the corneal epithelium. However, the oxidative activity and metabolic demand of the endothelial cell, to carry out transport function is five to six times higher compared to that of the epithelial cell. Atmospheric oxygen remains the predominant source of oxygen for the endothelium. Interruption in source of supply by limited oxygen transmissible contact lenses would eventually result in a shift toward anaerobic metabolism, a concurrent rise in the stromal levels of lactic acid and CO_2, and a subsequent drop in stromal pH [15]. Hypoxia further inhibits endothelial Na/K-ATPase. Acute reversible changes observed due to hypoxia result in stromal swelling, endothelial dysfunction, and endothelial blebbing. Chronic hypoxia would eventually result in irreversible endothelial polymegathism and pleomorphism [14].

1.4.6.4 Advanced Corneal Ectasia

Acute corneal hydrops is caused by the acute disruption of Descemet's membrane in corneal ectasia, resulting in compromised barrier function of the Descemet's membrane. This results in fluid uptake by the overlying corneal stroma, causing focal corneal edema of acute hydrops. Healing occurs by EnMT mediated by growth factors. Ensuing scar is largely dependent on extent of Descemet's membrane rupture.

1.5 Limbus: Anatomical Considerations and Response to Wound Healing

Limbus is a highly vascular zone of transition between the cornea and sclera, comprising of reservoir of pluripotent stem cells. The limbal cells are present in two compartments, namely proliferative and non-proliferative. The proliferative compartment houses stem cells that amplify in a transient manner. The post mitotic and terminally differentiated cells constitute the non-proliferative compartment. The "palisades of Vogt" are basement membrane undulations, which provide enhanced vascularity and surface area for adhesion, and protection until the cells are called into action [2].

Peripheral cornea, owing to its proximity to the limbus and conjunctival lymphoid tissue, displays a unique characteristic. Thus, limbal infections, vascular inflammatory disorders, collagen vascular disorders, local degenerations, and neoplastic diseases may affect the peripheral cornea in a distinctive way. Circulating immune complexes in the blood, in the patients with collagen vascular disease, could deposit at the ends of limbal vessels by virtue of their size and the retentive molecular sieving properties of the cornea.

Limbal stem cells along with corneal epithelium act as a barrier thereby preventing migration of the conjunctival epithelial cells over the cornea, keeping a check on conjunctivalization of the cornea. Ocular surface conditions that cause a loss of limbal stem cells (e.g., ocular cicatricial pemphigoid, SJS, and alkali burns) result in conjunctival epithelium growing over the cornea [10].

It is hence prudent to examine the wound healing response of limbus in corneal emergencies; particularly in the following situations:

1.5.1 Stevens–Johnson Syndrome

The exact pathophysiology of SJS is unknown. Majority of cases of SJS are attributable to a delayed hypersensitivity reactions to a drug or its metabolite. The drug in question or its metabolite is processed by keratocytes and presented to CD8 cytotoxic T cells via the major histocompatibility (MHC) class I complex [11]. The primed cytotoxic T cells initiate the signaling cascade and ensuing severe inflammatory reaction, involving small blood vessels and epithelium.

1.5.2 PUK

It is a destructive inflammation of the juxtalimbal corneal stroma. The pathophysiology implicated in PUK is mediated via both humoral and cell-mediated pathways [2]. Deposition of circulating immune complexes, inflammatory response to corneal antigens, and hypersensitivity reactions to exogenous antigens are other mechanisms involved in the pathogenesis of PUK.

1.6 Corneal Innervation and Applied Aspects

The cornea is one of the densely innervated tissues in the body [2, 42]. Corneal neuronal plexuses are integral to normal physiological functioning of corneal layers including tissue vitality and tissue repair. There are two principles set of nerve segments responsible for corneal innervation, namely sensory and autonomic sympathetic systems [42]. Corneal sensory nerves are primarily derived from the ciliary branches of the ophthalmic division of trigeminal nerve. Deep peripheral stroma is penetrated by the corneal nerve fibers radially and which then course anteriorly, resulting in the formation of a terminal sub-epithelial plexus [2]. The myelination of the nerve fibers is quickly lost, within a short distance from their entry point into the cornea, from where they penetrate Bowman's layer, and eventually terminate at the winged-cell layer of the corneal epithelium. Any breach in the superficial corneal epithelium exposes the terminal nerve endings and results in severe ocular pain and lacrimation in conditions with epithelial defects [2, 42].

Corneal innervation also plays an important role in wound healing. The dense sensory innervation of trigeminal origin contains the substance P, which is a sensory neurotransmitter, and regulates plasma extravasation, histamine release from mast cells, and vasodilatation [42]. Depletion of neuropeptides from sensory nerve terminals delays the healing rate of corneal wounds. Recent studies have shown that IGF-1 and substance P containing eyedrops administration could be an effective treatment in cases with persistent epithelial defects, especially in individuals with diabetic neuropathy or neurotrophic keratopathy [43].

For the maintenance of corneal integrity, the presence of corneal sensations is vital. Abnormalities such as trauma, infection, surgery, or inflammation could adversely affect the corneal sensation. Loss of sensation often results in disruption of the normal corneal integrity. Persistent epithelial defects or delayed corneal wound healing are frequently seen in patients with a reduced corneal sensation, such as those with herpes simplex or herpes zoster virus as well as in diabetes mellitus. Furthermore, frank corneal ulceration has been documented to occur in anesthetized eyes and in the rare instances of topical anesthetic abuse. These observations emphasize the role of neural regulation in the maintenance and repair of the corneal epithelium [2, 42].

1.7 Corneal Vascular System

Corneal avascularity is a prominent factor, which renders the cornea transparent. Although the normal cornea is devoid of blood vessels, but there is an important bearing of hematological factors over corneal metabolism and wound healing. The anterior ciliary artery, a branch of ophthalmic artery, constitutes limbal vascular arcade that anastomoses with blood vessels derived from the facial branch [2]. The cornea is, therefore, supplied by both the internal and external carotid systems. Oxygen is primarily supplied via diffusion from the tear film and the aqueous as well as limbal blood vessels. When the transparent corneal stroma is perforated by new abnormal vessels from the limbus, it results in loss of corneal transparency. Corneal neovascularization may result from inflammation associated with conditions such as trauma, microbial infection, chemical burns, or from LSC deficiency and can cause visual impairment [2].

1.8 Conclusion

Human cornea is undoubtedly a marvel in human body. A detailed understanding of anatomical and pathophysiological aspects of tissue damage in corneal emergencies is of great importance to elucidate the disease process and subsequent complications. Additionally, it is imperative to understand the complexities of cellular and biochemical pathways that coordinate the corneal wound healing response. Delving into the details of cellular events of corneal inflammation, its consequences, corneal wound healing, and the outcome of healing response is important in initiating appropriate therapeutic interventions and overall prognosis of patients. It is crucial that ophthalmologists acknowledge the importance of this firm and resilient, yet vulnerable tissue while performing medical and surgical interventions.

Key Points

- Corneal layers have specific function in maintaining the anatomical and physiological integrity, thereby combating the pathology.
- Corneal emergencies can be a cause of permanent damage to anatomical and physiological integrity of cornea, leading to opacification and scar formation
- Cellular and molecular events play an important role in wound healing of epithelium, stroma, and endothelium.
- The epithelial healing is consequent to migration and differentiation of LSC without undergoing transformation to different cell types.
- Stromal wounds heal with transformation of stromal keratocytes to fibroblasts and myofibroblasts.
- Corneal endothelium heals by cell migration and spreading, and endothelial–mesenchymal transformation, however cell proliferation plays a secondary role.
- With the lowest regenerative capacity the wound healing response of endothelium differs from other layers.
- Corneal avascularity and dense innervation have special implications in wound healing response to such emergencies.

Acknowledgement Figures drawn by Dr. Sajith Haridas.

References

1. Sridhar MS. Anatomy of cornea and ocular surface. Indian J Ophthalmol. 2018;66(2):190–4.
2. Krachmer JH, Mannis MJ, Holland EJ, editors. Cornea: fundamentals, diagnosis and management. 4th ed. Philadelphia: Elsevier Mosby.

3. Uchino Y. The ocular surface glycocalyx and its alteration in dry eye disease: a review. Invest Ophthalmol Vis Sci. 2018;59(14):57–62.
4. Feizi S. Corneal endothelial cell dysfunction: etiologies and management. Ther Adv Ophthalmol. 2018;10
5. Ljubimov AV, Saghizadeh M. Progress in corneal wound healing. Prog Retin Eye Res. 2015;49:17–45.
6. Saghizadeh M, Kramerov AA, Svendsen CN, Ljubimov AV. Concise review: stem cells for corneal wound healing. Stem Cells. 2017;35(10):2105–14.
7. Wilson SE, Mohan RR, Ambrosio R Jr, Hong J, Lee J. The corneal wound healing response: cytokine-mediated interaction of the epithelium, stroma, and inflammatory cells. Prog Retin Eye Res. 2001;20(5):625–37.
8. Yu FS, Yin J, Xu K, Huang J. Growth factors and corneal epithelial wound healing. Brain Res Bull. 2010;81(2-3):229–35.
9. Wilson SE. Corneal myofibroblast biology and pathobiology: generation, persistence, and transparency. Exp Eye Res. 2012;99(1):78–88.
10. Sacchetti M, Rama P, Bruscolini A, Lambiase A. Limbal stem cell transplantation: clinical results, limits, and perspectives. Stem Cells Int. 2018;2018:8086269. Published 2018 Oct 11.
11. Oakley AM, Krishnamurthy K. Stevens Johnson syndrome (toxic epidermal necrolysis). 2017. Available from: https://europepmc.org/article/nbk/nbk459323. Last accessed on Apr 2020
12. De Araujo AL, Gomes JÁ. Corneal stem cells and tissue engineering: Current advances and future perspectives. World J Stem Cells. 2015;7(5):806.
13. Xue M, Jackson CJ. Extracellular matrix reorganization during wound healing and its impact on abnormal scarring. Adv Wound Care (New Rochelle). 2015;4(3):119–36.
14. Liesegang TJ. Physiologic changes of the cornea with contact lens wear. Eye Cont Lens. 2002;28(1):12–27.
15. Bruce AS, Brennan NA. Corneal pathophysiology with contact lens wear. Surv Ophthalmol. 1990;35(1):25–58.
16. Naderan M, Jahanrad A, Balali S. Histopathologic findings of keratoconus corneas underwent penetrating keratoplasty according to topographic measurements and keratoconus severity. Int J Ophthalmol. 2017;10(11):1640–6.
17. Cheung IM, McGhee CN, Sherwin T. A new perspective on the pathobiology of keratoconus: interplay of stromal wound healing and reactive species-associated processes. Clin Exp Optom. 2013;96(2):188–96.
18. Brightbill FS. Corneal surgery: theory, technique and tissue. 4th ed. Elsevier; 2009.
19. Baldwin HC, Marshall J. Growth factors in corneal wound healing following refractive surgery: a review. Acta Ophthalmol Scand. 2002;80(3):238–47.
20. Moshirfar M, Desautels JD, Walker BD, Murri MS, Birdsong OC, Hoopes PC. Mechanisms of optical regression following corneal laser refractive surgery: epithelial and stromal responses. Med Hypothesis Discov Innov Ophthalmol. 2018;7(1):1.
21. Ashby BD, Garrett Q, Willcox MD. Corneal injuries and wound healing—review of processes and therapies. Austin J Clin Ophthalmol. 2014;1(4):1017.
22. Dua HS, Gomes JA, Singh A. Corneal epithelial wound healing. Br J Ophthalmol. 1994;78(5):401.
23. Walko G, Castañón MJ, Wiche G. Molecular architecture and function of the hemidesmosome. Cell Tissue Res. 2015;360(2):363–78.
24. Gurumurthy S, Iyer G, Srinivasan B, Agarwal S, Angayarkanni N. Ocular surface cytokine profile in chronic Stevens-Johnson syndrome and its response to mucous membrane grafting for lid margin keratinisation. Br J Ophthalmol. 2018;102(2):169–76.
25. Di Pascuale MA, Espana EM, Liu DT, Kawakita T, Li W, Gao YY, Baradaran-Rafii A, Elizondo A, Raju VK, Tseng SC. Correlation of corneal complications with eyelid cicatricial pathologies in patients with Stevens–Johnson syndrome and toxic epidermal necrolysis syndrome. Ophthalmology. 2005;112(5):904–12.
26. Eslani M, Baradaran-Rafii A, Movahedan A, Djalilian AR. The ocular surface chemical burns. J Ophthalmol. 2014;2014:196827.

27. Kuwabara T, Perkins DG, Cogan DG. Sliding of the epithelium in experimental corneal wounds. Invest Ophthalmol Vis Sci. 1976;15(1):4–14.
28. Yao L, Li ZR, Su WR, Li YP, Lin ML, Zhang WX, Liu Y, Wan Q, Liang D. Role of mesenchymal stem cells on cornea wound healing induced by acute alkali burn. PLoS One. 2012;7(2):e30842.
29. Sharma N, Vajpayee RB. Corneal ulcers diagnosis and management. 1st ed. India: Jaypee; 2008.
30. Yagci A. Update on peripheral ulcerative keratitis. Clin Ophthalmol. 2012;6:747–54.
31. Chow CY, Foster CS. Mooren's ulcer. Int Ophthalmol Clin. 1996;36(1):1–3.
32. Dana MR, Qian Y, Hamrah P. Twenty-five-year panorama of corneal immunology: emerging concepts in the immunopathogenesis of microbial keratitis, peripheral ulcerative keratitis, and corneal transplant rejection. Cornea. 2000;19(5):625–43.
33. Bukowiecki A, Hos D, Cursiefen C, Eming SA. Wound-healing studies in cornea and skin: parallels, differences and opportunities. Int J Mol Sci. 2017;18(6):1257.
34. Shu DY, Lovicu FJ. Myofibroblast transdifferentiation: The dark force in ocular wound healing and fibrosis. Prog Retin Eye Res. 2017;60:44–65.
35. Loh IP, Fan Gaskin JC, Sherwin T, McGhee CNJ. Extreme Descemet's membrane rupture with hydrops in keratoconus: Clinical and histological manifestations. Am J Ophthalmol Case Rep. 2018;10:271–5.
36. Obata H, Tsuru T. Corneal wound healing from the perspective of keratoplasty specimens with special reference to the function of the Bowman layer and Descemet membrane. Cornea. 2007;26:S82–9.
37. Yang AY, Chow J, Liu J. Corneal innervation and sensation: the eye and beyond. Yale J Biol Med. 2018;91(1):13–21.
38. Hori J. Mechanisms of immune privilege in the anterior segment of the eye: what we learn from corneal transplantation. J Ocul Biol Dis Inform. 2008;1(2-4):94–100.
39. Takeuchi M, Alard P, Verbik D, Ksander B, Streilein JW. Anterior chamber-associated immune deviation-inducing cells activate T cells, and rescue them from antigen-induced apoptosis. Immunology. 1999;98(4):576–83.
40. Dana MR, Dai R, Zhu S, Yamada J, Streilein JW. Interleukin-1 receptor antagonist suppresses Langerhans cell activity and promotes ocular immune privilege. Invest Ophthalmol Vis Sci. 1998;39(1):70–7.
41. Zavala J, Hernández-Camarena JC, Loya-García D, Tamez A, Valdez-García JE. Wound healing in the corneal endothelium. 2017. Available from: https://www.researchgate.net/publication/322116530_Wound_healing_in_the_corneal_endothelium. Last accessed on Apr 2020
42. Marfurt CF, Cox J, Deek S, Dvorscak L. Anatomy of the human corneal innervation. Exp Eye Res. 2010;90(4):478–92.
43. Versura P, Giannaccare G, Pellegrini M, Sebastiani S, Campos EC. Neurotrophic keratitis: current challenges and future prospects. Eye Brain. 2018;10:37–45.

Epidemiology and Risk Factors

2

Prashant Bhartiya, Deepak Soni, Rituka Gupta, and Bhavana Sharma

2.1 Introduction

Corneal emergencies are commonly encountered entities that can be a potential cause of visual and structural deprivation. Cornea is the most exposed part of the eye and is commonly involved in injuries, infections, and systemic diseases. The symptoms may vary from minor pain or blurring to severe pain and total loss of vision. Certain emergencies like recurrent corneal erosion syndrome may present with extreme pain and discomfort but have limited potential for severe vision loss if managed adequately. However, other corneal emergencies like mechanical/chemical injuries, microbial keratitis, postsurgical causes, advanced corneal ectasias, etc. can be associated with significant visual impairment. Knowledge regarding their epidemiological determinants and risk factors can guide in designing preventive strategies, appropriate treatment, and timely referral.

The commonest cause of corneal emergency presenting for acute intervention has been reported to be a mechanical injury. Causative factors which have been identified include corneal abrasions, foreign bodies, laceration, and perforation. Most serious corneal injuries are caused by blunt objects, large sharp objects, small flying particles, or burns. Ocular emergency cases constitute approximately 3% of all emergency department visits, 80% of such cases of trauma involve corneal injury [1, 2].

Globally, approximately 1.6 million people get blind from eye injuries, 2.3 million with bilateral visual impairment, and 19 million with unilateral vision loss [3]. Age group comprising 18–45 years constitutes nearly one-half (48%) of all reported

P. Bhartiya
Suprabhat Healthcare & Cornea Labs and Surgical Centre, Indore, Madhya Pradesh, India

D. Soni · R. Gupta · B. Sharma (✉)
All India Institute of Medical Sciences, Bhopal, Madhya Pradesh, India
e-mail: head.ophtho@aiimsbhopal.edu.in

B. Sharma, J. S. Titiyal (eds.), *Corneal Emergencies*,
https://doi.org/10.1007/978-981-16-5876-1_2

eye injuries. In addition, subjects of less than 18 years constitute 25% of cases while 27% occur in people aged 46 years and older. Males are at four times greater risk of eye injury than females [4]. 40–60% higher risk of ocular injury is seen in Black people as compared to white people [5].

2.2 Minor Corneal Emergencies

Minor corneal emergencies include corneal abrasions, foreign body, recurrent corneal erosions, and phototoxicity, of which a major proportion is constituted by corneal abrasions and foreign bodies.

2.2.1 Epidemiology

Corneal abrasions are common corneal emergencies of all age groups with a higher incidence seen in working-age groups. Automotive industry workers in the age group of 20 and 29 years have been reported to have the highest incidence of eye injuries [6]. In a study in the USA, the most common injury to the eye was abrasion (44.4%), followed by foreign body (30.8%) [6]. Recurrent corneal erosions usually present with acute episodes of pain and foreign body sensation on first opening the eyes in the morning. The patient, usually a young female, between 30 and 40 years of age is so incapacitated that the activities of daily living are not possible during the acute event. Incidence of recurrent corneal erosion is more frequently seen in females than in males [7]. Recurrent corneal erosions usually have a bilateral presentation and present after the fourth decade but certain anterior corneal dystrophies, such as Reis-Buckler's and lattice dystrophies can present as painful recurrent erosions in early childhood.

2.2.2 Risk Factors

Direct trauma to the ocular surface, foreign bodies, and contact lens wear are the main risk factors associated with corneal abrasions. Various mechanisms which predispose the eye for direct trauma include fingernail injury, injury by plant branches, animal claws, and chemical splashes.

A foreign body such as dust, rust, or glass particle stuck under the eyelid can also lead to corneal abrasion. Recurrent corneal erosion can occur either post corneal trauma or spontaneously. Epithelial basement membrane dystrophy, diabetes mellitus, focal mechanical trauma to the corneal epithelium, and surgical trauma of the corneal epithelium are important risk factors for recurrent corneal erosions. Common associations which predispose the eye for recurrent corneal erosions include rosacea, blepharitis, and dry eye disease. Most of the risk factors are preventable, treatable and the recurrences can be managed with minimal or no loss of vision.

2.3 Corneal Lacerations and Penetrating Injuries

Spectrum of corneal injuries can range from minor injuries to major vision and eye threatening trauma. Corneal laceration is a partial- or full-thickness injury to the cornea while penetrating injuries involve the full thickness of the cornea. There may be associated injuries which may include iridodialysis, hyphema, lens dislocation and cataract formation, vitreous hemorrhage or retinal detachment depending on the severity of the injury. Various types of injuries affecting the cornea have been reported as in Table 2.1 [8–10].

2.3.1 Epidemiology

Incidence of mechanical trauma with associated ocular involvement in the Indian population has been reported to be 57 cases per 10,000 in a year [11]. Penetrating eye injury can occur in individuals of any age, but data from USEIR demonstrate that the mean age of the patient with ocular injury is 29 years, with nearly 60% being younger than 30 years of age [12]. Moreover, penetrating injury is the leading cause of unilateral visual loss in children. The male sex has been found to be more prone to ocular injuries ranging from 63 to 77.4% [13]. Pediatric ocular trauma study from central India revealed a mean age of 8.74 ± 3.93 years with males being more commonly involved. Children from rural areas were observed to have a 1.5 times higher risk of ocular injuries than children from urban areas [13]. While with reference to socioeconomic status, higher prevalence was observed among the lower socioeconomic group [13]. Interestingly, Black and Hispanic races have a 40–60% higher risk of ocular injury as compared to the white race and are at more than twice the risk of sustaining impaired vision from the injury [14]. Incidences of trauma have been correlated with an increase in temperature, thus more likely in warmer months particularly swimming pool chemicals and refrigerants, suggesting a seasonal dependent exposure.

Table 2.1 Types of injuries affecting the cornea

Types of trauma associated with corneal emergencies:
• Occupational injuries with metals, like Chisel and Hammer injury, Screwdriver or instrumental injury • Domestic injuries like Road traffic accidents and Falls • Occupational or Domestic injuries with chemicals • Farming injury, Thorn injury • Childhood injuries like Scissor point injuries Fireworks Bow and Arrow injury Chemical injury (e.g., chuna packet injury)

2.3.2 Risk Factors

Corneal laceration and penetrating injuries may occur when high-speed projectile objects such as saws, stone, angle grinder, or pounding metal objects hit the cornea with an adequate force causing a breach in the cornea layers. Common causes of corneal lacerations are fingernails, air-bag deployment, fireworks, explosions, blunt force trauma, and pellets. Young adults in the working-age group are mostly involved in occupational injuries or domestic injuries while working with metallic objects, moving items, or by assaults. While elder ones are more prone to falls and the risk of ocular injury is more in operated patients especially post keratoplasty. Firecracker injuries are one of the commonly seen causes of childhood corneal trauma particularly during religious festivals [15]. In a retrospective study to document the profile of ocular firework injuries in children during the festive season of Diwali in Southern India, corneal trauma constituted more than 50% of cases [15]. Sports-related injuries have been seen to be commoner amongst children aged 5–14 years and a majority of them involve the cornea. The commonest cause of trauma in such cases has been reported to be wooden and sharp objects including bow and arrows, broken toys, and playtime activities [10, 13].

2.4 Microbial Keratitis

Corneal ulcers are common medical emergencies presenting to an ophthalmologist, which can lead to surgical emergencies like corneal perforation and sloughing.

2.4.1 Epidemiology

The incidence of microbial keratitis varies largely between geographical locations depending on the climatic conditions. The reported incidence varies from 10/lakh-persons/year in the USA to 799/lakh-persons/year in Nepal, the average age of patients being 45 years [16, 17]. However, the average age may vary according to risk factors as in contact lens users where age incidence may be low as opposed to ocular surface disease where the same may be high. The average age may also vary significantly according to infection type. In bacterial and viral keratitis, the average age is higher as compared to *Acanthamoeba* keratitis. This low average age could be due to the predisposition of younger age group CL wearers to *Acanthamoeba*.

Bacterial keratitis is the most common form of microbial keratitis, accounting for 90–95% of cases with the highest reported cases in temperate climate regions. A large study from India reported a male-to-female ratio of 2.25:1 with patients mostly in the middle age (30–40 years) at a tertiary care hospital [18]. Female preponderance in the incidence of microbial keratitis has been reported by Ibrahim et al. [19] Keratitis in patients aged 18 years and younger has been reported to be associated more with trauma (48.3%) and in young adults with contact lens wear (64%) [20]. A study from Taiwan reported a peak incidence of microbial keratitis between the ages of 18 and 40 years [21]. Bimodal incidence in the age distribution has been reported and attributed to contact lens-related keratitis, corneal trauma in the younger group, and predisposing ocular surface diseases, eyelid diseases in the older group [22]. A higher incidence of keratitis among housewives (21.3%), followed by farmers (16.6%), laborers (14.6%), and carpenters (10.6%) has been reported by Tiwari et al. [23].

Seasonal variation in microbial keratitis has been reported by various authors. A study from Pennsylvania reported increased incidence during spring and decreased incidence during winter [24]. In South India, fungal keratitis peaked in July and January without any significant trend in bacterial keratitis [25]. In France, severe keratitis occurred more in periods of heatwaves during summer time [26].

Significant variability exists between the incidence of pathological agents within India. In a study from South India by Lin et al., fungal infections accounted for 63% of all cases of microbial keratitis, while bacterial etiology resulted in only 35.7%. On the contrary, 65.1% and 34.9% were the proportions of bacterial and fungal infections, respectively, in a study from Ahmadabad in western India [23, 25]. Filamentous fungi such as *Fusarium* and *Aspergillus spp.* contributes to the majority of fungal keratitis in India. In a study from Southern India, the most common fungal pathogens were *Fusarium* (47.1%) and *Aspergillus* (16.1%) [27]. While in another study from South India the most common fungal species isolated were *Fusarium* (37.2%) and *Aspergillus* (30.7%) [28]. In studies from other developing countries, the prevalence of fungal ulcer ranged from 5 to 60% of microbial corneal ulcers [29–31]. In temperate regions, Fungi cause keratitis in about 6% of patients but figure more prominently in tropical regions [32].

2.4.2 Risk Factors

Microbial keratitis is rare in absence of predisposing factors. In India, microbial keratitis is ten times more common than in the USA [33]. This difference is believed to be due to risk factors such as humid climate and corneal trauma. Ocular trauma, contact lens use, tear film abnormalities, use of topical steroid medications, ocular surgery, and neurotrophic keratopathy are some of the common predisposing factors associated with bacterial and mycotic keratitis. Globally predisposing factors for microbial keratitis vary tremendously with geographical location. In the USA, contact lens wear has emerged as a major risk factor for microbial keratitis and non-surgical trauma constitutes only 27% of cases whereas non-surgical trauma accounted for 48.6–65.4% of all corneal ulcers in the developing countries of Nepal and India [27, 34]. The agrarian population or manual laborers are at a higher risk of corneal ulcer with trauma being the most common risk factor. The Hong Kong Keratitis Study Group studied 223 cases in 1997–1998, the main risk factors were history of ocular surface disease followed by trauma, and the most prevalent causative bacteria were *Pseudomonas* [35]. Bullous keratopathy is a significant risk factor for the development and progression of corneal ulcer. Luchs and associates reported that approximately 4.7% of patients with bullous keratopathy had a corneal ulcer during a 10-year period [36].

The microbial etiology pattern also differs geographically. Early diagnosis of mycotic keratitis is a pre-requisite for adequate treatment, it involves familiarity with predisposing risk factors. Ocular trauma particularly with vegetative materials is the most common inciting factor in addition to other predisposing factors like ocular surface diseases, lacrimal sac pathologies, use of topical and systemic steroids, contact lens use, immune-compromised status, and humid climatic conditions. Ocular trauma, heat and sunlight, menstruation, stress, infectious disease, and immunocompromised states are considered as predisposing factors for severe disease and reactivation of viral keratitis.

Diabetes Mellitus (DM) is an important risk factor for microbial keratitis. They have been shown to have higher infections than non-diabetic counterparts [37, 38]. DM is postulated to cause damage to the corneal barrier function and impaired epithelial healing thus increasing the susceptibility to infection. Topical use of anti-glaucoma agents has been described as a risk factor for microbial keratitis [39]. Microbial keratitis associated with HIV is descriptive of incidence of ulcerative keratitis in human immunodeficiency virus-positive patients as 238.1 per 100,000 person-years [40].

2.5 Corneal Perforations

Corneal perforations are grave ocular emergencies with myriad causes such as trauma, infection, autoimmune and ocular diseases. Severe keratitis, either infective or non-infective can lead to thinning and consequent corneal perforation. Microbial keratitis constitutes a major cause of corneal perforation.

2.5.1 Epidemiology

Young adults in the working age group are mostly involved in occupational injuries or domestic injuries while working with metallic objects, moving items, or by assaults. Identifiable predisposing factors of perforation in microbial keratitis are mean age of 40–44.8 years, male sex, rural residence, outdoor manual occupation are associated with risk of corneal perforation [41].

2.5.2 Risk Factors

Outdoor manual work, ocular trauma particularly with a history of organic matter, and illiteracy are well-established risk factors associated with a higher likelihood of perforated corneal ulcers especially in developing countries [19, 27]. In an Indian study, ocular trauma was seen to be associated with over 90% of mycotic ulcers and more than 50% of these were from vegetative injuries [42]. Tree branches, paddy grains, and thorns were the commonest agricultural matter implicated in these cases.

Failure to implement standard therapy at first contact, delay in initiation of definitive treatment, and absence of use of fortified antibiotics has been mentioned as a treatment-related risk factor for corneal perforation. In a study from South India, primary treatment failure (i.e., progressive worsening of the ulcer despite maximal medical treatment) or infiltrate size >14 mm^2 or associated hypopyon at presentation were observed as major risk factors associated with corneal perforations [43].

Other risk factors include alcohol use, vision less than counting fingers at presentation, central corneal ulcers, iatrogenic trauma during corneal foreign body removal or surgery, peripheral ulcerative keratitis, neurotrophic keratitis, and pellucid marginal degeneration. Fungal keratitis constitutes a special group of microbial keratitis with a higher risk for corneal perforations. The Mycotic Ulcer Treatment Trial (MUTT II) identified three major risk factors for developing a perforation or a need for TPK in cases with fungal keratitis as hypopyon at presentation, presence of a posterior infiltrate, or a larger geometric size of the infiltrate [44].

2.6 Acute Chemical Injuries

Ocular chemical injuries produce extensive damage to the ocular surface, cornea, anterior segment, and limbal stem cells resulting in a guarded visual prognosis. Chemical injuries occur commonly in domestic as well as industrial places. More than 60% of chemical injuries occur in workplace accidents, 30% occur at home, and 10% are the result of an assault [45]. Chemical injuries constitute 11.5–22.1% of all ocular injuries [46].

2.6.1 Epidemiology

The incidence of burns to the eye has been reported to be 10.7 per 100,000 population and such cases represent an estimated 10% of ocular trauma treated in emergency [47]. Studies from the UK and Germany indicate males aged 16–25 years to be affected more by chemical injuries [2, 48]. A study of severe chemical eye injuries in China found that nearly 70% of patients hospitalized for chemical burns were the result of alkali agents, including lime and sodium hydroxide (NaOH). Ethnicity, culture, geographic influence, and the types of chemicals used frequently are the important determinants of outcome (Table 2.2) [49].

In a retrospective study to analyze the epidemiology of chemical injuries, industrial trauma has been observed to contribute almost double to total cases of chemical ocular burn in comparison to household injuries [50]. Young people in the age group of 20–40 years are more likely to be involved in such injuries. Males are three times more prone to chemical injuries as compared to females [51, 52]. However, McGwin et al. observed eye injuries from chemicals and compounds to be more common among females (19.5%) than males (10.6%) [53]. In recent past, automotive battery acid burns have emerged as a common cause of ocular chemical injury. Bursting of chuna packets can cause severe ocular alkali burns in children as has been reported

Table 2.2 Types of chemicals frequently associated with corneal injuries

Chemical substance (formula)	Available as
Alkali	
Ammonia (NH_3)	Fertilizers, Refrigerants, Chemical Reagents
Potassium Hydroxide (KOH)	Caustic Potash
Lye (NaOH)	Drain Cleaners
Lime ($Ca(OH)_2$)	Chuna, Whitewash, Cement, Plaster and Mortar
Magnesium Hydroxide ($Mg(OH)_2$)	Fireworks like Sparklers and Flares
Acid	
Hydrochloric Acid (HCl)	Chemical Reagents, Toilet Cleaner
Sulfuric Acid (H_2SO_4)	Battery Acid, Dairy Agent
Acetic Acid (CH_3COOH)	Glacial Acetic Acid, Vinegar
Hydrofluoric Acid (HF)	Industrial Reagent in Glass Polishing
Sulfurous Acid (H_2SO_3)	Fruit or Vegetable Preservative, Bleach

by Agarwal et al. [54]. Children have been reported to be affected by household cleaning agents and leading causes of injury from consumer products among this age group [55].

2.6.2 Risk Factors

Various chemicals have been implicated such as alkalis, acids, or neutral agents [56]. Common agents of acidic ocular burns include sulfuric, hydrochloric, hydrofluoric, and battery acids while common alkaline agents include calcium hydroxide, cement or lime, sodium hydroxide (present in oven cleaners and drain cleaners), chlorine bleach (sodium hypochlorite), and ammonia products. Alkalis are the most common and with the most damaging potential as they are found more commonly in building materials and cleaning agents. Other common agents include solvents/paints, detergents, antipersonnel sprays, adhesives, bleach, automotive battery acid, plaster, and ammonia. A unique form of chemical injury is seen mostly in children in the Indian subcontinent by *Chuna*. *Chuna* or calcium hydroxide is a common source of chemical injury as it is readily available domestically in all parts of India [55]. The child usually gets injured by a projectile of large quantities of the material directly into the eye while pressing the packet. Workers in chemical factories and agricultural industries are at greater risk for ocular chemical injuries because of higher chances of accidental exposure. The use of extremely caustic solutions such as ammonia has been documented in assaults. Rare incidences of injury by uncommon agents like super glue also have been reported [57].

2.7 Emergencies Associated with Corneal Transplantation

Corneal transplantation is one of the most successful forms of human solid-tissue transplantation. Immunological rejections are the main contributing factor for higher failure rates in penetrating keratoplasty leading to graft failure, followed by late endothelial failure and ocular surface disorders.

2.7.1 Epidemiology

Fairer prognosis of graft survival has been reported in the younger age group ranging between 21 and 40 years as opposed to older patients according to a study on Australian eyes [58]. Male recipients have been observed to have a higher risk of graft failure as compared to females [59].

2.7.2 Risk Factor

Postoperative patients especially post keratoplasty are prone to ocular damage following even trivial trauma. Other factors may predispose such patients to emergency situations like the use of topical steroids, reactivation of herpes simplex infection, etc. Loose suture (pain and foreign body sensation) and rejection (decreased vision) as other common causes for emergency visits [60]. Graft infection is usually associated with loose sutures. Loose sutures or removal of sutures can lead to infections as well as precipitate graft rejection. The major risk factors for graft infection other than loose sutures are persistent epithelial defects (PED) and the presence of ocular surface disorders. Other diagnoses noted in the emergency visits were wound leak, corneal abrasion, corneal ulcer, flat anterior chamber, uveitis, high intraocular pressure, and endophthalmitis [60].

Most of the graft infections are caused by *Staphylococcus epidermidis* species [61]. Fungal infections can either recur or can occur due to long-term steroid use. Similarly, Herpes Simplex keratitis can recur in the host graft junction and many a time may be indistinguishable from graft rejections. Patients with corneal vascularization have a higher risk of rejection. Other factors include a previous keratoplasty, pre-existing herpes simplex keratitis, uveitis, synechiae, or increased surgical manipulation leading to excessive postoperative inflammation. Poor compliance to medications particularly steroids is also a known risk factor for graft rejection.

Allograft rejection is a major cause of corneal graft failure, necessitating prompt diagnosis and treatment. At least 10% of graft failures are due to graft rejection. Most of the patients with graft rejection have risk factors and the patients with high-risk criteria need to be counseled regarding the predisposition. Patients with corneal vascularization have a higher risk of rejection and can get an earlier onset than those without vascularization. The severity can be quantified in terms of quadrants involved with more than two quadrants of deep stromal vascularization considered as "High Risk." Other factors include a previous keratoplasty, pre-existing herpes simplex keratitis, uveitis, synechiae, or increased surgical manipulation leading to excessive postoperative inflammation.

2.8 Acute Graft Rejection

Acute graft rejection is a complex immunological process. It occurs when the host's immune system recognizes alloantigen from the corneal graft leading to an immune response against the graft which could lead to rejection. One of the major postoperative complications following keratoplasty is immunological rejection and one of the main causes of corneal graft failure.

2.8.1 Epidemiology

The incidence of graft rejection differs widely depending on the type of transplantation and the presence of risk factors for rejection. Incidences of graft rejection are lower in endothelial keratoplasty as compared to penetrating keratoplasty. Williams et al. reported that the failure of the graft due to irreversible rejection was 28% for penetrating keratoplasty, 1.7% for deep anterior lamellar keratoplasty, 13% for Descemet Stripping Endothelial Keratoplasty (DSEK), and 9% for Descemet Membrane Endothelial Keratoplasty (DMEK) [62]. In penetrating keratoplasty graft rejection rate ranges from 2.3 to 68% while in DMEK incidence has been reported to have a rejection rate as low as 0.7% at 1 year in one series [63, 64]. According to the Cornea Donor Study, 23% of subjects reported at least one rejection episode and 37% of the eyes with a rejection had graft failure reported in a 5-year follow-up [65]. Infants have a higher risk of graft rejection as compared to adults. Female recipients have a higher probability of rejection as compared to males. No racial predilection has been reported in cases of acute graft rejection.

2.8.2 Risk Factor

A younger recipient age group, history of previously failed penetrating keratoplasty, ocular comorbidities like herpetic eye disease, the presence of ocular inflammation, deep stromal vascularization, anterior synechiae, history of glaucoma, systemic metabolic disorders like diabetes are the most established risk factors for acute graft rejection. The indication per se of keratoplasty and the concurrent surgical procedures being performed also affects the risk of rejection. Poor compliance with immunosuppression therapy is associated with higher rates of graft rejection. The donor factors like donor age, gender, race, ABO blood type compatibility, method of cornea retrieval, and timing of use of the graft are not directly correlated to a higher risk of graft failure according to the Cornea Donor Study [66, 67].

2.9 Post-surgical Corneal Wound Dehiscence

Post-surgical corneal wound dehiscence is an important complication after keratoplasty. It could result in graft failure due to direct damage to the endothelial cells or as a consequence of secondary inflammation.

2.9.1 Epidemiology

The incidence of traumatic wound dehiscence after PK is reported between 1.3 and 2.6% [68]. A large review of wound dehiscence found that only 3.2% had dehiscence in DALK cases. In studies, the 50–60 years age group has been reported to be more susceptible for postsurgical corneal wound dehiscence. Males are more prone to traumatic corneal wound dehiscence as compared to females. No racial predilection has been reported [69].

2.9.2 Risk Factors

Trauma is the most common risk factor for corneal wound dehiscence. Other risk factors include early suture removal, infection, and graft–host junction disparity. Socially and physically active lifestyles of men attribute them to being more prone to traumatic wound dehiscence. Graft indications such as keratoconus, corneal scar, and herpes simplex keratitis are also found to be at greater risk for postsurgical traumatic wound dehiscence. The risk of postsurgical corneal wound dehiscence is less in endothelial grafts, as a small corneoscleral limbal incision is being used for graft placement.

Long-term steroid usage, elevated intraocular pressure, and multiple grafts are the most important risk factors for graft dehiscence. Suture techniques including continuous suture removal and suture material like nylon with lower tissue reactivity are associated with a higher risk of wound dehiscence [69]. Neglect of intraoperative factors like head positioning and flap irrigation and post-operative use of eye shield, preventive measures are also considered significant risk factors for early postoperative wound dehiscence.

2.10 Contact Lens-Associated Corneal Emergency

Contact lens-induced keratitis is one of the most serious complications seen to be associated with poor contact lens wear practices. Sterile corneal infiltrates, corneal neovascularization, corneal warping, edema, corneal de-epithelization are the other complications of contact lens usage.

2.10.1 Epidemiology

In a study from Hongkong, the annual incidence of infectious keratitis was reported as 3.4 per 10,000 in contact lens wearers [70]. Due to increasing rates of contact lens usage, the annual incidence of infectious keratitis in the developed world has been increased up to 2–11 per 100,000 per year [71]. Most patients are in the age group between 20 and 29 years [72]. Contact lens-associated corneal infiltrative events (CIE) are more common in younger lens wearers. Male sex is associated with about a 1.4-fold greater risk for developing a CIE [73] while higher socioeconomic status is reported to have a 2.7–4.1-fold increased risk of infectious keratitis and CIE [74]. The incidence of corneal ulceration in contact lens wearers has been reported to be 130.4 per 100,000 person-years [75].

2.10.2 Risk Factor

Lack of lens hygiene practice, overnight use of lenses, exposure to contaminated water, lens cases or both are significant risk factors for the development of contact lens-induced keratitis and subsequent risk of corneal ulcerations. Silicone hydrogel materials have double the risk of keratitis as compared to poly-HEMA-based hydrogel materials. The keratitis risk increases by four- to eightfold during extended wear due to Lens bioburden [76]. Patients with a higher level of ametropia, smokers, previous history of contact lens-induced keratitis are at higher risk of developing corneal infiltrative events.

2.11 Peripheral Ulcerative Keratitis

Peripheral ulcerative keratitis is a devastating ocular inflammation of the peripheral part of cornea. Peripheral ulcerative keratitis is usually associated with a systemic illness. A high index of suspicion and a thorough systemic evaluation are necessary to rule out the underlying cause.

2.11.1 Epidemiology

A study from England reported an incidence of peripheral ulcerative keratitis (PUK) as 3 per million per year [77]. PUK caused by Mooren ulcer is commoner in males as compared to females. Age is variable and dependent on the associated risk factor with no racial predilection reported.

2.11.2 Risk Factors

The most common risk factors associated with PUK are connective tissue disorders and vasculitis like rheumatoid arthritis, polyarteritis nodosa, inflammatory bowel disease, systemic lupus erythematosus, relapsing polychondritis, progressive systemic fibrosis, ANCA vasculitides, granulomatosis with polyangiitis, and

Churg–Strauss syndrome. The commonest among them is rheumatoid arthritis, which has been observed to be present in 34–42% of PUK patients. Ocular factors like exposure, bad ocular surface, and infections like herpes simplex or herpes zoster are local risk factors. Apart from systemic associations, local ocular infectious conditions (e.g., herpes simplex keratitis, fungal keratitis), noninfectious entities (e.g., Mooren ulcer, marginal keratitis), and systemic infectious diseases (e.g., hepatitis, syphilis, tuberculosis) are important causative factors. Additionally, it can be triggered by environmental factors in genetically susceptible individuals [78]. Associations have also been reported among Mooren's ulcer, helminthiasis, and ocular injuries [79, 80].

2.12 Emergency in Advanced Corneal Ectasia

Corneal ectasia includes conditions characterized by progressive thinning and bulging of the cornea and can lead to moderate to severe impairment of vision. It includes keratoconus, pellucid marginal degeneration, Terrien's marginal degeneration, keratoglobus , and ectasias following surgery.

2.12.1 Epidemiology

The prevalence of keratoconus ranges from 0.5 to 2.3 per 1000 population in Western countries according to Rabinowitz, while worldwide the prevalence of keratoconus is 1.38 per 1000 [81]. The mean age is reported as 18–24 years in Asian countries. A higher prevalence is seen in males as compared to females. The prevalence of keratoconus in Asian populations is about four times higher than other ethnic populations with the highest prevalence reported in the Mediterranean region and the Middle East, including Iran [82]. Pellucid marginal degeneration is a rare disorder, more common in 20–40 years males and is characterized by inferior corneal thinning.

2.12.2 Risk Factor

One of the most important risk factors for keratoconus is eye rubbing in addition to positive family history. Risk factors for ectasia consequent to post-refractive surgery include both surgery and patient-specific characteristics, such as topographic and tomographic abnormalities, younger age, thinner preoperative corneas, and residual stromal beds, high myopia, and higher percentage tissue altered. Additionally, genetic predisposition has been evaluated for corneal ectasia, and various genes and inflammatory biomolecular markers related to corneal biomechanical integrity have been implicated.

2.13 Stevens–Johnson Syndrome

Stevens–Johnson Syndrome (SJS) is a devastating although rare condition affecting the ocular surface. It is a severe, immunological reaction, usually to drugs, and is associated with widespread destruction of the epidermis and mucous membrane.

2.13.1 Epidemiology

The incidence of SJS is approximately 1–6 cases per million persons per year, and the overall mortality rate is 20–25% [83]. It has been reported that Asian patients are at a twofold higher risk of SJS compared with Caucasians. One case-control study reported that, of all the medicines that precipitate SJS, the antibacterial sulfonamides had an excess risk of 4.5 cases/million exposed people per week [84].

2.13.2 Risk Factor

Human leukocyte antigen (HLA) types may predispose patients to adverse drug reactions. HLA-B*1502 allele has a strong association with carbamazepine-induced SJS in the Han Chinese population. The presence of HLA-B*1502, HLA-C*0602, or HLA-C*0801 alleles has been associated with trimethoprim/sulfamethoxazole-induced SJS [85]. The risk factors for developing SJS are radiotherapy, collagen vascular disease, transplantation, and herpes infection. Drugs are implicated for most of the cases, with sulphonamides still the leading agent, but nearly 40% of cases do not have any identifiable cause. About 50–80% of patients with SJS have been observed to have ocular involvement in the acute phase. Pre-existing ocular surface disturbance and immunological activity are the risk factors that may cause corneal melting and can lead to perforation.

2.14 Vitamin A Deficiency and Xerophthalmia

Vitamin A deficiency (VAD) is a major health problem mainly in developing countries like ours. As per WHO guidelines, if the prevalence of Bitot's spots among the under 6-year age group children is 0.5% or more, it indicates a significant disease burden. It is usually seen in ages 1–4 years and such children have a high risk of not only visual morbidity but also mortality.

2.14.1 Epidemiology

Globally, the incidence of xerophthalmia has been estimated at 350,000 cases annually; however, a major proportion from this cohort of children who have VAD severe enough to cause bilateral corneal melting, perforation, and blindness have very high mortality rate within the first year of becoming blind. To report an accurate estimate of the incidence of xerophthalmia is difficult owing to the synergy of VAD and measles infection that usually results in xerophthalmia and the multifactorial etiology of corneal disease. The WHO estimated that about 254 million children have Vitamin A deficiency and 2.8 million children have Xerophthalmia [86]. In population-based surveys from the past decade, some of the lowest estimates of serum VAD have been obtained in China with the highest estimates in areas of South and Southeast Asia including India where deficiency is almost universal in some of the areas surveyed. The incidence of xerophthalmia in many parts of the world has been declining over the previous few decades. The reason could be because of mass supplementation with vitamin A, various national level prevention programs, and improvements in the availability of foods containing vitamin A.

2.14.2 Risk Factors

Preschool children with comparatively higher requirements for growth and with low body store of vitamin A are susceptible to VAD and hence xerophthalmia in addition to neonates and pregnant women with relatively increased demand of vitamin A. Peak prevalence of xerophthalmia have been observed around 3–4 years of age [87]. Africans are four times more susceptible to VAD and xerophthalmia in comparison to South-East Asians. Rural habit, poor infant feeding practices, several infections, including measles, diarrhea, and respiratory tract infection, systemic diseases, parenteral illiteracy, inappropriate antenatal care and economically stressed communities are other risk factors associated with VAD and xerophthalmia.

2.15 Conclusion

A systematic and careful documentation and screening of risk factors helps in finding the etiology in corneal emergencies. Trauma is the leading cause of corneal emergencies. It could be a minor injury, and especially if associated with the vegetative matter may be associated with devastating fungal infection leading to corneal perforation and even phthisis. Detection of rare causes like vitamin A deficiency, Stevens–Johnson syndrome, etc., if diagnosed and treated early can prevent significant morbidity and even mortality.

Key Points

- All age groups can present with corneal emergencies, with trauma being the most common risk factor.
- Children are prone to diseases like Vitamin A deficiency, trauma, and chemical injury especially with chemicals like Chuna (lime).
- Fungal infections are common in Agrarian occupations
- Drug reactions, steroid abuse and systemic predisposition need to be carefully screened for.

References

1. Hong J, Qiu T, Wei A, Sun X, Xu J. Clinical characteristics and visual outcome of severe ocular chemical injuries in Shanghai. Ophthalmology. 2010;117(12):2268–72.
2. McGwin G, Xie A, Owsley C. Rate of eye injury in the United States. Arch Ophthalmol. 2005;123(7):970–6.
3. MacEwen CJ. Ocular injuries. J R Coll Surg Edinb. 1999;44(5):317–23.
4. Kuhn F, Mester V, Berta A, et al. Epidemiology of severe eye injuries: the United States Eye Injury Registry (USEIR) and the Hungarian Eye Injury Registry (HEIR) [in German]. Ophthalmologe. 1998;95(5):332–43.
5. Katz J, Tielsch JM. Lifetime prevalence of ocular injuries from Baltimore eye survey. Arch Ophthalmol. 1993;111(11):1564–8.
6. McGwin G, Owsley C. Incidence of emergency department-treated eye injury in the United States. Arch Ophthalmol. 2005;123(5):662–6.
7. Suri K, Kosker M, Duman F, Rapuano CJ, Nagra PK, Hammersmith KM. Demographic patterns and treatment outcomes of patients with recurrent corneal erosions related to trauma and epithelial and bowman layer disorders. Am J Ophthalmol. 2013;156(6):1082–7.e2.
8. Beshay N, Keay L, Dunn H, Kamalden TA, Hoskin AK, Watson SL. The epidemiology of Open Globe Injuries presenting to a tertiary referral eye hospital in Australia. Injury. 2017;48(7):1348–54.
9. Saxena R, Sinha R, Purohit A, Dada T, Vajpayee RB, Azad RV, et al. Pattern of pediatric ocular trauma in India. Indian J Pediatr. 2002;69:863–7.
10. Singh S, Sharma B, Kumar K, Dubey A, Ahirwar K. Epidemiology, clinical profile and factors, predicting final visual outcome of pediatric ocular trauma in a tertiary eye care center of Central India. Indian J Ophthalmol. 2017;65:1192–7.
11. Shukla B. Epidemiology of ocular trauma. 1st ed. New Delhi: Jaypee; 2002. p. 21.
12. Kuhn F, Morris R, Witherspoon CD, Mann L. Epidemiology of blinding trauma in the United States Eye Injury Registry. Ophthalmic Epidemiol. 2006;13(3):209–16.
13. Saxena R, Sinha R, Purohit A, Dada T, Vajpayee RB, Azad RV. Pattern of paediatric ocular trauma in India. Indian J Pediatr. 2002;69(10):863–7.
14. Katz J, Tielsch JM. Lifetime prevalence of ocular injuries from Baltimore eye survey. Arch Ophthalmol. 1993;111(11):1564–8.
15. John D, Philip SS, Mittal R, John SS, Paul P. Spectrum of ocular firework injuries in children: A 5-year retrospective study during a festive season in Southern India. Indian J Ophthalmol. 2015;63(11):843–6.
16. Erie JC, Nevitt MP, Hodge DO, et al. Incidence of ulcerative keratitis in a defined population from 1950 through 1988. Arch Ophthalmol. 1993;111:1665–71.
17. Upadhyay MP, Karmacharya PC, Koirala S, et al. The Bhaktapur eye study: ocular trauma and antibiotic prophylaxis for the prevention of corneal ulceration in Nepal. Br J Ophthalmol. 2001;85:388–92.
18. Gopinathan U, Sharma S, Garg P, Rao GN. Review of epidemiological features, microbiological diagnosis and treatment outcome of microbial keratitis: Experience of over a decade. Indian J Ophthalmol. 2009;57:273–9.
19. Ibrahim YW, Boase DL, Cree IA. Epidemiological characteristics, predisposing factors and microbiological profiles of infectious corneal ulcers: the Portsmouth corneal ulcer study. Br J Ophthalmol. 2009;93(10):1319–24.
20. Al-Ghafri A, Al-Raisi A. The epidemiology of nonviral microbial keratitis in a tertiary care center in Muscat, Oman. Oman J Ophthalmol. 2018;11(3):213.
21. Koh YY, Sun CC, Hsiao CH. Epidemiology and the estimated burden of microbial keratitis on the health care system in Taiwan: A 14-year population-based study. Am J Ophthalmol. 2020;220:152–9.
22. Bourcier T, Thomas F, Borderie V, Chaumeil C, Laroche L. Bacterial keratitis: predisposing factors, clinical and microbiological review of 300 cases. Br J Ophthalmol. 2003;87(7):834–8.

23. Tewari A, Sood N, Vegad MM, Mehta DC. Epidemiological and microbiological profile of infective keratitis in Ahmedabad. Indian J Ophthalmol. 2012;60(4):267.
24. Ni N, Nam EM, Hammersmith KM, Nagra PK, Azari AA, Leiby BE, Dai Y, Cabrera FA, Ma JF, Lambert CE Jr, Honig SE, Rapuano CJ. Seasonal, geographic, and antimicrobial resistance patterns in microbial keratitis: 4-year experience in eastern Pennsylvania. Cornea. 2015;34(3):296–302.
25. Lin CC, Prajna L, Srinivasan M, Prajna NV, McLeod SD, Acharya NR, Lietman TM, Porco TC. Seasonal trends of microbial keratitis in South India. Cornea. 2012;31(10):1123.
26. Labeille-Poizat É, Cornut PL, Poli M, Feldman A, De Bats M, Sebilleau V, Cheggour M, Denis P, Burillon C. Caractéristiques cliniques et microbiologiques des patients atteints de kératite infectieuse sévère en période caniculaire [Clinical and microbiological features of severe infectious keratitis during heatwaves]. J Fr Ophtalmol. 2013;36(9):732–9. French.
27. Srinivasan M, Gonzales CA, George C, et al. Epidemiology and aetiological diagnosis of corneal ulceration in Madurai, south India. Br J Ophthalmol. 1997;81:965–71.
28. Gopinathan U, Garg P, Fernandes M, et al. The epidemiological features and laboratory results of fungal keratitis: a 10-year review at a referral eye care center in South India. Cornea. 2002;21:555–9.
29. Ormerod LD. Causation and management of microbial keratitis in subtropical Africa. Ophthalmology. 1987;94:1662–8.
30. Xie L, Zhong W, Shi W, et al. Spectrum of fungal keratitis in north China. Ophthalmology. 2006;113:1943–8.
31. Upadhyay MP, Karmacharya PC, Koirala S, et al. Epidemiologic characteristics, predisposing factors, and etiologic diagnosis of corneal ulceration in Nepal. Am J Ophthalmol. 1991;111:92–9.
32. Toshida H, Kogure N, Inoue N, et al. Trends in microbial keratitis in Japan. Eye Contact Lens. 2007;33(2):70–3.
33. Gonzales CA, Srinavasan M, Whitcher JP, et al. Incidence of corneal ulceration in Madurai district, South India. Ophthalmic Epidemiol. 1996;3:159–66.
34. Ormerod LD, Hertzmark E, Gomez DS, et al. Epidemiology of microbial keratitis in Southern California. A multivariate analysis. Ophthalmology. 1987;94:1322–33.
35. Lam DS, Houang E, Fan DS, Lyon D, Seal D, Wong E. Incidence and risk factors for microbial keratitis in Hong Kong: comparison with Europe and North America. Eye. 2002;16(5):608–18.
36. Luchs JI, Cohen EJ, Rapuano CJ, Laibson PR. Ulcerative keratitis in bullous keratopathy. Ophthalmology. 1997;104(5):816–22.
37. Hine JL, de Lusignan S, Burleigh D, et al. Association between glycaemic control and 23 common infections in people with Type 2 diabetes: a cohort study. Diabet Med. 2017;34(4):551–7.
38. Dan J, Zhou Q, Zhai H, Cheng J, Wan L, Ge C, Xie L. Clinical analysis of fungal keratitis in patients with and without diabetes. PLoS One. 2018;13(5):e0196741.
39. Lin A, Rhee MK, Akpek EK, et al. Bacterial keratitis preferred practice pattern(R). Ophthalmology. 2019;126(1):P1–55.
40. Jeng BH, Gritz DC, Kumar AB, Holsclaw DS, Porco TC, Smith SD, Whitcher JP, Margolis TP, Wong IG. Epidemiology of ulcerative keratitis in Northern California. Arch Ophthalmol. 2010;128(8):1022–8.
41. Titiyal JS, Negi S, Anand A, Tandon R, Sharma N, Vajpayee RB. Risk factors for perforation in microbial corneal ulcers in north India. Br J Ophthalmol. 2006;90(6):686–9.
42. Bharathi MJ, Ramakrishnan R, Vasu S, et al. Epidemiological characteristics and laboratory diagnosis of fungal keratitis. A three-year study. Indian J Ophthalmol. 2003;51:315–21.
43. Chidambaram JD, Venkatesh Prajna N, Srikanthi P, Lanjewar S, Shah M, Elakkiya S, Lalitha P, Burton MJ. Epidemiology, risk factors, and clinical outcomes in severe microbial keratitis in South India. Ophthalmic Epidemiol. 2018;25(4):297–305.
44. Prajna NV, Krishnan T, Rajaraman R, et al. Predictors of corneal perforation or need for therapeutic keratoplasty in severe fungal keratitis: a secondary analysis of the mycotic ulcer treatment trial II. JAMA Ophthalmol. 2017;135(9):987–91.

45. Morgan SJ. Chemical burns of the eye: causes and management. Br J Ophthalmol. 1987;71(11):854–7.
46. Sharma N, Kaur M, Agarwal T, Sangwan VS, Vajpayee RB. Treatment of acute ocular chemical burns. Surv Ophthalmol. 2018;63(2):214–35.
47. Ramirez DA, Porco TC, Lietman TM, Keenan JD. Ocular injury in United States Emergency Departments: seasonality and annual trends estimated from a nationally representative dataset. Am J Ophthalmol. 2018;191:149–55.
48. Blackburn J, Levitan EB, MacLennan PA, Owsley C, McGwin G Jr. The epidemiology of chemical eye injuries. Curr Eye Res. 2012;37(9):787–93.
49. Hemmati H, Colby KA. Treating acute chemical injuries of the cornea. Cornea Ophthalmic Pearls. 2012;43–5.
50. Kuckelkorn R, Makropoulos W, Kottek A, Reim M. Retrospective study of severe alkali burns of the eyes. Klin Monbl Augenheilkd. 1993;203:397–402.
51. Bunker DJ, George RJ, Kleinschmidt A, Kumar RJ, Maitz P. Alkali-related ocular burns: a case series and review. J Burn Care Res. 2014;35(3):261–8.
52. Kuckelkorn R, Kottek A, Schrage N, Reim M. Poor prognosis of severe chemical and thermal eye burns: the need for adequate emergency care and primary prevention. Int Arch Occup Environ Health. 1995;67(4):281–4.
53. McGwin G Jr, Hall TA, Seale J, Xie A, Owsley C. Consumer product-related eye injury in the United States, 1998-2002. J Safety Res. 2006;37:501–6.
54. Agarwal T, Vajpayee RB, Sharma N, Tandon R. Severe ocular injury resulting from chuna packets. Ophthalmology. 2006;113(6):961.e1.
55. McKenzie LB, Ahir N, Stolz U, Nelson NG. Household cleaning product-related injuries treated in US emergency departments in 1990-2006. Pediatrics. 2010;126(3):509–16.
56. Hall AH. Epidemiology of ocular chemical burn injuries. In: Chemical ocular burns. Berlin: Springer; 2011. p. 9–15.
57. Knight IJ. Mistaken eye drops and subsequent instillation of superglue. Eye (Lond). 2001;15:663.
58. Williams KA, Roder D, Esterman A, et al. Factors predictive of corneal graft survival: report from the Australian Corneal Graft Registry. Ophthalmology. 1992;99:403–14.
59. Sit M, Weisbrod DJ, Naor J, Slomovic AR. Corneal graft outcome study. Cornea. 2001;20:129–33.
60. Bamashmus MA, Al-Akily SA, AlAkhalee HA, Al-Nuseriy KO. Emergency visits after corneal transplantation in Yemen. Oman J Ophthalmol. 2017;10(3):193–7.
61. Vajpayee RB, Boral SK, Dada T, Murthy GV, Pandey RM, Satpathy G. Risk factors for graft infection in India: a case-control study. Br J Ophthalmol. 2002;86(3):261–5.
62. Williams K, Keane M, Coffey N, et al. The Australian Corneal Graft Registry 2018 Report. 2018. p. 1–409
63. Panda A, Vanathi M, Kumar A, Dash Y, Priya S. Corneal graft rejection. Surv Ophthalmol. 2007;52(4):375–96.
64. Guerra FP, Anshu A, Price MO, Giebel AW, Price FW. Descemet's membrane endothelial keratoplasty: prospective study of 1-year visual outcomes, graft survival, and endothelial cell loss. Ophthalmology. 2011;118(12):2368–73.
65. Stulting RD, Sugar A, Beck R, Belin M, Dontchev M, Feder RS, et al. Effect of donor and recipient factors on corneal graft rejection. Cornea. 2012;31(10):1141–7.
66. Wu EI, Ritterband DC, Yu G, et al. Graft rejection following Descemet stripping automated endothelial keratoplasty: features, risk factors, and outcomes. Am J Ophthalmol. 2012;153:949–58.
67. Dunn SP, Stark WJ, Stulting RD, et al. The effect of ABO blood incompatibility on corneal transplant failure in conditions with low-risk of graft rejection. Am J Ophthalmol. 2009;147:432–8.e3.
68. Steinberg J, Eddy M-T, Katz T, et al. Traumatic wound dehiscence after penetrating keratoplasty: case series and literature review. Eur J Ophthalmol. 2012;22:335–41.

69. Das S, Whiting M, Taylor HR. Corneal wound dehiscence after penetrating keratoplasty. Cornea. 2007;26(5):526–9.
70. Lam DS, Houang E, Fan DS, et al. Hong Kong Microbial Keratitis Study Group. Incidence and risk factors for microbial keratitis in Hong Kong: comparison with Europe and North America. Eye. 2002;16(5):608–18.
71. Erie JC, Nevitt MP, Hodge DO, et al. Incidence of ulcerative keratitis in a defined population from 1950 through 1988. Arch Ophthalmol. 1993;111(12):1665–71.
72. Kinota S, Wong KW, Biswas J, et al. Changing patterns of infectious keratitis: overview of clinical and histopathologic features of keratitis due to Acanthamoeba or atypical Mycobacteria, and of infectious crystalline keratopathy. Indian J Ophthalmol. 1993;41(1):3–14.
73. Morgan PB, Efron N, Brennan NA, et al. Risk factors for the development of corneal infiltrative events associated with contact lens wear. Invest Ophthalmol Vis Sci. 2005;46:3136–43.
74. Stapleton F, Keay L, Edwards K, et al. The incidence of contact lens-related microbial keratitis in Australia. Ophthalmology. 2008;115:1655–62.
75. Jeng BH, Gritz DC, Kumar AB, Holsclaw DS, Porco TC, Smith SD, Whitcher JP, Margolis TP, Wong IG. Epidemiology of ulcerative keratitis in Northern California. Arch Ophthalmol. 2010;128(8):1022–8.
76. Steele KR, Szczotka-Flynn L. Epidemiology of contact lens-induced infiltrates: an updated review. Clin Exp Optom. 2017;100(5):473–81.
77. McKibbin M, Isaacs JD, Morrell AJ. Incidence of corneal melting in association with systemic disease in the Yorkshire Region, 1995-7. Br J Ophthalmol. 1999;83(8):941–3.
78. Lee HJ, Kim MK, Wee WR, Oh JY. Interplay of immune cells in Mooren ulcer. Cornea. 2015;34(9):1164–7.
79. Zelefsky JR, Srinivasan M, Kundu A, Lietman T, Whitcher JP, Wang K, Buyse M, Cunningham ET Jr. Hookworm infestation as a risk factor for Mooren's ulcer in South India. Ophthalmology. 2007;114(3):450–3.
80. Srinivasan M, Zegans ME, Zelefsky JR, Kundu A, Lietman T, Whitcher JP, et al. Clinical characteristics of Mooren's ulcer in South India. Br J Ophthalmol. 2007;91(5):570–5.
81. Rabinowitz YS. Keratoconus. Surv Ophthalmol. 1998;42:297–319.
82. Georgiou T, Funnell C, Cassels-Brown A, O'Conor R. Influence of ethnic origin on the incidence of keratoconus and associated atopic disease in Asians and white patients. Eye. 2004;18(4):379–83.
83. Rzany B, Mockenhaupt M, Baur S, et al. Epidemiology of erythema exsudativum multiforme majus, Stevens-Johnson syndrome, and toxic epidermal necrolysis in Germany (1990-1992): structure and results of a population-based registry. J Clin Epidemiol. 1996;49(7):769–73.
84. Roujeau JC, Kelly JP, Naldi L, et al. Medication use and the risk of Stevens-Johnson syndrome or toxic epidermal necrolysis. N Engl J Med. 1995;333(24):1600–7.
85. Kongpan T, Mahasirimongkol S, Konyoung P, et al. Candidate HLA genes for prediction of co-trimoxazole-induced severe cutaneous reactions. Pharmacogenet Genomics. 2015;25(8):402–11.
86. West KP Jr. Extent of vitamin A deficiency among preschool children and women of reproductive age. J Nutr. 2002;132(9 Suppl):2857S–66S.
87. Paranjpe R, Manade V, Kulkarni N, Oza S, Khandelwal M. Prevalence of xerophthalmia and coverage of vitamin A prophylaxis programme in slums of rural and urban communities amongst children less than 6 years of age. Indian J Clin Exp Ophthalmol. 2019;5(4):466–9.

Requisites of Cornea Clinic and Casualty Services to Manage Corneal Emergencies

3

Pranita Sahay and Prafulla K. Maharana

3.1 Introduction

Corneal blindness is the fourth leading cause of blindness globally (5.1%) as per World Health Organization [1].The major causes of corneal blindness include corneal trauma, vitamin A deficiency, infectious keratitis, congenital disease, and use of traditional medicine or home remedies, which often harm the eye rather than relieve pain or improve eyesight [2, 3]. In developing countries, corneal scars (28.1%) and active keratitis (12.2%) often contribute a major proportion of this burden [4].

Corneal trauma is the most significant cause of unilateral loss of vision in developing countries, and up to 5% of all bilateral blindness has been attributed to direct ocular trauma [1]. Xerophthalmia and ophthalmia neonatorum were important causes of corneal blindness in children [2]. Besides these conditions some rare conditions that could lead to corneal blindness include acute corneal hydrops, corneal graft failure, toxic keratitis, and congenital corneal abnormalities.Most of these cases present to the ophthalmic casualty services or cornea clinic as an acute emergency with the complaint of acute vision loss that needs immediate assessment and management [5–11]. A major factor that decides the outcome in such conditions is the delay in treatment in seeking a cornea consult or a lack of logistics such as instruments and devices. Hence, it is important that both the ophthalmic casualty services and cornea clinic have adequate facilities to appropriately investigate and manage these patients, as any delay in treatment may affect the final visual outcome and result in life-long visual handicap.

P. Sahay
Department of Ophthalmology, Lady Hardinge Medical College, New Delhi, India

P. K. Maharana (✉)
Dr Rajendra Prasad Centre for Ophthalmic Sciences, All India Institute of Medical Sciences, New Delhi, India

B. Sharma, J. S. Titiyal (eds.), *Corneal Emergencies*,
https://doi.org/10.1007/978-981-16-5876-1_3

3.2 Clinic Setup

The cornea clinic or ophthalmic casualty service must have every basic stuff to manage acute emergencies. The first thing while planning to set up a cornea emergency set up is working space. Ideally, there should be separate designated spaces/rooms for initial assessment and triage; basic examination such as slit lamp, non-contact tonometry, visual acuity; and interventions such as saline wash for chemical injury, tissue adhesive and bandaged contact lens application for management of small corneal perforation, and foreign body removal. Every corneal emergency service must have an access to a fully equipped operation room (OR) prepared to take up cases under local as well as general anesthesia.

3.2.1 Equipment and Manpower

Ideally, every corneal emergency service must have a triage room to start with. An expert nursing staff, and an intern or ophthalmology resident for initial assessment and segregation of patients depending on the urgency of intervention should man the triage room. The examination and investigation room should have all the investigative tools required for evaluation of patients presenting with corneal emergencies including visual acuity assessment chart, photo slit lamp biomicroscope, indirect ophthalmoscope, non-contact tonometer, ultrasound B scan (8–10 Hz), anterior segment optical coherence tomography (ASOCT), and pachymeter (Table 3.1). Slit lamp anterior segment photography serves as an important tool for objective documentation of microscopic and obscure details of the transparent,

Table 3.1 Investigative tools required in ophthalmic emergency services and cornea clinic

S. No.	Investigative Tools	Purpose
1	Visual acuity assessment chart	Baseline visual acuity assessment and counseling as well as prognostication of the patients
2	Slit lamp biomicroscope (preferably with camera)	Baseline detailed ocular examination and documentation with slit lamp photography (if possible)
3	Indirect ophthalmoscope	Fundus examination
4	Non-contact tonometer	Assessment of intra-ocular pressure as often the patients may have an epithelial defect where contact procedure like applanation tonometry is contraindicated
5	Ultrasound B scan (8–10 Hz)	Posterior segment evaluation as media is often haze in these cases
6	Anterior segment optical coherence tomography	For detailed assessment of cornea as well as anterior chamber details
7	Pachymeter	For assessment of corneal thickness especially in cases of graft rejection for further monitoring of response to treatment

translucent, and opaque structures of the ocular tissue. Ultrasound B scan imaging assists in the evaluation of the posterior segment of the eye specially in cases with non-transparent media as well as for the integrity of the posterior lens capsule. ASOCT provides qualitative and quantitative assessment of the anterior segment. Advantages of the ASOCT include the non-contact capture system that causes minimal discomfort in corneal emergency patients while providing high-resolution cross-sections images of the anterior segment. ASOCT is very helpful in cases with poor corneal clarity for detailed evaluation of cornea as well as the anterior chamber.Measurement of corneal thickness using pachymeter is especially useful in evaluation of cases with corneal emergencies secondary to refractive or transplantation procedures. An expert optometrist and a cornea fellow should be there, round the clock, for performing any investigation and appropriate examination.

It is prudent to equip the emergency room with an autoclave for emergency sterilization specially of surgical instruments. Additionally, adequate provision of biomedical waste disposal should be ensured with training of medical and support staff for efficient conduction of biomedical waste disposal.

Visual acuity assessment is necessary in all cases followed by detailed slit lamp examination. Media is often hazy hence indirect ophthalmoscopy or ultrasound B scan is required in most cases for posterior segment evaluation. Cases presenting with graft rejection require a baseline pachymetry assessment to document treatment response after starting systemic steroid therapy (Table 3.2).

Management of cases with corneal emergencies often necessitates the multidisciplinary approach. Integration of ancillary departments including microbiology, radiology, anesthesia, plastic surgery, and pediatrics is necessary to deal with prompt referral and urgent systemic evaluation and management. This kind of multidisciplinary approach often speeds up the evaluation and treatment process which is a pre-requisite for dealing with corneal emergencies.

3.2.2 Consumables

The consumable items that should be available for assessment of patients include fluorescein strips, Schirmer strips, 23/26/30-gauge needle, Kimura spatula, glass slides, cotton tipped applicators, culture plates [blood agar, chocolate agar, Sabouraud dextrose agar (SDA)], and litmus paper. The uses of these items have been highlighted in Table 3.3. Apart from this, hand gloves, hand wash, and alcohol-based hand sanitizer for maintaining hand hygiene in between examination of two patients is essential. Therapeutic procedures that can be performed in the ophthalmic emergency outpatient department (OPD) include application of tissue adhesive with bandage contact lens in cases of small corneal perforation [12]. Hence, keeping a cyanoacrylate glue and bandage contact lens in stock can be beneficial. Also, availability of fibrin glue facilitates bedside application of amniotic membrane graft especially in cases of acute Steven–Johnson Syndrome with ocular involvement [13].

Table 3.2 List of equipment and consumables required for performing minor procedure in casualty OPD for corneal emergencies

S. no.	Minor procedures	Equipment and consumables required
1	Corneal scraping	1. Slit lamp biomicroscope 2. Eye drop Proparacaine 3. Eye speculum 4. 23-gauge needle/15 number blade/Kimura spatula 5. Culture media—Blood agar, chocolate agar, SDA agar, Nutrient broth 6. Glass slides
2	Corneal foreign body removal	1. Slit lamp biomicroscope 2. Eye drop Proparacaine 3. Eye speculum 4. 26-gauge needle and 2 ml syringe
3	Saline wash in acute chemical injury of eye	1. Eye drop Proparacaine 2. Litmus paper 3. Dessmarres retractor 4. Plain forceps 5. IV stand 6. Normal saline bottles 7. Eye speculum
4	Corneal gluing	1. Eye drop Proparacaine 2. Eye speculum 3. 30-gauge needle and a 2 ml syringe 4. N-butyl-cyanoacrylate glue 5. Bandage contact lens
5	Corneal suture removal	1. Eye drop Proparacaine 2. Eye speculum 3. 26-gauge needle and 2 ml syringe 4. McPherson forceps

A sterile intervention room or minor OT well equipped with the facility of autoclaving and medical waste disposal system is a basic pre-requisite required to facilitate immediate interventions while dealing with corneal emergency cases

Table 3.3 Consumable items required in ophthalmic emergency services and cornea clinic

S. no.	Consumables	Purpose
1	Fluorescein strips	Better assessment of epithelial defects on slit lamp examination after staining with fluorescein
2	23-gauge needle and Kimura spatula	Performing corneal scraping in cases of corneal ulcer
3	Glass slides	Preparing smears of obtained specimen from corneal scraping
4	Blood agar, Chocolate agar, Sabouraud dextrose agar	Direct plating of the obtained specimen from corneal scraping Direct plating improves sensitivity of culture test
5	26/30-gauge needle	For removal of superficial corneal foreign body
6	Litmus paper	For checking the pH of tear in cases of chemical injury

3.2.3 Drugs

Medicines required in emergency include antiseptic ophthalmic solutions (such as povidone-iodine 10% w/v and 5% w/v), topical anesthetic eye drops (such as proparacaine 0.5%), fortified antibiotics, sodium citrate 20%, sodium ascorbate 20%, injectable dexamethasone, methylprednisolone and mannitol, tablet acetazolamide, normal saline, and balanced salt solution (Table 3.4). In-house availability of these essential drugs reduce the lag between diagnosing a patient and initiating therapy in cases presenting with corneal emergency conditions especially corneal ulcer, chemical injury, and acute graft rejection [10, 11].

3.2.4 Instruments

Surgical instruments that are often required while assessing these patients include an eye speculum, McPherson forceps, Lims forceps, globe holding forceps, and Desmarres retractor. The eye speculum, preferably self-retaining with locking system, is essential for performing corneal scraping in cases of keratitis and saline wash in patients presenting with chemical injury, McPherson for removing loose corneal sutures and Desmarres for double eversion of lid in cases of chemical injury, and visualizing the fornix to rule out impacted chuna/foreign particles [11, 14–16].

Table 3.4 Medicines required in ophthalmic emergency services and cornea clinic

S. no.	Medicines	Purpose
1	Eyedrop Proparacaine (0.5%)	Corneal anesthesia prior to corneal scraping, foreign body removal, and saline wash
2	Topical Fortified antibiotics (Cefazolin 5%, Tobramycin 1.3%, Vancomycin 5%)	For prescription in cases of moderate-severe corneal ulcer The injectable preparation should be available and fortified drops should be prepared fresh before dispensing as they have short shelf life
3	Topical Antibiotics (Moxifloxacin, Gatifloxacin, Tobramycin)	For use following contact procedures, following minor procedures
4	Topical mydriatics and cycloplegics (Tropicamide, Phenylephrine, Homatropine)	For pain relief and detailed examination
5	Topical sodium citrate 20% Topical sodium ascorbate 20%	For prescription in cases of chemical injury Should be prepared fresh
6	Injectable dexamethasone, and methylprednisolone	For management of patients presenting with acute graft rejection
7	Normal saline	For saline wash in cases of chemical injury
8	Injection Mannitol and Tablet acetazolamide	For prescription in cases presenting with high intra-ocular pressure

3.3 Procedures Performed in OPD

3.3.1 Corneal Scraping

Corneal scarping is performed in cases of corneal ulcer and has both diagnostic and therapeutic implications. To perform this procedure the following items are required and should be kept together as a kit for performing the procedure

- *Eye drop Proparacaine* for topical anesthesia prior to performing this procedure
- *Eye speculum* for proper exposure of the corneal ulcer and avoiding blinking of the eye during the process of corneal ulcer scarping
- *23-gauge needle/15 number blade/Kimura spatula for scraping the corneal ulcer*
- Blood agar/chocolate agar/SDA agar for direct plating of the obtained scraping specimen
- Nutrient broth in cases where bacterial culture media is not available for direct plating
- Glass slides for smear preparation from the obtained corneal scraping specimen

3.3.2 Corneal Gluing

Corneal gluing is performed in cases with severe corneal thinning, impending corneal perforation, small corneal perforation (without iris plugging the wound), and descemetocele for providing tectonic support. To perform this procedure, the following items are required:

- Sterile intervention room or minor OT
- *Eye drop Proparacaine* for topical anesthesia prior to performing this procedure
- *Eye speculum* for proper exposure and avoiding blinking of the eye during the procedure
- *30-gauge needle* and a *2 ml syringe* for application of *cyanoacrylate glue*
- N-butyl-cyanoacrylate glue for sealing the site of perforation or thinning
- *Bandage contact lens* for application at the end of procedure for improving patient's post-operative comfort

3.3.3 Saline Wash in Acute Chemical Injury

Immediate wash off the chemicals from the eye is the primary treatment for all cases presenting with ocular chemical injury. The following items are required for performing a saline wash

- *Eye drop Proparacaine* for topical anesthesia prior to performing this procedure
- Litmus paper for checking pH of the eye before and after saline wash

- Dessmarres retractor for double eversion of the lid to inspection and remove impacted particles of the chemical agent from the fornixes
- Plain forceps to remove the impacted chemicals like chuna particles
- IV stand and Normal saline bottles (at least 2 l) for irrigating the ocular surface
- Eye speculum for proper exposure of the ocular surface during saline wash

3.3.4 Corneal Foreign Body Removal

Patients often present with superficial corneal foreign body following trauma at workplace. Management includes removal of superficial corneal foreign body on the slit lamp while deeply buried foreign bodies require removal in the theater under an operating microscope. The following items are required for removal of superficial corneal foreign bodies

- *Eye drop Proparacaine* for topical anesthesia prior to performing this procedure
- *Eye speculum* for proper exposure of the ocular surface and avoiding blinking of the eye during the procedure
- *26-gauge needle* and *2 ml syringe* for removal of the foreign body.

3.3.5 Corneal Suture Removal

Patients with loose sutures and suture site infiltrate, commonly seen in cases that have undergone keratoplasty, require urgent removal of sutures to avoid complications like graft infection and rejection. The following items are required for performing corneal suture removal

- *Eye drop Proparacaine* for topical anesthesia prior to performing this procedure
- *Eye speculum* for proper exposure of the ocular surface and avoiding blinking of the eye during the procedure
- *26-gauge needle* and *2 ml syringe* for cutting the suture
- McPherson forceps for removing the suture.

3.4 Conclusion

In nutshell, availability of basic ophthalmic equipment, instruments, consumable items, and medicines can help in smooth functioning of the ophthalmic casualty services and cornea clinic with timely and optimal management of cases presenting with corneal emergency. Also, many cases may require an urgent surgical intervention and hence the cornea clinic/casualty services should have an adjacent ophthalmic OT for managing these cases.

Key Points

- Corneal emergencies require prompt intervention for best outcome
- It includes traumatic corneal laceration, graft rejection, corneal ulcers, acute hydrops, and chemical injury to the eye
- The cornea clinic and casualty services should be adequately equipped to investigate and treat these cases
- Equipment required include visual acuity assessment chart, slit lamp biomicroscope, indirect ophthalmoscope, non-contact tonometer, ultrasound B scan (8–10 Hz), anterior segment optical coherence tomography (ASOCT), and pachymeter
- Consumables required include fluorescein strips, Schirmer strips, 23/26/30 gauge needle, Kimura spatula, glass slides, cotton tipped applicators, culture plates, and litmus paper
- Drugs required for managing these cases include topical anesthetic eye drops (such as proparacaine 0.5%), fortified antibiotics, sodium citrate 20%, sodium ascorbate 20%, injectable dexamethasone, methylprednisolone and mannitol, tablet acetazolamide, normal saline, and balanced salt solution
- Minor procedures performed in cornea clinic and casualty services include corneal scraping, corneal foreign body removal, corneal gluing, saline wash, and suture removal
- Instruments required to perform these procedures should be available for use
- Cases requiring major procedures need an OT setup for further management; hence, the casualty services should have an adjacent OT setup.

References

1. Whitcher JP, Srinivasan M, Upadhyay MP. Corneal blindness: a global perspective. Bull World Health Organ. 2001;79(3):214–21.
2. Gupta N, Tandon R, Gupta SK, Sreenivas V, Vashist P. Burden of corneal blindness in India. Indian J Community Med. 2013;38(4):198–206.
3. Sahay P, Saluja G, Maharana PK, Titiyal JS. Topical ayurvedic ointment-induced chemical injury presenting as bilateral acute keratitis. BMJ Case Rep. 2017;20:2017.
4. Garg P, Krishna PV, Stratis AK, Gopinathan U. The value of corneal transplantation in reducing blindness. Eye (Lond). 2005;19(10):1106–14.
5. Maharana PK, Sharma N, Nagpal R, Jhanji V, Das S, Vajpayee RB. Recent advances in diagnosis and management of mycotic keratitis. Indian J Ophthalmol. 2016;64(5):346–57.
6. Maharana PK, Sharma N, Vajpayee RB. Acute corneal hydrops in keratoconus. Indian J Ophthalmol. 2013;61(8):461–4.
7. Austin A, Lietman T, Rose-Nussbaumer J. Update on the management of infectious keratitis. Ophthalmology. 2017;124(11):1678–89.
8. Fujikawa A, Mohamed YH, Kinoshita H, Matsumoto M, Uematsu M, Tsuiki E, et al. Visual outcomes and prognostic factors in open-globe injuries. BMC Ophthalmol. 2018;18(1):138.
9. Kohanim S, Palioura S, Saeed HN, Akpek EK, Amescua G, Basu S, et al. Acute and chronic ophthalmic involvement in Stevens-Johnson syndrome/toxic epidermal necrolysis—a comprehensive review and guide to therapy. II. Ophthalmic disease. Ocul Surf. 2016;14(2):168–88.

10. Panda A, Vanathi M, Kumar A, Dash Y, Priya S. Corneal graft rejection. Surv Ophthalmol. 2007;52(4):375–96.
11. Sharma N, Kaur M, Agarwal T, Sangwan VS, Vajpayee RB. Treatment of acute ocular chemical burns. Surv Ophthalmol. 2018;63(2):214–35.
12. Rana M, Savant V. A brief review of techniques used to seal corneal perforation using cyanoacrylate tissue adhesive. Cont Lens Anterior Eye. 2013;36(4):156–8.
13. Jain R, Sharma N, Basu S, Iyer G, Ueta M, Sotozono C, et al. Stevens-Johnson syndrome: The role of an ophthalmologist. Surv Ophthalmol. 2016;61(4):369–99.
14. Aishwarya A, Gupta P, Tiwari US. Wire lid retractor—a new use of wire eye speculum. Indian J Ophthalmol. 2019;67(3):391–2.
15. Leck A. Taking a corneal scrape and making a diagnosis. Community Eye Health. 2009;22(71):42–3.
16. Gupta N, Tandon R. Investigative modalities in infectious keratitis. Indian J Ophthalmol. 2008;56(3):209–13.

4 Diagnostic and Therapeutic Approach in Management of Corneal Emergencies

Dhruv Kamra and Anubha Rathi

4.1 Introduction

Corneal emergencies account for a vast majority of cases presenting to the emergency department. Corneal abrasions and foreign bodies in the external eye are the most frequently encountered ocular emergencies [1]. The severity of these conditions may vary depending on the underlying pathology, time to presentation, and various other local and systemic factors. Corneal emergencies need utmost care and precision in handling as they can be potentially vision-threatening. This chapter highlights the various corneal emergencies and the basic history taking skills along with the diagnostic and therapeutic approach that must be kept in mind while managing these potentially serious corneal conditions.

4.2 History Taking

In any case of ***ocular trauma***, it is vital to obtain a detailed history to make the correct diagnosis and plan your management accordingly. A good history should include the following:

4.2.1 Assess Systemic Status

History of loss of consciousness, vomiting, or nasal bleed following trauma warrants a proper neurological assessment including Glasgow Coma Score (GCS) and neuroimaging.

D. Kamra · A. Rathi (✉)
The Cornea Institute, L V Prasad Eye Institute, Hyderabad, Telangana, India

B. Sharma, J. S. Titiyal (eds.), *Corneal Emergencies*,
https://doi.org/10.1007/978-981-16-5876-1_4

4.2.2 Determine the Mechanism of Injury

- Blunt or penetrating
- Material—vegetative matter, metallic foreign bodies, chemicals (acids or alkali), thermal injuries, etc.
- The velocity of impact/projectile
- Workplace-related injury, rule out assault, road traffic accidents, as these may be medico-legal cases

4.2.3 Symptoms

- Diminution of vision—sudden or gradual; painless or painful
- Pain, redness, watering, and photophobia
- Foreign body sensation
- Bleeding

4.2.4 Medical History

- Tetanus immunization status
- Diabetes, hypertension, and other systemic illness
- Bleeding disorders

4.2.5 Treatment History

- Medical—h/o use of any topical eye drops or oral antibiotics in the recent past
- Surgical—h/o previous surgery or trauma in the affected eye
- In cases of chemical injury, it is essential to ask if a thorough eyewash was done immediately following the injury.

In cases of ***corneal ulcers***, history taking is important to ascertain the inciting agent or risk factors that may be associated with the development of the ulcer. One must ask for any history of:

- **Trauma**—organic or non-organic material
- **Duration of symptoms**
- **Contact lens wear**—type of contact lenses (rigid or soft), wearing schedule, and contact lens hygiene. It is also important to ask for a history of sleeping with contact lenses on (especially in cases of non-extended wear lenses) and taking bath in a pond or swimming pool with contact lenses on.
- **Systemic diseases**
  - Collagen vascular diseases may be associated with dry eye disease, PUK, and sterile corneal melts. Take a history of joint pain.

  - Immunocompromised state—DM, HTN, alcoholism
- **Treatment**—self-medication with home remedies, use of topical steroids, or other ayurvedic eye drops.
- **History of recurrent episodes in the same eye**—may be suggestive of viral etiology.

Post corneal transplant emergencies need to be assessed with case-specific history taking which includes:

- Suture-related problems—patient may complain of foreign body sensation, pain, and watering in cases of loose, broken sutures or due to un-buried knots.
- Acute graft rejection—patient usually presents with blurring of vision, redness, and discomfort. It is important to check for compliance of the patient toward the use of topical steroids.
- Wound dehiscence—important to ask for history of trauma
- Post-PK glaucoma—dull aching pain associated with a unilateral headache
- Graft infiltrate—patients usually complain of pain, excessive tearing, discharge, photophobia, and redness. It is vital to enquire about any history of trauma, contact lens wear, or bath in a pond.

Post-refractive surgery corneal emergencies also demand specific history taking pertaining to the underlying condition. Some patients may present with symptoms of foreign body sensation, discomfort, and dryness after LASIK surgery. This may point toward post-refractive surgery Dry eye disease. It is important to ask the patient whether they had similar complaints prior to the surgery as dry eye disease is a relative contraindication to LASIK. Post LASIK ectasia patients may present to the clinic with a history of gradually progressive diminution of vision. It is of utmost importance to differentiate myopic regression from ectasia, as retreatment in the latter can result in worsening of visual outcomes by facilitating the progression of ectasia. Preoperative topography/tomography maps if available must be assessed in such cases.

Corneal emergencies associated with ***advanced corneal ectasia*** may present with:

- Acute Hydrops—Patient usually presents with sudden onset of pain, watering, photophobia, and reduced visual acuity. It is important to ask for a history of eye rubbing or other skin allergies and to obtain any previous topography scans of the same eye and the opposite eye.
- Corneal perforation—this may occur either spontaneously or following minor trauma in cases of advanced ectatic conditions.

Stevens–Johnson syndrome is another major corneal emergency. It is an autoimmune blistering disorder affecting the skin and mucous membranes. The acute stage of SJS occurs during the first 2 weeks after the onset of symptoms; however, the patient is usually admitted to the hospital for intensive medical care and rarely ever presents to an ophthalmologist during this phase. The patient may however present in the subacute stage with c/o pain, photophobia, watering and redness in both eyes. It is therefore important to ask for a detailed history of drug intake (especially sulfa drugs, anti-epileptics, and allopurinol), hospitalization or admission in the intensive care unit, history of fever and skin rash preceding the sudden onset of eye redness (conjunctivitis), history of mouth ulcers, any peeling of skin, or disfigurement/falling of nails.

4.3 Clinical Examination

4.3.1 Visual Acuity

In all cases of corneal emergencies, it is important to assess the vision at presentation in both eyes as this not only gives us an idea regarding the severity of the injury or disease but also helps to prognosticate the outcome. This may be done using a simple Snellen's chart for assessing distant vision and a Jaeger eye chart for near vision. However, in cases where the vision is severely diminished, such as corneal trauma, one may have to record vision as finger counting, hand movements, or perception of light and projection of rays. Visual assessment may be deferred in cases of chemical injuries, where an immediate wash is of utmost importance. It is essential to keep a record of the vision at each visit in all cases of corneal emergencies, more so in cases of corneal trauma as this may have medico-legal implications.

4.3.2 Systemic Examination

Some patients presenting with an ocular emergency may have associated systemic features that should be looked for on examination. These include:

- Skin rashes, blisters, peeling of skin, mouth and genital ulcers, distortion, or loss of nails in cases of acute SJS.
- Joint deformities in cases of PUK associated with Rheumatoid arthritis.
- Corneal ectasias may be associated with various syndromes having peculiar deformities or systemic abnormalities that need to be evaluated.

4.3.3 External Examination

- **Face and peri-orbital region**—The face and periorbital region should be examined carefully for any wounds or chemical burns in all cases of ocular trauma. In cases of acute Stevens–Johnson syndrome, rashes and peeling of skin may be noted on the face along with other parts of the body.
- **Ocular alignment and motility**—may be affected in cases of orbital bone fractures or injuries involving the third, fourth, and sixth cranial nerves.

- **Palpation**—of the facial and orbital bones for crepitus and for any discontinuity of the orbital rim may help in clinically diagnosing orbital bone fractures.
- **Pupil:**
  - Size: may be enlarged due to damage to the iris sphincter muscles incurred during ocular trauma.
  - Shape: may be altered in cases of iris tissue prolapse through a corneal wound or perforation.
  - Reactivity: may be non-reactive to light either because of injury to the optic nerve or because of traumatic mydriasis. Swinging flashlight examination should be done to illicit any relative afferent pupillary defect and both direct as well as consensual light reflexes should be assessed in all cases of ocular trauma.

4.3.4 Slit Lamp Examination

4.3.4.1 Lids

Lids should be evaluated for edema, ecchymosis, tears, lacerations (with or without tissue loss), and canalicular involvement in all cases of ocular trauma. Eyelid burns (superficial or deep), tissue loss, and charring of lashes may be seen in cases of acute thermal or chemical injuries and can lead to cicatricial entropion or ectropion upon healing. The lids must be everted in all cases of chemical injury (especially lime injury) in order to reveal the offending chemical agent which might be stuck to the tarsal conjunctiva and even lodged in the fornices; therefore, a double eversion of the lid should be done and the chemical agent should be thoroughly removed with irrigation. SJS patients may present with varied lid findings depending on the time of presentation. In the initial few weeks, there may be lid edema, erythema, crusting, and lid margin ulceration. Lid eversion may reveal conjunctival membranes or pseudomembranes as well. With time, chronic lid changes may result in trichiasis, lid margin keratinization, and distichiasis.

Lids of all patients presenting with a corneal ulcer should be examined for trichiasis, lagophthalmos, entropion, ectropion as these may pose as predisposing factors for corneal infection.

4.3.4.2 Conjunctiva

Conjunctiva needs to be examined carefully by slit-lamp evaluation for:

- Conjunctival congestion (diffuse or circumciliary), chemosis, tears, subconjunctival hemorrhage, and any foreign body lodged in tarsal conjunctiva in all cases of ocular trauma
- Conjunctival epithelial defects and for any chemical agent stuck to the tarsal conjunctiva in all cases of chemical injury
- Conjunctival membranes and ulceration in cases of SJS

4.3.4.3 Sclera

It is important to look for any scleral tear or rupture in all cases of ocular trauma. Subconjunctival hemorrhage, conjunctival congestion, and chemosis may sometimes preclude a detailed examination of the sclera and an occult scleral tear may be missed. In cases where the posterior border of the subconjunctival hemorrhage cannot be made out (extends posteriorly beyond the equator), intracranial bleed, orbital roof fracture, skull base fracture, or posterior scleral tear should be suspected.

Focal or diffuse redness or violaceous discoloration of the sclera along with nodules or scleral necrosis are signs of scleritis that may be associated with peripheral ulcerative keratitis (PUK) whereas scleral abscess and ulcers may be noted in cases of sclerokeratitis.

4.3.4.4 Cornea

In all cases of penetrating corneal injuries, the cornea should be examined under the slit-lamp to evaluate the wound size, configuration (linear, stellate, lamellar, irregular), involvement of the limbus or extension into the sclera, any uveal tissue or vitreous prolapse, or any embedded corneal foreign bodies. Seidel's test and forced Seidel's test may be helpful in distinguishing between partial-thickness/sealed corneal tears and full-thickness corneal tears.

With regards to some of the other corneal emergencies, it is essential to do a complete slit lamp examination of the cornea evaluating each layer in detail:

Epithelium

Epithelial defect: can be detected by fluorescein staining and its size should be measured in all cases of acute SJS, chemical injuries, corneal ulcers, PUK, and in post-PK grafts.

Superficial punctate keratitis: punctate fluorescein staining may be noted in cases of dry eye disease (associated with PUK), SJS, chemical injuries (mild to moderate), contact lens wearers, and corneal grafts in patients having lid abnormalities or poor ocular surface.

Stroma

Infiltrate:

- Size—can be measured either horizontally and vertically or in terms of the largest diameter of the infiltrate and the longest perpendicular to it.
- Depth—optical slit beam may be used to estimate the depth of the infiltrate (anterior, mid, or posterior stromal).
- Color—yellowish, gray, white, brown (pigmented in cases of Dematiaceous fungi)
- Margins—well defined or ill defined, regular or irregular, feathery, tentacles, pinhead lesions.
- Associated epithelial defect and its size
- Edges of the ulcer—sloping, rounded, elevated, heaped up, or overhanging.
- Satellite lesions—number and location.

- A few clues to differentiate between a sterile and infective infiltrate include location which is usually central in infectious infiltrates and the presence of mucopurulent discharge. Presence of symptoms, anterior chamber reaction or lid edema also suggest infective etiology of the infiltrate [2].

Scar:

- The presence of footprint scars in patients presenting with recurrent episodes of redness may hint toward a viral etiology.
- Multiple small scars with/without pigments may be seen in factory workers presenting with embedded corneal foreign bodies (iron).
- Faint nebular scars may be noted in contact lens wearers who have had previous episodes of Contact lens-related peripheral ulcers (CLPU).
- Superficial stromal scars or apical scarring may be seen in cases of advanced keratoconus

Thinning:

- Peripheral thinning associated with sterile peripheral corneal melt may be seen in cases of PUK.
- Central thinning is more likely to be seen in cases of keratoconus
- Thinning and perforation due to stromal necrosis may be seen in infectious keratitis (Fig. 4.1).

Corneal edema: may be seen in ocular emergencies such as hydrops, corneal ulcers, HSV keratitis, graft rejection, and chemical injuries. It may be focal or diffuse.

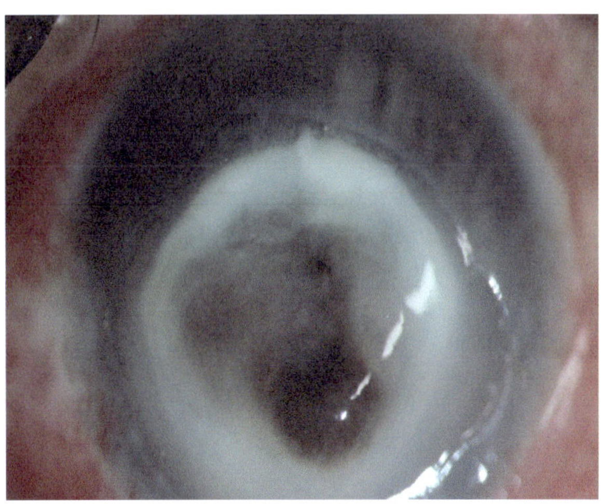

Fig. 4.1 Clinical photograph of the eye showing a perforated corneal ulcer with surrounding corneal infiltrates and thinning

Vascularization may be seen in cases of:

- SJS, graft rejection, chemical injuries, and PUK—due to the ongoing inflammation.
- Microbial keratitis—especially in cases of recurrent HSV stromal keratitis.
- Contact lens wearers (soft contact lens >Rigid Gas Permeable lenses (RGP)—due to hypoxia
- Broken or loose sutures in post-PK grafts may also incite vascularization.

Descemet Membrane

Breaks and detachment—may most often be seen on slit lamp examination in cases of acute hydrops and corneal penetrating injuries.

Descemetocele—Is bulging of the Descemet membrane in an area of extreme focal corneal thinning with just the DM remaining. It is an ominous sign of impending perforation and may be seen in cases of sterile corneal melts (PUK associated with RA), advanced ectasia, and corneal ulcers.

Endothelium

Keratic precipitates: these are inflammatory cells that deposit on the endothelium of the cornea. Fresh KPs usually appear white, rounded, and glistening whereas old KPs are usually pigmented, faded with crenated irregular margins. KPs may be seen in cases of:

- HSV endothelitis—usually appear focally with overlying stromal edema (Disciform keratitis)but can be diffusely spread over the endothelium as well.
- Microbial keratitis—Intense AC inflammation due to microbial invasion of the cornea may lead to the formation of KPs.
- Graft rejection—The linear arrangement of KPs in a post-PK corneal graft (Khodadoust line) is pathognomic of endothelial graft rejection (Fig. 4.2).

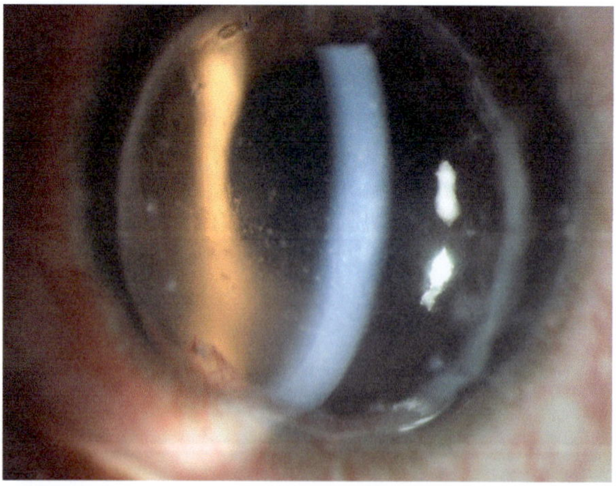

Fig. 4.2 Clinical photograph of the eye showing acute graft rejection post penetrating keratoplasty with graft edema and keratic precipitates on the endothelium

Endoexudates—These are a collection of inflammatory cells that may be seen attached to the endothelium and are commonly witnessed in cases of microbial keratitis (more often in fungal keratitis).

4.3.4.5 Anterior Chamber (AC)

It should be examined carefully in most cases of ocular emergencies for the following:

- **Depth**—The AC may be shallow or flat in cases of penetrating corneal injuries, corneal perforations, and in post-PK grafts with wound leak (low IOP) or pupillary block (high IOP). The AC may appear deeper as compared to the other eye in cases of angle recession and lens dislocation/subluxation due to blunt trauma.
- **AC reaction (cells)**—a 1 × 1 mm slit beam of maximum illumination can be used to view and count cells in the AC, which are then graded according to the SUN classification system (Table 4.1). These cells are mainly comprised of leucocytes (mainly PMNs) and indicate the level of inflammation in the AC. It is a common finding in cases of blunt corneal injury, corneal ulcers, chemical injuries and is one of the earliest signs of graft rejection. Intense AC reaction may lead to the collection and deposition of leucocytes inferiorly to form a hypopyon. The hypopyon is sterile and mobile in most cases except for fungal keratitis wherein the invasion of fungal filaments into the AC gives rise to a fixed, infected hypopyon.
- **Hyphema**—the choroid and iris contain a rich vascular complex, therefore injury to the ciliary body or iris is one of the major causes of hyphema in cases of blunt ocular trauma. Hyphema is usually classified based on the proportion of the AC it occupies (Table 4.2).
- **Exudates**—large clumps of exudates may be seen in the AC in a few cases of microbial keratitis, especially fungal keratitis (Fig. 4.3).

4.3.4.6 Iris

The iris has a rich network of blood vessels, the endothelial cells of which comprise the blood-aqueous barrier. Any injury or inflammation of the iris tissue leads to a

Table 4.1 Standardization of Uveitis Nomenclature, 2005 (SUN) grading of anterior chamber cells and flare

Cells in field (1 mm × 1 mm slit beam)	Grade of AC cells	Grade of AC flare
<1	0	0 None
1–5	0.5+	
6–15	1+	1+ Faint
16–25	2+	2+ Moderate (iris lens details clear)
26–50	3+	3+ Marked (iris lens details hazy)
50+	4+	4+ Intense (severe aqueous haze)

AC, anterior chamber

Table 4.2 Grading of hyphema based on the extent of fill in the anterior chamber

Grade of hyphema	Extent of anterior chamber fill
0 (Microhyphema)	Circulating RBCs seen
I	<33% fill
II	33–50% fill
III	>50% fill
IV	100% fill, eight ball hyphema

RBC, red blood cell

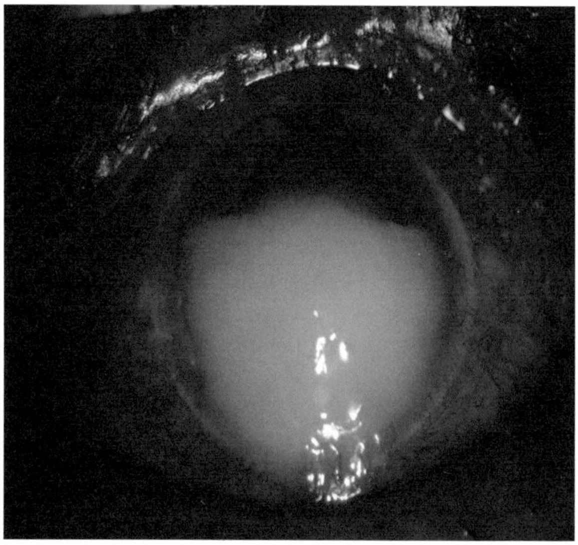

Fig. 4.3 Clinical photograph of the eye showing a case of fungal keratitis with an anterior chamber full of exudates

disruption of this blood-aqueous barrier and results in AC reaction. The iris should be examined under a slit lamp for the following:

- **Prolapsed iris tissue**—Most cases of penetrating corneal injury present as a corneal tear with prolapsed iris tissue. It is important to check the viability of this iris tissue on table. An avascular, necrotic, friable iris tissue that does not bleed on touch is mostly non-viable and should be excised rather than being reposited back into the AC.
- **Holes and foreign bodies**—In cases of penetrating corneal injuries especially by small-sized, high-velocity objects such as iron particles and shrapnel, it is important to look for these foreign bodies carefully as these may be lodged in the iris tissue. Also, the presence of iris holes in such kinds of injuries should raise the suspicion of an intraocular foreign body.
- **Sphincter tears**—Blunt trauma can cause damage to the sphincter pupillae muscle of the iris that may render the pupil non-reactive to light and result in traumatic mydriasis, it may also lead to a distortion of the pupil shape.

- **Atrophy**—Sectoral iris atrophy may be seen in cases of Herpes zoster keratouveitis, whereas patchy iris atrophy is more often associated with HSV keratouveitis.
- **Peripheral anterior synechiae (PAS)**—post-keratoplasty patients may present with peripheral anterior synechiae resulting from extensive AC inflammation or shallow AC. Extensive PAS may result in angle closure leading to a high IOP.

4.3.4.7 Lens

In all cases of ocular trauma, it is important to examine the lens for any anterior lens capsule (ALC) breach, traumatic cataract, zonular dialysis, and foreign body on the ALC or intralenticular foreign body. The absence of lens may indicate posterior dislocation of the lens and it is important to do a thorough fundus examination in such cases. In cases of blunt trauma, a pigmented ring known as the Vossius ring may be seen on the ALC. Trauma to the lens by vegetative matter raises the likelihood of developing a lens abscess, which may appear as a yellowish coagulum in the pupillary area and is often associated with endophthalmitis.

4.3.4.8 Intraocular Pressure (IOP)

Measurement of IOP may be deferred in cases of penetrating corneal injuries; however, it is important to measure the IOP in all cases of blunt trauma. Although Goldmann applanation tonometer is the gold standard for measuring IOP, it might not be possible to use applanation methods in cases presenting with epithelial defects or infiltrates, in such cases non-contact tonometry is preferred. The following ocular emergencies may be associated with a significant change in IOP:

- *Blunt trauma*—Intense AC reaction, hyphema, damage to the trabecular meshwork, or intumescent lens leading to pupillary block may all contribute to a rise in IOP following blunt ocular trauma. A decrease in IOP might be observed due to the disruption of the ciliary body attachment to the scleral spur leading to a ciliary body cleft. It is vital to do a gonioscopy in all cases of blunt trauma to look for angle recession, ciliary body clefts, and blood in the Schlemm's canal. Hypotony may also be noted in cases of occult scleral tear and retinal detachment.
- *Chemical injury*—IOP may be elevated in cases of chemical injury due to direct damage to the trabecular meshwork and angle structures by the offending chemical agent, intense AC inflammation leading to obstruction of the TM by leucocytes and fibrin or it can occur secondary to the use of topical steroids. Hypotony on the other hand may occur due to direct chemical injury to the ciliary body or secondary to anterior segment ischemia.
- *Post corneal transplant*—raised IOP in a post keratoplasty eye can be due to multiple factors ranging from retained viscoelastic, intense AC inflammation, hyphema, distortion of the angle (long and tight sutures), and collapse of the trabecular meshwork (especially in aphakic eyes) to pupillary block in the early post-op period. In the late post-op period, raised IOP may be attributed to extensive peripheral anterior synechiae, ghost cells, vitreous in AC, and prolonged use of steroids. In post-Descemet stripping endothelial keratoplasty (DSEK) cases

elevated IOP in the initial few days may be due to pupillary block caused by air going behind the iris in the absence of a peripheral iridectomy. Late IOP rise may be due to steroid response, angle crowding, or peripheral anterior synechiae.

4.3.4.9 Fundus

Fundus should be examined with the help of an indirect ophthalmoscope and a 20D lens wherever possible. In cases of ocular trauma, it is important to look for any retinal detachment, associated retinal breaks, dislocated lens or IOL, vitreous hemorrhage, vitreous exudates, intraocular foreign bodies, and status of the optic disc (pallor/edema). Patients with corneal ulcers may also have associated endophthalmitis; therefore, evaluation of the posterior segment either by indirect ophthalmoscopy (if possible) or by B-scan is necessary in all cases of corneal ulcers.

4.4 Diagnostic Approach

4.4.1 Fluorescein Stain

Fluorescein stain is one of the simplest diagnostic techniques which can be used by an ophthalmologist. All one needs is a fluorescein strip and a slit lamp having a cobalt blue filter. Fluorescein absorbs light of wavelengths between 485 and 500 nm (blue light falls within this range), this then causes it to emit a greenish light (longer wavelength and lower energy). The intact corneal epithelium prevents the corneal stroma to absorb the dye; and no staining is seen if the epithelium is intact. Hence fluorescein may be utilized in the following ocular emergencies:

- Corneal ulcers—to measure the size of the epithelial defect, which in turn helps in monitoring the response to treatment. To identify dendritic or geographic ulcers in cases of HSV keratitis.
- Chemical injuries—helps in identifying superficial punctuate keratitis in cases of mild chemical injuries. In moderate to severe chemical injuries, it helps in measuring the size of the corneal epithelial defect and in identifying conjunctival epithelial defects, which in turn help in the grading of chemical injuries, management strategy, and prognostication.
- Corneal tears—some corneal tears appear to be self-sealed on slit lamp examination; however, performing a Siedel's test or a forced Siedel's test may reveal an open wound.
- PUK—helps in demarcating the zone of activity (no overlying epithelium) within the peripheral thinned-out cornea in cases of Mooren's or PUK related to autoimmune diseases.
- Stevens–Johnson syndrome—In the acute phase, this test may be done bedside with the help of an indirect ophthalmoscope having a blue light. The fluorescein helps to stain any corneal and conjunctival epithelial defects. In the later stages of SJS, it may also help in identifying areas of lid margin keratinization.

- Contact lens associated emergencies—stains epithelial defects in cases of contact lens associated infective keratitis (CLIK) and contact lens-induced peripheral ulcer (CLPU).
- Post-PK grafts—it helps to identify any non-healing or persistent epithelial defects, epithelial rejection (elevated, undulating fluorescein-stained rejection line), and loose sutures (dye accumulates beneath the loose suture).
- Post-LASIK—in cases of epithelial ingrowth, fluorescein stain may help in staining the area of an epithelial fistula or may pool in a retracted or elevated flap edge via which the epithelial ingrowth is occurring.

4.4.2 X-Ray

X-ray of the skull can help reveal skull and orbital bone fractures and metallic foreign bodies. It is a relatively inexpensive and quick investigative modality in cases of ocular trauma.

4.4.3 CT-Scan

A thin slice CT-scan of the PNS, orbit, and brain with 0.5 mm cuts in the axial, coronal and sagittal plane can be used in cases of ocular trauma to detect soft tissue injuries and orbital wall fractures, optical canal fractures, radiolucent intra-ocular foreign bodies (exact location) and can pick up signs of occult globe rupture such as a change in globe contour, loss of globe volume ("flat tire sign") and presence of intraocular air. Contrast-enhanced CT can be used in cases of suspected vascular injury.

4.4.4 MRI

MRI can be used in cases of suspected intra-ocular wooden foreign bodies as these may be missed on CT scan; however, MRI is contraindicated in cases of metallic foreign bodies. It can also be used in suspected cases of traumatic optic neuropathy where T2 prolongation is visualized as increased signal intensity in the injured optic nerve.

4.4.5 B-Scan

High-frequency ultrasound (10 Mhz) is used in brightness mode scan to produce two-dimensional images of the posterior segment. It is a quick and non-invasive test that can provide information that may be missed by indirect ophthalmoscopy such as the size and location of a foreign body and is particularly useful in ocular emergencies where ophthalmoscopy may be obscured, such as large corneal ulcers, vitreous hemorrhage, vitreous exudates, dense cataracts, corneal edema (in post-PK graft rejection, hydrops), open globe injuries and in closed globe injuries with hyphema or cataractous lens obscuring the view. The gain may be adjusted to a higher level, so that weaker signals are more easily visualized (vitreous opacities, posterior vitreous detachment, small foreign bodies, etc.) and vice-versa so that stronger signals are more easily visualized (masses, tumors, retinal detachment, etc.) and the weaker signals may become absent. B-scan may be utilized in the following ocular emergencies:

- Ocular trauma—to identify posterior segment pathologies such as retinal detachment, vitreous exudates (suspected endophthalmitis), vitreous hemorrhage, choroidal or scleral rupture (in occult globe rupture), non-radio-opaque and radio-opaque foreign bodies (especially useful for identifying wooden or glass foreign bodies missed on CT scan) and dislocated lens/IOL. In cases of open globe injuries, one can either defer the B-scan till after the primary wound repair or should be very gentle while performing the scan.
- Corneal ulcers—in all cases of microbial keratitis where the infiltrate and surrounding stromal edema precludes indirect ophthalmoscopy, one must do a B-scan to rule out any associated endophthalmitis. In cases of long-standing perforated corneal ulcers, a B-scan may reveal choroidal detachments.

4.4.6 Ultrasound Biomicroscopy (UBM)

Ultrasound Biomicroscopy (UBM) uses a much higher frequency of 35–100 Mhz as compared to A-scan or B-scan and hence provides a better resolution. It may be used to view the anterior segment structures such as the iris, anterior chamber angle, scleral spur, ciliary body, lens, zonules, anterior and posterior chamber thereby helping to identify intra-ocular foreign bodies embedded in the angle, zonular deficiency, cyclodialysis, angle recession (tear between the circular and long muscle layers of the ciliary body), and posterior capsular status in cases of ocular trauma.

4.4.7 Anterior Segment OCT (AS-OCT)

Anterior Segment OCT (AS-OCT) is a non-contact, quick, and relatively easy to use imaging technique that provides high-quality, cross-sectional images of the anterior segment structures. It may be used in the following ocular emergencies:

- Acute hydrops—to identify Descemet membrane breaks (size, rolled or flat margins) and detachment (depth, size, location), which further helps in management and prognostication. It can also identify epithelial edema, stromal edema (corneal thickness), and intrastromal fluid clefts.
- Corneal Foreign bodies—to localize the exact location and depth at which the foreign body is lodged (Fig. 4.4)

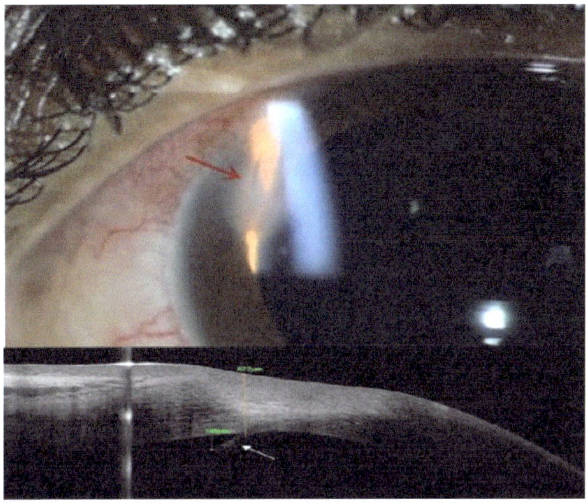

Fig. 4.4 Clinical photograph of the eye showing a bee sting embedded in the cornea with surrounding stromal edema Anterior segment Optical coherence tomography (ASOCT) from the area shows its extent into the anterior chamber

- Post-PK grafts—to view the posterior graft host junction and its alignment in suspected areas of wound dehiscence. It can also be used to view any peripheral anterior synechiae and their extent. In cases of acute graft rejection, posterior corneal surface undulations may be noted, whereas in chronic graft rejection stromal thickening with a smooth posterior corneal surface is usually seen.
- Post-DSAEK—any graft detachment, interface fluid, residual DM, graft edema, or wrong graft orientation may be picked up on AS-OCT.
- Post-LASIK—to identify any interface debris or fluid, micro or macrostriae, interface infiltrates, epithelial ingrowth, and to pick up any abnormalities in flap alignment.

4.4.8 In-Vivo Confocal Microscopy (IVCM)

In-vivo confocal microscopy (IVCM) is a non-invasive imaging and diagnostic modality which allows morphological and quantitative analysis of the various layers of the cornea. It has a lateral resolution of 1–2 μm and an axial resolution of 25–27 μm. It has the added advantage of imaging through moderately opaque tissues (corneal scars, infiltrates, edema). It may be used in corneal emergencies such as:

- Corneal ulcers—especially in suspected fungal or acanthamoeba keratitis since delayed diagnosis of these infections is common due to the time delay of corneal cultures and slow-growing fungi and Acanthamoeba. IVCM can identify acanthamoeba cysts and trophozoites as well as fungal filaments and can also be used to measure the depth of invasion and to monitor response to treatment.
- Limbal stem cell deficiency—IVCM can be used to image the corneoscleral junction and help in detecting early changes of LSCD in cases of SJS and chemical injuries.

- Post-LASIK—IVCM aids in evaluating flap-related complications and describe changes in corneal nerves and sublayers. It can image flap interface as well as Bowman layer's microfolds. It can also be used to study corneal wound healing after refractive surgery [3].

4.4.9 OCT Angiography (OCTA)

OCT angiography (OCTA) is a rapid, non-invasive imaging technique that can identify the anatomy of the ocular vasculature based on the measurement of erythrocyte flow. It may be used in cases of acute chemical injuries to identify and monitor the recovery of limbal ischemia by looking at both the conjunctival and intrascleral vessels.

4.4.10 Corneal Topography

Corneal topography plays an important role in differentiating myopic regression from post-LASIK ectasia after LASIK surgery. An increase in irregular astigmatism accompanied by focal steepening (often inferiorly) usually points toward ectasia, whereas myopic regression usually has a regular topography.

4.4.11 Microbiology

Microbiology plays a vital role in identifying the causative organism in most cases of microbial keratitis be it a graft infiltrate, perforated corneal ulcer, or a post-LASIK interface infection. Scrapings are taken from the base and edge of the ulcer (in cases of post-LASIK interface keratitis, the flap is lifted and scrapings are taken) and sent for smear (Gram stain, KOH mount, and in suspected cases of Nocardia or atypical mycobacteria, acid-fast staining is also done) and culture (blood agar, chocolate agar, non-nutrient agar, Sabouraud dextrose or potato dextrose agar and brain–heart infusion). In cases of deep stromal infiltrates which are not amenable to scraping, a corneal biopsy may be done to obtain samples from the infiltrate. Treatment is commenced on the basis of the smear report and may be changed once the culture report identifies the growth of the causative organism, which usually takes 2–3 days in cases of bacterial infection and can take up to 2 weeks or more in cases of fungi.

4.5 Therapeutic Approach

All ocular emergencies need not require early surgical intervention, and some may not need intervention at all. Table 4.3 lists the various corneal emergencies and the appropriate time for surgical intervention recommended for each of these.

Table 4.3 List of various corneal emergencies and the appropriate time to surgical intervention recommended

Early intervention	Late intervention	No surgical intervention
Full-thickness corneal tear	Sealed corneal tear with traumatic cataract	Partial-thickness corneal tear, sealed corneal tear (Siedel's negative)
Chemical injuries (Roperhall grade 3–4)	Chemical injuries (grade 2–3)	Chemical injuries (grade 1)
Corneal infiltrate involving the limbus (especially fungus), perforated corneal ulcer	Corneal ulcer not responding to medications, infiltrate approaching the limbus	Corneal ulcer responding to medications
Hydrops—large DM break with rolled margins, Deep DM detachment	No improvement in corneal edema or DM reattachment even after 36 weeks	Hydrops—small DM breaks, shallow detachments
Post-PK wound dehiscence, wound leak		
Stevens–Johnson syndrome with epithelial defect		
Active PUK with severe thinning, PUK with perforation	PUK not responding to medications	Mildly active/Inactive PUK with minimal thinning
Post-LASIK infectious keratitis, DLK (stage 3, 4), Epithelial ingrowth (severe, affecting vision)	DLK stage 2 not responding to medications	PISK, CTK, Epithelial ingrowth (mild, peripheral)

DM, descemet membrane; PK, penetrating keratoplasty; PUK, peripheral ulcerative keratitis; DLK, diffuse lamellar keratitis; PISK, pressure-induced stromal keratitis; CTK, central toxic keratopathy

4.5.1 Acute Chemical Injury

Chemicals, be it acid or alkali, can cause significant damage to the ocular surface and lead to activation of the inflammatory cascade. The inflammation contributes to various sequelae in the presence of an epithelial defect by promoting stromal melting which in turn inhibits the epithelial healing process, in a kind of vicious cycle. Hence, the primary aims of treating acute chemical injuries are:

1. To completely remove the inciting agent/chemical from the eye—the extent of damage and inflammation not only depends on the type of chemical but also depends on the contact time, hence it is important to irrigate the eye thoroughly to dilute and remove the offending agent from the eye and normalize the pH (checked by litmus paper or pH paper). It is mandatory to evert the eyelids and double evert the upper lid to examine the fornices and tarsal conjunctiva for any residual adherent chemical (especially in cases of lime injury), all the residual adherent particles along with the necrotic conjunctival tissue must be removed even if it requires excision of the conjunctiva.

2. Reducing inflammation and promoting epithelial healing—topical steroids are started within the first week following injury and although continuing steroids beyond the first 2 weeks may accelerate stromal melting, in cases of ongoing inflammation where the epithelial defect does not heal within the first 2 weeks despite using a bandage contact lens, an amniotic membrane graft (AMG) may be applied and topical steroids continued. Topical lubricants also help to promote epithelialization and help in diluting and washing away the inflammatory mediators. A topical antibiotic should be used in the presence of an epithelial defect in order to prevent secondary infection.
3. Minimizing ischemia—scleral ischemia may be detrimental to epithelial healing and can also lead to coagulative necrosis and stromal ulceration or melting. One may observe areas of ischemia for a few days (especially of less than 3 clock hours) and serial OCT angiographies may be employed to objectively identify areas of ischemia and see their progression or regression over time. Persistence or worsening of ischemia may require tarsorrhaphy and tenonplasty to re-establish vascularity.
4. Control intraocular pressure—a high IOP may lead to corneal edema and in turn delay epithelial healing. Topical antiglaucoma drugs may be employed to maintain a normal IOP.
5. Reduce exposure—burns to the adnexal tissue including the lids can lead to tissue loss and contractures which may result in the inability to close the eyelids, the resultant corneal exposure further delays epithelial healing and therefore a tarsorrhaphy or lid repair is mandatory in such cases.

4.5.2 Stevens–Johnson Syndrome

SJS is an immune-mediated mucocutaneous disease that leads to sloughing of the skin and mucosal surfaces, including that of the ocular surface. It is most often triggered by medication and less commonly due to an infection, hence it is of utmost importance to try and find out which medication was the inciting agent so that it is avoided in the future. The degree of inflammation and damage to the ocular surface in the acute phase determines the severity of the chronic sequelae of SJS; therefore, it is very important to intervene as early as possible in the acute phase of SJS.

The main objectives of treatment during the acute phase are to reduce surface inflammation, promote epithelialization, and prevent secondary infection. An overview of the management protocol is outlined below:

1. Any mucous, debris, or membranes should be removed thoroughly with saline flushes, cotton swabs, or jewelers' forceps.
2. In cases of conjunctival hyperemia alone—aggressive treatment with topical steroids, antibiotics, and lubricants should be initiated. It is essential to follow up with these patients daily to look for any lid margin changes or corneal and conjunctival epithelial defects.
3. In cases of corneal, conjunctival, or lid margin defects—A large amniotic membrane should be applied over the whole ocular surface and should include the

tarsal conjunctiva and lid margins as well. This may be achieved with the help of a symblepharon ring or infant feeding tube which helps to keep the amniotic membrane in place. An additional tarsorrhaphy helps in keeping the AMT in situ and prevents mechanical damage due to blinking. In hospitalized patients, bedside AMT may be performed under sedation and may need to be repeated several times as the ongoing inflammation may lead to a disintegration of the AMT after a few weeks.

4.5.3 Corneal Ulcer

A detailed history, clinical and microbiological examination as mentioned earlier is of utmost importance in diagnosing and managing a corneal ulcer. Treatment can be initiated based on the smear findings and may be changed as and when the culture reports are available. A few key points to remember during the management of corneal ulcers are listed below:

- In cases of bacterial infection (noted on smears), empirical therapy with two antibiotics covering for Gram-positive and Gram-negative bacteria can be initiated. These antibiotics are usually fortified preparations with higher drug concentrations and need to be stored at a cool temperature and used within a week from formulation. One may shift to monotherapy once the culture and sensitivity reports are available. In cases of small peripheral ulcers, fluoroquinolones may be used for monotherapy as they are more convenient; can be kept for longer than a week, do not require special formulation, and have a broad spectrum of activity including both Gram-positive and Gram-negative bacteria. Initially, all antibiotics are started as half-hourly or hourly instillation and the frequency may be gradually reduced based on the clinical response to treatment. Once a significant response to medications is observed, topical steroids may be added judiciously to minimize stromal scarring.
- Close follow-up, preferably daily or at least once every 3 days, is important to understand the progression and clinical response to treatment. In cases of worsening, one should search for potential causes of poor response such as concomitant lid abnormalities not allowing epithelialization, poor blood sugar control in diabetics, possibility of mixed infection, poor compliance to medications, etc.
- In cases of negative smear and culture reports—it is important to ask for prior use of antibiotics and if the patient was already using antibiotics, it may be a good idea to give a drug holiday of at least 48–72 h before re-scraping the ulcer. It is also important to think of non-infectious causes of corneal ulcers in such cases.
- In cases of fungal keratitis, the most used first-line antifungal is Natamycin 5% eye drops. The use of steroids is absolutely contraindicated. Oral antifungals may be indicated in:
  - Perforated/impending perforation
  - Deep ulcers (involving >2/3rd stromal depth): intrastromal Amphotericin B or voriconazole may also be used in deep stromal infiltrates not responding to topical or oral antifungals.

  - Large ulcers (>6 mm in diameter)
  - Scleral involvement
  - Associated endophthalmitis
- The management of viral keratitis varies depending on its presentation, whether it is epithelial, stromal, both or associated with uveitis. This shall be discussed further in the respective chapter on corneal ulcers.
- A strong level of suspicion is needed to diagnose cases of acanthamoeba keratitis. History of taking bath in a pond/swimming pool or use of contact lenses should make one suspicious of acanthamoeba. Scrapings taken for KOH mount may reveal double-walled cysts on microscopy and growth on non-nutrient agar with E. coli overlay confirms the presence of acanthamoeba. Treatment usually involves the use of biguanides such as PHMB and antiseptic agents such as chlorhexidine. Acanthamoeba may lead to severe inflammation and there are specific indications where topical steroids may be used in such cases.
- Indications for therapeutic keratoplasty:
  - Large corneal ulcers not showing any response to treatment
  - Infiltrate involving the limbus or approaching the limbus despite maximal medications
  - Deep infiltrates not responding to topical or oral medications
  - Large central perforation not amenable to tissue adhesives
- Supplementary treatment may involve: the use of cycloplegic drugs to reduce ciliary spasm and resultant pain, oral analgesics to reduce pain, repeated debridement of plaques in cases of fungal keratitis to increase drug penetration and facilitate faster resolution

4.5.4 Peripheral Ulcerative Keratitis

Peripheral ulcerative keratitis presents with a crescent-shaped stromal inflammation involving the juxtalimbal cornea associated with thinning and an overlying epithelial defect. It may have an infective or non-infective (more common) etiology. Infective PUK may be treated similarly on the lines of a corneal ulcer as discussed above. However, non-infective causes of PUK share a common pathogenic mechanism of immune-mediated inflammation, and therefore immunosuppression forms the mainstay of treatment in such cases. PUK is most often associated with autoimmune diseases of which rheumatoid arthritis is the most common, hence systemic immunosuppression with oral steroids, cytotoxic agents (methotrexate, azathioprine, mycophenolate mofetil, cyclophosphamide, etc.), and/or biological agents (infliximab, rituximab, etc.) is essential in treating systemic disease as well as ocular manifestations such as scleritis and PUK. Local ocular treatment of PUK involves the use of lubricants (as most of these autoimmune diseases also lead to dry eye and to wash away the inflammatory mediators), topical antibiotics (to prevent secondary infection), and topical steroids (to reduce surface inflammation). The surgical management includes resection of the perilimbal conjunctiva surrounding the area of PUK.

Tissue adhesive may be applied over an area of thinning to provide more tectonic support and can be used to seal small (<3 mm) perforations. Larger areas of stromal melting or perforation may require penetrating keratoplasty in the form of lamellar or full thickness crescentic patch grafts.

A step ladder approach for immunosuppression based on the severity of involvement (number of quadrants of peripheral corneal involvement, percentage stromal loss, impending or frank perforation), laterality, and age of the patient may be used for treating Mooren's ulcer.

4.5.5 Contact Lens-Related Emergencies

These include microbial keratitis (MK), contact lens-induced acute red eye (CLARE), contact lens-induced peripheral ulcer (CLPU), and infiltrative keratitis (IK). In all the above cases, contact lenses should be immediately discontinued and in cases of microbial keratitis, the contact lens, its case and cleansing solution along with the corneal scrapings should be sent for a microbiological workup and the management should be similar to that of a corneal ulcer as described earlier. In cases of CLARE, CLPU (may add prophylactic antibiotic) and IK discontinuation of contact lenses, use of lubricants, and close observation are sufficient for resolution. Whenever there is a doubt in differentiating CLPU from MK it is always advisable to scrape the lesion and send for microbiological confirmation.

4.5.6 Corneal Hydrops

Corneal hydrops may be seen in patients with advanced ectatic disorders of the cornea such as keratoconus, pellucid marginal corneal degeneration (PMCD), and keratoglobus.

Spontaneous resolution of hydrops without any surgical intervention usually takes around 2–4 months; therefore, hydrops may be managed conservatively with topical lubricants, hypertonic saline eye drops (to withdraw fluid from the stroma), topical steroids (to reduce inflammation and neovascularization), and cycloplegics to reduce pain. However, the use of intracameral gases such as SF6 and C3F8 helps speed up recovery by mechanically reattaching DM to the posterior stroma and by preventing further percolation of aqueous into the stroma. In cases of large stromal clefts or where the gas bubble migrates intrastromally, compression sutures may be used along with gas injection. Although the final visual outcome is similar to conservative or surgical management, intracameral gas injection usually hastens recovery by 1–2 months. However, it is important to note that intracameral gas injection may not offer any benefits in cases of PMCD and keratoglobus as the DM break and detachment is too peripheral in PMCD and too large in cases of keratoglobus.

Once the corneal edema resolves the corneal surface usually flattens, which might lead to an improvement in visual acuity and allow for better contact lens fitting; however, cases of dense central corneal scarring may require corneal transplants in the form of DALK or PK.

4.5.7 Post-PK Emergencies

Patients who undergo corneal transplantation in the form of penetrating keratoplasty may face numerous complications in both the early and late postoperative periods. A few of these complications require immediate attention and are listed below:

1. Suture related—loose or broken sutures can be picked up by fluorescein staining and should be removed. If there is an associated wound leak (positive Siedel's test) on the removal of the suture, a new suture should be applied. The presence of an infiltrate with an overlying epithelial defect near at the suture end is characteristic of a stitch abscess; corneal scraping should be taken and treatment should be initiated accordingly. However, a stitch abscess must be differentiated from immune-related suture infiltrates, which are multiple grayish white dot-sized infiltrates along the length of the suture without any overlying epithelial defect; these may be treated by simply stepping up topical steroids.
2. Graft infiltrate—any infiltrate in the graft should be managed along the lines of corneal ulcer management mentioned earlier. In case a therapeutic keratoplasty was done for corneal infection, it is important to differentiate a new infiltrate from recurrence. In cases of recurrence, the infiltrate usually starts in the host and straddles the graft-host junction spreading to the donor graft. If the recurrence is not brought under control with medications, then a repeat keratoplasty may be required with a larger graft.
3. Persistent epithelial defect—the donor surface usually epithelises completely by 1 week postoperatively; however, in certain situations epithelial defects may persist. It is important to preoperatively assess all the factors that may delay or impede epithelialization of the graft and address these appropriately. For example, lid problems, such as entropion, ectropion, trichiasis, lagophthalmos, or blepharitis, should be corrected. If tear production is deficient, punctal occlusion should be considered. In conditions, such as ocular pemphigoid, Stevens–Johnson syndrome, and chemical injuries, limbal stem cell transplantation along with AMT and tarsorrhaphy should be considered along with penetrating keratoplasty. Postoperative management of persistent epithelial defects involves the use of preservative-free lubricants, AMT, and tarsorrhaphy. It is important to start a topical broad-spectrum antibiotic in order to prevent secondary graft infection.
4. Post PK glaucoma—a raised IOP on the first postop day may be due to retained viscoelastic which usually clears within 24–48 h. Another common cause of early postoperative glaucoma is a pupillary block which may be relieved by using eye drops to dilate the pupil, in cases where this fails, a peripheral laser iridotomy or surgical peripheral iridectomy may be indicated. Post-PK glaucoma may also occur secondary to prolonged use of topical steroids, which can

be controlled by using topical AGMs and switching over to softer steroids like loteprednol or fluorometholone. The formation of extensive peripheral anterior synechiae may also lead to angle closure and rise in IOP, this may be brought under control with the help of topical and systemic AGMs and a peripheral iridotomy. In cases of post PK glaucoma not responding to maximal antiglaucoma medication, surgical intervention in the form of transscleral cyclophotocoagulation (TSCPC) or Ahmed glaucoma valve may be considered.

5. Wound dehiscence—any trauma to a post-PK eye may result in the graft host junction giving way, resulting in wound dehiscence. Such situations require urgent surgical intervention to reappose the graft host junction with sutures and prevent dreadful complications such as endophthalmitis and expulsion of intraocular contents.
6. Allograft rejection—it is vital to pick up signs and symptoms of allograft rejection early, so that treatment can be initiated in time to reverse the episode of rejection and prevent subsequent graft failure. The mainstay of treatment is steroids; a single intravenous methylprednisolone (IVMP) 500 mg pulse dose may be given in cases of severe reaction, while stepping up the frequency of topical steroids to hourly instillation. Oral steroids are also implicated in reversing an episode of rejection and topical cyclosporine or tacrolimus may be added for long-term immunosuppression to prevent further episodes of rejection.

4.5.8 Post-refractive Surgery Corneal Emergencies

- These include: Microbial keratitis—early-onset infections are usually caused by Gram-positive cocci, whereas late-onset infections may be due to atypical mycobacteria or fungi. LASIK flaps should be lifted, and scrapings should be taken from the stromal bed for smear and culture. The flap bed should be irrigated with fortified antibiotics and topical antibiotics should be started based on the smear report. In non-responsive infections, the flap may need to be amputated to facilitate antibiotic penetration.
- DLK—aggressive use of topical steroids (hourly administration) should be initiated. This may be combined with oral steroids for stage 2 and 3 DLK. Flap lift and irrigation may be required in some cases of stage 2 DLK and all cases of stage 3 and 4 DLK.
- PISK—The most important step in the management of PISK is to differentiate it from DLK by careful slit lamp examination to look for interface fluid and IOP measurements. IOP should be measured both centrally and peripherally with Goldmann applanation or tonopen. Once the diagnosis of PISK is confirmed, steroids should be stopped and antiglaucoma medications should be initiated until the interface fluid resolves.
- CTK—is self-limiting and treatment is not required; however, it is important to distinguish it from stage 4 DLK.
- Epithelial ingrowth—majority of the mild cases not affecting visual acuity may be managed by just observation. However, in moderate to severe cases involving

the visual axis, initial surgical treatment involves flap lift, removal of epithelial cells from the under surface of the flap and the stromal bed using a blade and replacement of the flap without glue or sutures. In recurrent episodes, fibrin glue or flap sutures may be used to prevent further ingrowth. Another treatment modality involves the use of YAG laser targeted at the epithelial cells.

One of the most dreaded postoperative complications of LASIK is post-LASIK ectasia. It is of utmost importance to differentiate myopic regression from post-LASIK ectasia as enhancement surgery in the latter can lead to worsening of ectasia; therefore, critically reviewing the preoperative corneal topography and tomography maps as well as AS-OCT may help in outlining whether the patient had any preoperative risk factors (age, abnormal topography, corneal thickness, residual stromal bed thickness, etc.) for developing ectasia. The patient usually presents with a gradual diminution of vision which may be worse than his preoperative BCVA. An increase in irregular astigmatism accompanied by focal steepening (often inferiorly) on corneal topography usually clinches the diagnosis of post LASIK ectasia. Management of post LASIK ectasia can be conservative, minimally invasive, or invasive and includes RGP or scleral contact lenses, Collagen cross-linking (CXL), or keratoplasty.

The most common post-PRK complications are delayed epithelial healing and corneal haze. The former can be managed by prescribing frequent lubricants and applying a well-fit bandage contact lens. Most of the epithelial defects usually resolve within the first week. Delayed epithelial healing may increase the risk of secondary infections. Post-PRK corneal haze usually appears in the first few weeks or months following PRK, although late-onset haze may also occur. Post-PRK haze can be managed with topical steroids and adjunctive such as mitomycin C. Severe haze may need surgical intervention.

4.5.9 Corneal Perforation/Laceration

In all cases of corneal perforation, it is important to find out and treat the primary etiology behind the perforation. The management algorithm to be followed in cases of corneal laceration and perforation with tissue loss is summarized in Figs. 4.5 and 4.6. The causes of corneal perforation can broadly be classified into:

- Infective—In cases of corneal ulcers, the ongoing stromal infiltration, inflammation, and lysis may result in corneal perforation. It is important to take scrapings from the surrounding stromal infiltrate and send them for a microbiological workup to identify and treat the causative organism. Oral tetracyclines may be added to reduce collagenolysis and stromal lysis by their inhibitory action on MMPs produced by the infiltrating neutrophils.
- Non-infective—can be either traumatic perforations or may be related to autoimmune disease:

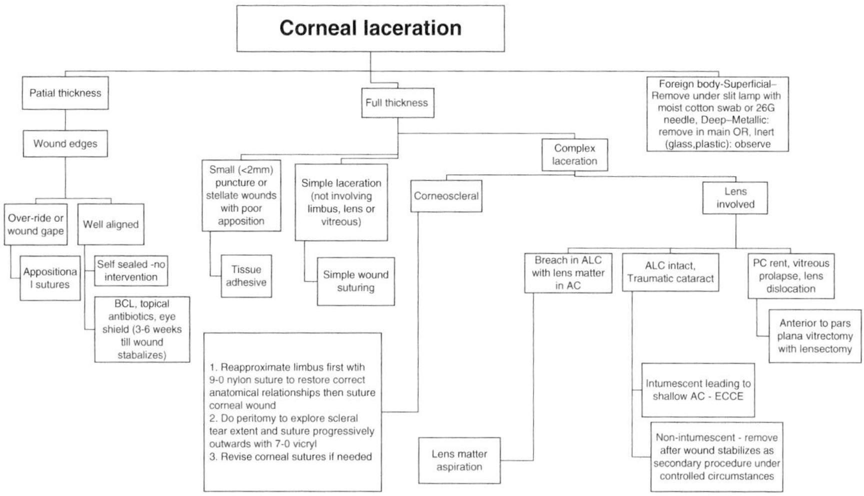

Fig. 4.5 The management algorithm for management of a corneal laceration

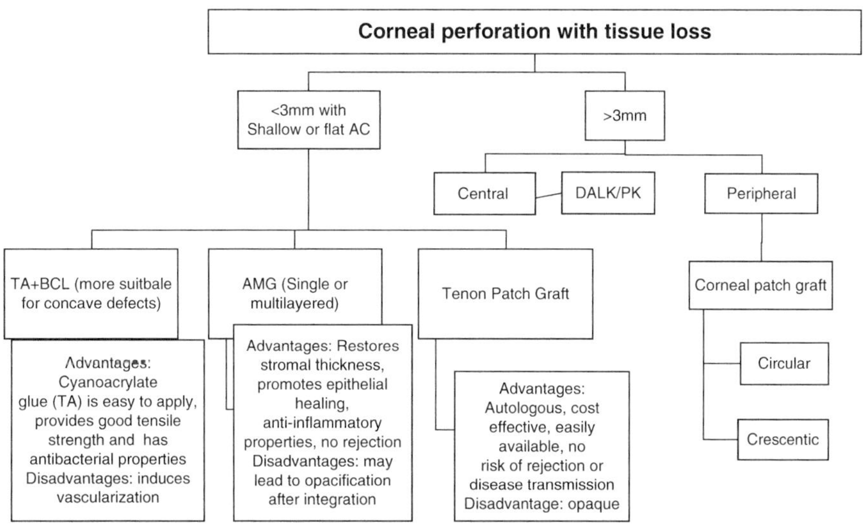

Fig. 4.6 The management algorithm for management of a corneal perforation with tissue loss

– Traumatic—small perforations may be closed directly using sutures, whereas larger perforations with tissue loss may require a corneal patch graft or PK.
– Autoimmune disease—perforations occurring in areas of severe peripheral thinning (like in PUK) or in eyes having severe dry eye should lead one to suspect an immune-mediated etiology. A complete systemic workup including blood tests should be advised to identify any collagen vascular diseases or autoimmune diseases that may have led to the corneal perforation. The main-

stay of treatment in such cases involves systemic immunosuppression by intravenous steroids, oral steroids, or steroid-sparing agents (cytotoxic agents, cyclosporine, and biological agents). Topical lubricants should be used to promote epithelial healing and to wash out the inflammatory mediators.

4.6 Conclusion

Corneal emergencies range from corneal foreign bodies to sight-threatening corneal ulcers. The diagnostic and therapeutic approach to each corneal emergency is different and has been described in this chapter.

Key Points

- Corneal emergencies are the most common ocular emergencies that present in the emergency room.
- Timely diagnosis and management are the key and help in saving sight as well as globe integrity.
- Detailed history taking and clinical examination including a comprehensive systemic workup is the first step in the management of a corneal emergency.
- Investigations such as fluorescein staining, X-Ray orbit, CT, MRI, Ultrasound B-scan, Ultrasound Biomicroscopy, ASOCT, Corneal topography, In vivo confocal microscopy, and OCT angiography can aid in diagnosis as well as case-specific management of these potential sight-threatening emergencies.
- Therapeutic approach to a corneal emergency is also case-specific and includes appropriate medical management or surgical treatment in the form of corneal perforation repair, use of tissue adhesives, and keratoplasty.

References

1. Channa R, Zafar SN, Canner JK, et al. Epidemiology of eye-related emergency department visits. JAMA Ophthalmol. 2016;134:312–9.
2. Stein RM, Clinch TE, Cohen EJ, et al. Infected vs. sterile corneal infiltrates in contact lens wearers. Am J Ophthalmol. 1988;105:632–6.
3. Perez-Gomez I, Efron N. Change to corneal morphology after refractive surgery (myopic laser in situ keratomileusis) as viewed with a confocal microscope. Optom Vis Sci. 2003;80:690–7.

Minor Corneal Emergencies

5

Nimmy Raj, Radhika Tandon, M Vanathi, Neiwete Lomi and Noopur Gupta

5.1 Introduction

Minor corneal emergencies are a frequent presentation to the general and ophthalmic emergency departments. These can involve traumatic corneal abrasions, corneal foreign body, photokeratitis, chemical injuries, contact lens-related problems and even microbial keratitis. Corneal abrasions and corneal foreign bodies are the commonest with an incidence of approximately 3 per 1000 persons and 2 per 1000 persons in the United States [1]. The patients usually present with a history of trauma followed by pain, tearing and foreign body sensation. The primary care for these cases by the general practitioner itself might suffice most of the time, but anxiety and mismanagement result in unwanted complications. Patching, topical antibiotics, cycloplegics and topical tear substitutes are the mainstay of treatment after establishing the diagnosis. Most of the cases resolve without any sequelae.

5.2 Corneal Abrasions

Traumatic corneal abrasions are amongst the commonest presentations of minor injuries to the cornea. They constitute almost 10% of the new cases presenting to the eye emergency department [2]. Corneal abrasion or corneal epithelial defect is defined as the loss of the surface epithelial layer of the cornea. A history of trauma is usually elicited.

N. Raj · R. Tandon · M. Vanathi · N. Lomi · N. Gupta (✉)
Dr Rajendra Prasad Centre for Ophthalmic Sciences, All India Institute of Medical Sciences, New Delhi, India

B. Sharma, J. S. Titiyal (eds.), *Corneal Emergencies*,
https://doi.org/10.1007/978-981-16-5876-1_5

5.2.1 Aetiology

Important causative factors are as follows:

- Mechanical trauma—self-induced or from others
- Contact lens related
- Trauma from outdoor activities (occupational/sports/recreation)
- Foreign body
- Chemical or flash burns

Accidental fingernail injuries are one of the most common causes of corneal abrasions. They are usually linear or geographic lesions(Fig. 5.1) [3]. As fingernails often harbour contaminants and microbes, there are increased chances of infection. Even though this mode of injury is quite common, there is a paucity of evidence in published literature. In a study conducted on 39 patients who completed 1 year follow-up, it was reported that long-term complications in the form of recurrent corneal erosion were seen in 15% of the patients and one patient developed corneal scarring with long-term effect on visual acuity with male gender (86%) and adult age group (43%) predominantly developing long-term complications [4]. In this series, no case of fingernail trauma developed a corneal infection, supporting the fact that prophylactic antibiotics play an important role in the management of minor corneal injuries [4].

Studies from different parts of the world have shown that occupational eye injuries constitute almost one-fourth of the total eye injuries. According to the 2008 Bureau of Labour Statistics analysis of workplace injuries, occupational eye injuries accounted for 62% of all facial injuries and it led to at least 1 day off from work [5].

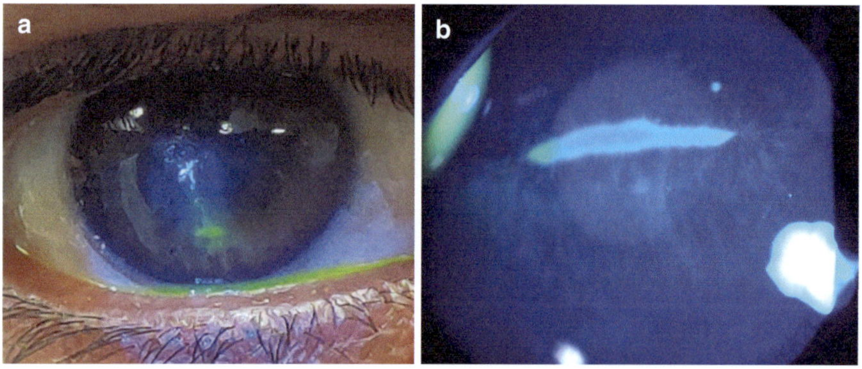

Fig. 5.1 Slit lamp photographs showing (**a**) peripheral and (**b**) central linear corneal abrasion following fingernail trauma in two patients

5.2.2 Clinical Features

The presenting signs and symptoms in a patient with corneal abrasion are highly non-specific (Table 5.1). The presentation will vary depending on the nature of the injury, and whether associated with a foreign body in situ. Superficial injuries tend to cause more symptoms and discomfort than the deeper ones due to exposure of the subepithelial nerve plexus in superficial injuries. The superficial corneal plexus gets exposed with even a mild abrasion leading to severe pain. A transient decrease in visual acuity is expected.

Signs can be elicited in each case if examined in detail and with a high index of suspicion (Table 5.2). Pupillary reaction can be a useful guide to assess the degree of involvement, a nonreacting or sluggish pupil should ring alarm with respect to the involvement of optic nerve. Miosis and circumcorneal congestion indicate traumatic iritis.

5.2.3 Complications

Even though majority of the corneal abrasions heal without any sequalae, if improperly treated can potentially develop long-term sight-threatening complications. A detailed clinical examination and removal of any foreign body with proper treatment are absolutely essential in any case of corneal injury. Complications that can arise include infectious microbial ulcers, recurrent erosion syndrome, traumatic iritis, residual scarring and opacity and consequent refractive error.

Table 5.1 Symptoms of corneal abrasion

- Acute ocular pain
- Redness
- Watering
- Foreign body sensation
- Sensitivity to light
- Varying degrees of diminution in vision

Table 5.2 Signs of corneal abrasion

- Congestion
- Photophobia
- Blepharospasm
- Reduced visual acuity
- Foreign body +/–
- Epithelial defect/ulcer with infiltrate
- Hyphema
- Hypopyon
- Abnormal pupillary reaction
- Other posterior segment involvement signs if any

5.2.4 Examination and Investigations

A detailed history of the mode of injury with a thorough clinical examination is mandatory in any case of ocular injury. Any history of high-velocity injury should urge the examiner to look for other associated signs in the eye. A systematic stepwise approach should always be followed by the primary care physicians to determine if any intervention is needed or referral to an ophthalmologist is needed (Fig. 5.2).

Following adjuncts should be readily available to perform a comprehensive eye examination: a Snellen visual acuity chart, torch light and binocular loupe, a direct

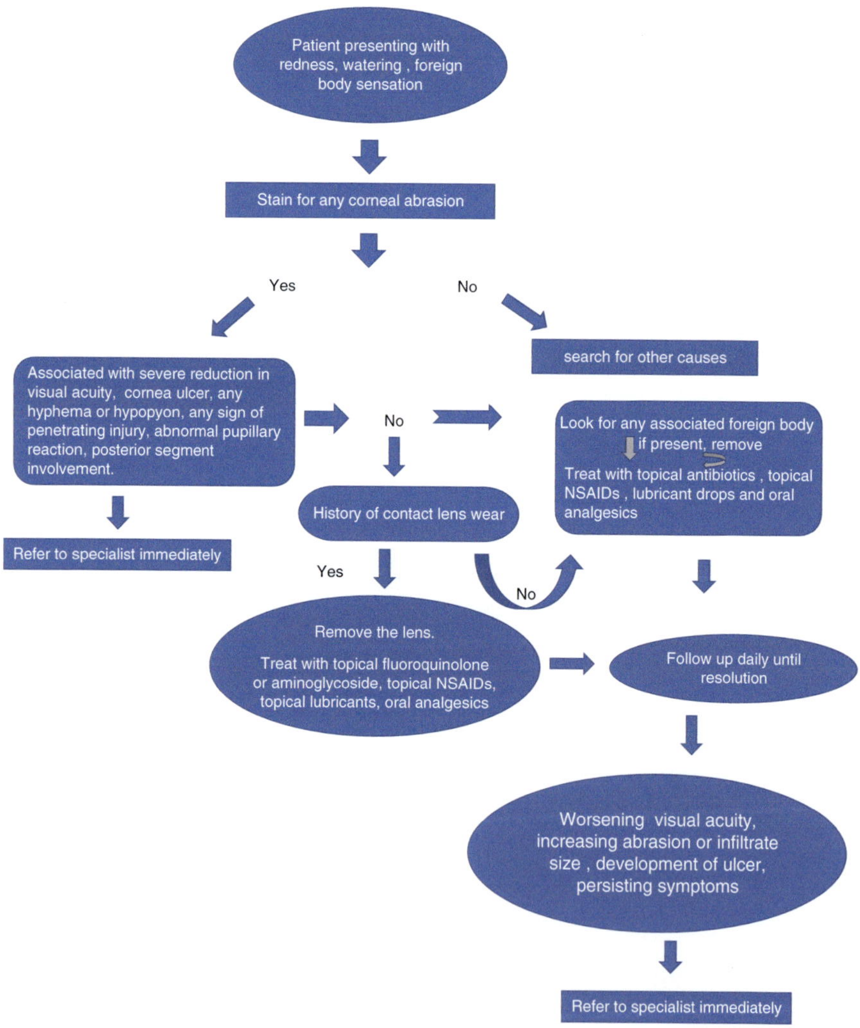

Fig. 5.2 Flow chart algorithm on general approach to a patient presenting with corneal abrasion

Table 5.3 Equipments required for examination of a case of corneal abrasion

1. Slit lamp with a cotton blue filter or a wood's lamp
2. Pen torch or a direct ophthalmoscope
3. Anaesthetic drops (proparacaine drops 0.5%)
4. Sodium fluorescein drops or strips
5. Topical antibiotic solution

ophthalmoscope, slit lamp, topical anaesthetic drops, and fluorescein strips (Table 5.3). Instillation of topical proparacaine like anaesthetic drops can make further examination easier especially if associated with severe photophobia and blepharospasm. A simple pen torchlight might not always be sufficient enough to detect an epithelial defect. This makes fluorescein dye drops or strips a necessary tool in diagnosing an occult epithelial defect. Fluorescein guided detailed slit lamp examination noting the size of the abrasion, its depth, any foreign body or any surrounding infiltrate. The eyelids should be everted and examined for any foreign body/giant papillae/concretions as that itself can cause corneal abrasion while blinking. Simple corneal abrasions are usually not associated with other deeper tissue involvement but detailed evaluation of the rest of the anterior segment should be done to rule out injury to other structures like the iris, traumatic cataract formation and also posterior segment involvement like commotio retinae, vitreous haemorrhage, retinal detachment, etc.

5.2.5 Management

It is important to manage every case of corneal abrasion carefully so as to prevent secondary infection and also to provide symptomatic relief to the patient. Even though minor abrasions of the cornea heal in most cases without any complication, there is a high risk of infection when the epithelial barrier is compromised. So, the mainstay of management involves prophylactic broad-spectrum antibiotics with lubricants to fasten healing. Usually, a fluoroquinolone like moxifloxacin (0.5%) or Gatifloxacin (0.3%) is preferred at least four times per day for 5–7 days along with carboxy methyl cellulose (0.5% or 1%) drops given six to eight times in the initial 2–3 days to fasten the process of re epithelisation. Even though there is an overwhelming lack of definitive treatment protocols in a case of corneal abrasion, most people follow the treatment as mentioned above.

Pain is another important concern in a case of corneal abrasion. Cycloplegic drops like homatropine 2% drops given four times/day are seen to be effective in relieving pain. Other means of pain control include the application of a bandage contact lens or pressure patching. Topical steroids should not be prescribed whenever an epithelial defect is present. Topical anaesthetic drops can aid in examination procedures but their extended use can have a deleterious effect on the cornea like delayed wound healing and ulcer formation.

Patching of the involved eye is an age-old treatment for traumatic corneal abrasions. It acts by reducing the discomfort caused by repeated blinking and friction between the lid and the abrasion. However, recent studies suggest that there is no added advantage of patching [6]. In a Cochrane review that included six studies from North America, five from Europe, and one from South America (Brazil) comparing the use of eye patches with no patching, it was found that in the first 24 h the people receiving patching is less likely to have a healed epithelial defect and may suffer from slightly more pain when compared to those with no patching given [7]. The other disadvantages include patient discomfort and disruption in binocular vision. Patching can reduce the oxygenation of cornea and the removal of metabolic waste products can get affected and the warm, moist environment by itself can act as a reservoir for infectious organisms [8]. Even though the role of patching remains controversial in the management of corneal abrasions, it can be extremely useful in cases of larger abrasions, paediatric patients and in mentally challenged adults [7].

5.3 Corneal Foreign Body

Corneal foreign bodies are usually comprised of sand or dust particles, but can also be vegetative material, stone, metallic, glass or wooden particles especially when the injury is inflicted in the workplace (Fig. 5.3). Farmers, construction and mechanical workers are mostly affected. Activities that pose more risk include grinding, hammering, drilling, and welding. Lack of protective eyewear and high-risk activities together contribute to such incidents. In a recent study from India, it was seen that 96% of the cases with corneal foreign body were patients in the age group ranging from 14 to 44 years, all of them being males. It was also reported that only 27% were wearing protective eye gear during these high-risk activities [9]. Hence, the need for more public education and stringent reinforcement of these guidelines is important.

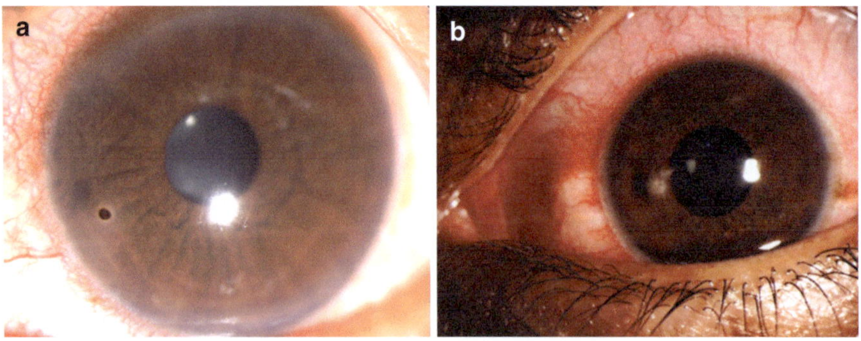

Fig. 5.3 Slit lamp photographs showing (**a**) metallic foreign body on the corneal surface and (**b**) wooden corneal foreign body embedded in anterior stroma with associated nebular corneal opacity

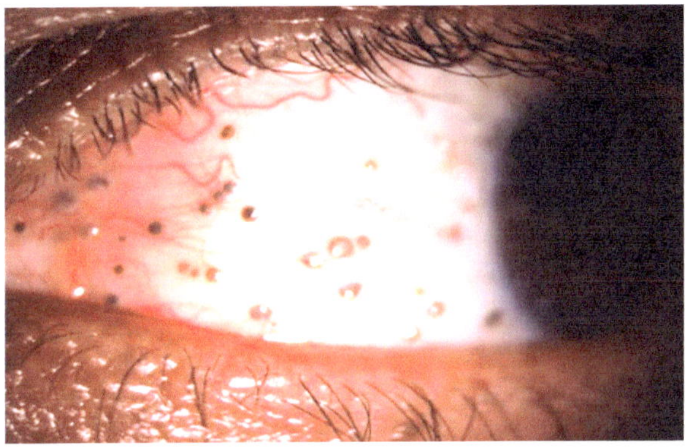

Fig. 5.4 Slit lamp image showing multiple pellets embedded in the conjunctiva in a case of gunshot injury

5.3.1 Clinical Features

Clinical features related to corneal foreign body are similar to that of corneal abrasion cases but with a history of foreign body fall into the eye and symptoms can include watering, pain, foreign body sensation, increased sensitivity to light and blurring of vision in the eye depending on the size of foreign body, site of injury (central or peripheral) and other associated injuries. In the case of high-velocity injuries like blast injuries, the presence of multiple foreign bodies over conjunctiva and adnexal areas should be looked for (Fig. 5.4). Signs will include the presence of a foreign body over the ocular surface with an associated epithelial defect, conjunctival congestion, localised corneal haze or oedema, anterior chamber reaction and iritis of varying extent. Posterior segment findings like vitreous haemorrhage, retinal detachment, commotio retinae, optic nerve avulsion, etc. should be looked for and ruled out.

5.3.2 Complications

With timely removal and adequate postoperative care including regular follow-up, most of the cases of corneal injury with a foreign body do not result in any complications. Infrequently, a corneal scar formation with sub-optimal vision gains especially in those cases with central rust ring, iritis, cataract, secondary glaucoma or endophthalmitis may occur.

5.3.3 Investigations

A detailed history of the mode of injury, duration since the occurrence, any associated injuries of the body, visual acuity assessment, slit lamp examination to assess the site, size, number of foreign bodies is absolutely essential. A thorough examination including upper eyelid eversion to look for any foreign body that has settled under the tarsal plate should be done. These inconspicuous foreign bodies can cause micro-trauma to the corneal layers with each blinking movement.

Additionally, anterior segment OCT and ultrasound biomicroscopy are helpful tools to delineate the shape, size and precise location of foreign bodies. However, UBM may be unsuitable in corneal tears, because of the pressure induced by the water bath and the risk of contamination [10]. AS-OCT provides detailed high-resolution images of cornea, at various depths thereby providing an accurate assessment of foreign body characteristics. Different types of foreign bodies show different reflectivity. Glass foreign bodies are well delineated with no internal reflectivity; wood exhibits moderate internal reflectivity while metal exhibits high anterior reflectivity with shadowing [11]. Foreign body composition determines the urgency of its removal and metallic foreign bodies require urgent removal [12].

The high resolution of AS-OCT is ideal for evaluating the depth and size of a foreign body in addition to extent of damage to surrounding tissue. It may thus guide the treatment choice and technique. Furthermore, Descemet's membrane integrity and the wound of entry can be utilised to plan surgical removal. If the Descemet's membrane is found to be intact with a foreign body impacted at a mid-stromal or superficial location and an evident wound of entry it can be removed through the anterior route, whereas when Descemet's membrane is breached and the foreign body is impacted at the deep stromal level it has to be removed via the anterior chamber using an air tamponade. AS-OCT can also guide on the potential risk of corneal perforation in event of corneal thinning due to damage incurred by a foreign body. Such cases may require corneal gluing with a bandage contact lens along with foreign body removal.

A fully dilated fundus examination to rule out co-existent injuries and also imaging to assess for any intraocular foreign body or intracranial foreign bodies, especially in cases of blast injuries, should be done. An ultrasound examination (a gentle one) might be necessary to look for vitreous haemorrhage or retinal detachment when the posterior segment visibility is compromised by hyphaemia or corneal oedema. Xrayorbit, B-scan ultrasound and non-contrast computed tomography of the head and orbit, wherever needed should be done to rule out the presence of intraocular or intracranial foreign bodies.

5.3.4 Management

A foreign body is usually present over the corneal surface (Fig. 5.5) or under the upper tarsal conjunctiva or in the upper or lower fornix. These are usually removed under topical anaesthesia using proparacaine 0.5% drops with either vigorous irrigation or on a slit lamp carefully using a 26 or 30G needle (Fig. 5.6) or small serrated ophthalmic forceps or even a moist cotton swab. An ophthalmic corneal burr, or spud, or more commonly called the "Alger brush" can also be used if available. It can be used to flick out the foreign body as it rotates, but it is more commonly used to get rid of the rust ring that a metallic foreign body leaves behind (Table 5.4).

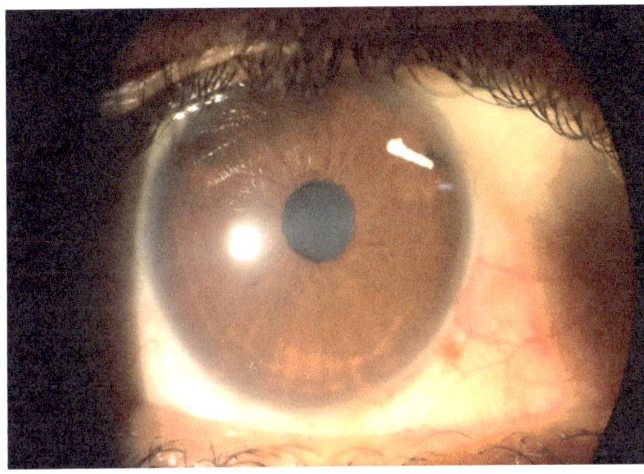

Fig. 5.5 Slit lamp image showing superficial wooden stick foreign body in a 28-year-old male patient

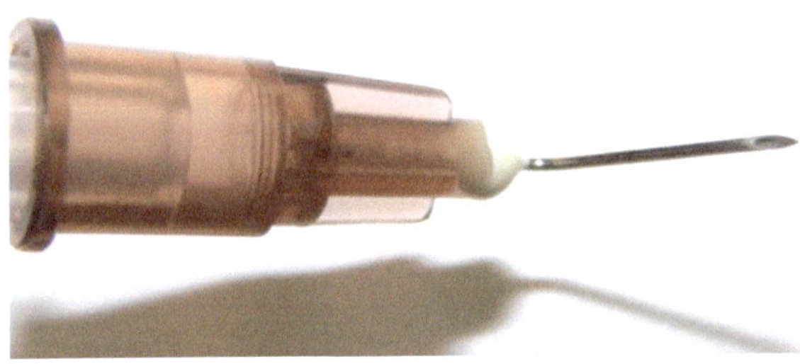

Fig. 5.6 External photograph demonstrating a bent 26-gauge needle that can be used to remove corneal foreign bodies

Table 5.4 Equipments needed for foreign body removal

1. Slit lamp with a cobalt blue filter or wood's lamp
2. Anaesthetic drops (proparacaine 0.5%)
3. Sodium fluorescein drops or strips
4. 26 Gauge needle, can use a bent one.
5. Sterile Cotton tipped applicator
6. Alger brush (if available)

All metallic foreign bodies regardless of the depth should be removed, as they may form a rust ring on reaction with the stromal tissue unlike the inert ones like glass or plastic which if cannot be removed easily, maybe carefully observed on regular follow-up visits. Smaller rust rings may resolve on their own with time and can be left alone, but larger ones, especially those located in the centre need to be removed as these have an impact on future vision, can hamper wound healing, or cause secondary iritis and stromal degeneration [13].

Following removal, the entry point should be checked for any aqueous leak using a fluorescent strip. If the seidel's test turns out to be positive, that is a visible leak or a lighter colour due to dilution of the dye by the aqueous humour, an overnight tight patching or tissue adhesive with bandage contact lens should be done depending on the clinicians' judgement and availability of resources in the emergency setting.

A foreign body embedded deeper in the cornea or extending into the anterior chamber needs removal under surgical microscope in an operation theatre. Any prolapsed uveal tissue might need excision or abscission depending on the duration of the injury. Wound is closed using interrupted 10-0 nonabsorbable sutures.

Postoperative treatment includes prophylactic topical and systemic broad-spectrum antibiotics (E/D Moxifloxacin 0.5% QID), lubricants (E/D CMC 0.5% 4–6 times/ day) and a mydriatic- cycloplegic (E/D Homatropine 2% 2–4 times/day) to alleviate ciliary spasm and related discomfort. Topical corticosteroids like Dexamethasone 0.1%, Fluorometholone 0.1% eye drop can be used to minimise postoperative inflammation and subsequent haze. However, steroid eye drops should be given only when the epithelial defect has healed. Macedo et al. [14] in his study reported that 90% of the bacterial culture-positive cases of corneal foreign bodies were sensitive to fluoroquinolone drops. Patching the eye, even though controversial and have not been seen to reduce the healing time or the degree of discomfort [6], is used commonly among Ophthalmologists. It can be tried especially in children and highly apprehensive adult patients to prevent further damage. It is contraindicated in contact lens wearers, as well as in cases of organic foreign bodies, as in these cases can increase the rate of infection. Systemic non-steroidal anti-inflammatory drugs in the form of tablet ibuprofen 200 or 400 mg BD or Diclofenac sodium 50 or 75 mg BD can be given in the initial 2–3 days, and if indicated, anti-glaucoma medication (E/D Timolol 0.5% or its combination with E/D brimonidine 0.2% BD) should be added. The follow-up schedule needs to be personalised on a case-by-case assessment based on the location, depth of the foreign body and associated ocular injuries.

Prognosis for vision is usually good. It can vary with the size, depth of involvement and nature of the foreign body involved. Peripheral and superficial ones have a very good prognosis with no long-term effect on visual acuity whereas central and deeper ones can be complicated and may need more frequent follow-up visits until they regain near-normal visual acuity. Prophylactic measures and appropriate education of the workers indulged in high-risk activities on the importance of wearing protective eye gear, about its appropriate fit, the seriousness of the injuries that can occur including the chances of complete loss of vision are of prime importance in preventing such injuries.

5.4 Recurrent Corneal Erosions

Recurrent corneal erosions are an important cause of ocular discomfort and can predispose the cornea to infections. Once it develops, medical treatment is enough for resolution in most cases. But in few patients, the treatment might fail and will result in recurrent erosions.

5.4.1 Aetiology

The majority of patients presenting with recurrent corneal erosions (RCE) give a history of trauma. When there is no obvious history of trauma, an underlying disorder like corneal dystrophies or ocular surface disease should be suspected and looked for. The incidence of recurrence was shown to be 1:150 cases following traumatic abrasion [15].

5.4.2 Aetiological Types

Recurrent erosions can be primary or secondary depending on whether the basement membrane complex abnormality is inherent or acquired. Primary would involve epithelial dystrophies like epithelial basement membrane dystrophy or map dot fingerprint dystrophy, Reis's buckler, lattice, granular or even stromal ones like macular dystrophy. Secondary causes are trauma, keratoconjunctivitis sicca, Salzmann nodular degeneration, herpetic infection, meibomian gland dysfunction where the basement membrane damage is acquired [16].

5.4.3 Clinical Features

The complaints are usually episodes of pain, discomfort, watering, increased sensitivity to light and associated blurring of vision typically on waking up in the morning. The history is usually one of the repeated episodes of ocular discomfort interspersed with periods of complete inactivity in a patient with or without a prior history of corneal injury or abrasion. These are usually seen in the central area due to the loose central epithelium getting displaced with the blinking of eye. The appearance of the affected cornea varies from loosely adherent and elevated epithelium, epithelial microcysts, or corneal epithelial defects, to stromal infiltrates and opacities [17, 18].

Two types have been described clinically- macro and micro erosions [19]. In the macro form, there is extensive involvement of the corneal surface and thus associated increased severity of symptoms and a prolonged period of recovery. Whereas the microform is one with a smaller area involved and less symptoms with rapid recovery and can be missed easily on examination.

5.4.4 Management

The treatment is usually in the form of mechanical debridement of the loose epithelium or removing the epithelium by using alcohol. Superficial corneal ablative procedures like Phototherapeutic Keratectomy may be performed with a reported success rate between 60 and 100% [20, 21]. For recalcitrant cases, a therapeutic bandage contact lens can be used. Techniques like anterior stromal puncture using 26 gauge needle, Nd:YAG laser treatment, micro diathermy can be used to promote scar tissue in the subepithelial layer and thereby promote epithelial stability.

5.5 Photokeratitis

Photokeratitis also known as snow blindness or welder's arc is another important reason for seeking treatment in the emergency department. It is caused by damage to the eye from direct exposure to ultraviolet rays. It is acute painful punctate keratopathy that occurs due to ocular surface damage.

5.5.1 Aetiology

Commonly implicated situations that can result in this condition are direct viewing of a solar eclipse, from tanning lamps or welding arcs. Sunlight reflection from sand, water, ice and snow all can lead to photokeratitis.

5.5.2 Clinical Features

Patients usually present with severe pain, watering and intolerance to light hours after the exposure. Other associated features include blurring of vision, headache, halos around lights. Multiple superficial punctate staining areas can be seen all over the cornea on slit lamp examination. This is a transient inflammatory reaction and tends to appear within 6 hours after exposure and the patient completely recovers in approximately 48 h without any long-term consequences [22].

5.5.3 Management

It is treated with eye patching, topical prophylactic antibiotics, lubricant drops and cycloplegics. Public education on avoiding direct sunlight exposure, wearing protective eye gears in the form of shades or goggles or UV (ultraviolet) resistant contact lenses to protect the cornea are important preventive public health measures to be reinforced.

5.6 Minor Chemical Injury

Chemical injury is another important cause of eye-related emergency. It accounts for 11.5–22.1% of traumatic ocular injuries with a majority of the victims being young males [23]. It is one amongst the common workplace-related injuries. A proper history can distinguish this from other differentials. It can be caused by both acid and alkali, chuna particle injury being the commonest [24]. Studies show alkali injuries to be more common than acid due to its extensive use both in industries and in household. Alkali injury is more dangerous as it penetrates more and results in severe forms of ocular injuries.

5.6.1 Clinical Features

Symptoms include pain, redness, watering, intolerance to light, irritation with foreign body sensation with a typical history of exposure to chemical agents either at home or at the occupational site. On examination, varying degrees of conjunctival and corneal involvement can be seen (Fig. 5.7). Area or clock hours of limbal ischemia and conjunctival involvement is to be clearly noted as the prognosis depends on the extent of limbus involved. Corneal injury can be superficial with an epithelial defect in cases of minor chemical injury. In cases of *chuna* particle injury, particulate material may be seen sticking to the area of involvement or in the fornices which need to be removed meticulously so as to curtail the exposure to the agent.

5.6.2 Management

The immediate management should be given within the first few minutes of the injury and involves copious irrigation of the ocular surface with any non-toxic liquid (tap water, normal saline, ringer's lactate or balanced salt solution) for a minimum of 30 min. pH should be checked from the cul-de-sac after every 5–10 min of irrigation and further irrigation to be done till pH reaches 7. A topical anaesthetic guided thorough examination of the ocular surface including all fornices by double eversion needs to be carried out after irrigation. Topical medications like antibiotic drops to prevent bacterial superinfection, topical steroid drops to control inflammation (needs to be tapered rapidly if epithelial defect present), sodium ascorbate and sodium citrate to minimise ulceration, cycloplegic drops like 2% homatropine for

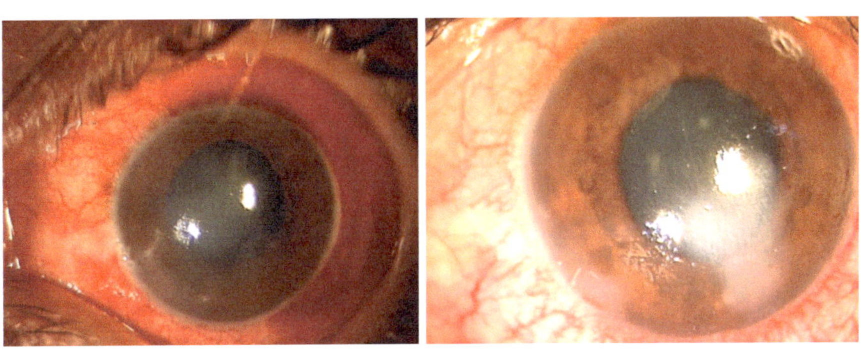

Fig. 5.7 Image of a case of acute chemical injury showing conjunctival and corneal involvement

pain relief, anti-glaucoma medications like brimonidine and timolol to tide over spikes in intraocular pressure along with measures to promote re-epithelization like supplementation of tear substitutes and application of bandage contact lens form the major crux of management. Oral tetracyclines which have anti-matrix metalloprotein activity along with vitamin C supplementation to promote collagen synthesis can help in controlling the disease activity in most cases. Other intermediate-term treatment modalities include debridement of the necrotic area with or without amniotic membrane transplantation, tissue adhesives like cyanoacrylate glue with BCL application for small corneal perforations and conjunctival or tenon advancement to improve the blood supply of the limbal area.

Prognosis can vary from case to case with the chemical agent involved, its concentration and volume, duration of exposure, location of involvement, delay in presentation to hospital and immediate management given. Minor forms can be treated with a good prognosis, unlike the grievous ones which can lead to limbal stem cell deficiency, severe ocular surface disease and permanent visual disability to the survivor. Effective preventive measures such as the use of protective eyewear and first aid methods should be reinforced in the public to reduce the morbidity of the condition.

5.7 Corneal Infections

5.7.1 Viral Keratitis

Herpes simplex virus (HSV) can have varying manifestations in the human eye ranging from epithelial, stromal, endothelial keratitis. HSV epithelial keratitis classically appears in a dendritic pattern with terminal bulbs or in a geographic pattern (Fig. 5.8a, b). Points in history taking that can point towards a probable HSV infection will be usage of topical or systemic steroids, immune deficiency states or recent episode of fever, with blistering in and around mouth & nose, hormonal

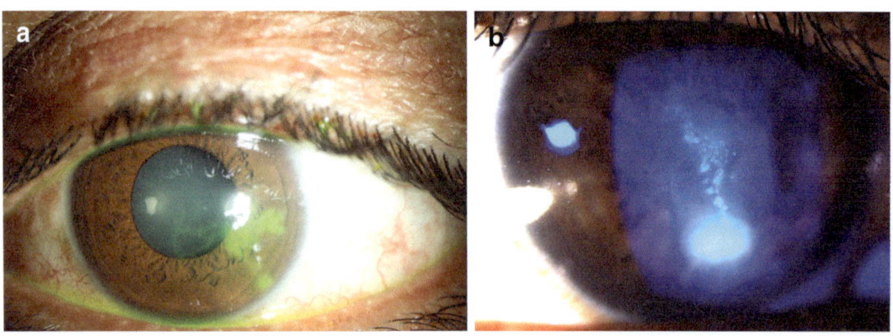

Fig. 5.8 Slit lamp photographs of a patient with (**a**) herpetic epithelial keratitis showing dendritic ulcer and (**b**) geographic pattern seen in viral epithelial keratitis after coalescing of the dendrites, both presenting with acute onset of painful, red eye to the ophthalmic emergency department

disturbances or UV or sunlight exposure. The patient most often typically gives a history of recurrent redness and pain with associated diminution of vision in the past.

5.7.1.1 Clinical Features

Symptoms are usually unilateral; although 1.3–12% of ocular HSV-1 is reported as bilateral [25]. Symptoms include photophobia, excessive tearing, pain, blurred vision, redness, irritation, foreign body sensation and painful blisters around the nose and mouth. On examination, the pattern of the ulcer can be either a dendritic one or a geographical one and characteristic finding of reduced corneal sensation is obtained in most cases. Epithelial involvement makes the patient more symptomatic rather than a deeper involvement like disciform keratitis. On staining the base of the ulcer which is composed of necrotic tissue takes up the fluorescein stain whereas the live virus laden marginal cells take up the rose Bengal stain. Associated stromal involvement in the form of stromal oedema, Descemet membrane folds can be present. In necrotizing stromal variant active stromal lysis can be seen. Endothelial involvement can be linear, disciform or diffuse with specified keratic precipitates seen in each pattern.

5.7.1.2 Management

Typical history of recurrent redness associated with diminution of vision combined with slit lamp findings and associated reduced sensation over cornea is almost conclusive of the diagnosis. HSV PCR in tear film can be done for confirmation. Treatment involves topical antiviral medications. Acyclovir and ganciclovir are selective antiviral agents (gets activated in virus-infected cells only) that are efficacious in managing HSV epithelial lesions [26].

5.8 Miscellaneous

5.8.1 Contact Lens-Related Minor Emergencies

More than 140 million people all over the world wear contact lenses [27]. Clinicians in emergency care set up should be able to identify contact lens associated ocular conditions like a corneal abrasion, ocular pain and discomfort, inability to remove contact lens and also the sight-threatening ones like microbial keratitis. Discomfort usually arises after prolonged wear or in patients with a tight fit which typically gets relieved by discontinuing its use. In a study by Aslam et al., it was found that 12% of corneal abrasion cases were contact lens related [28].

5.8.1.1 Risk Factors

The factors that predispose to corneal injury in contact lens wearers are [29, 30]:

- Poor hand hygiene
- Soft contact lens wear
- Extended/overnight wear

- Male gender
- Smoking
- Poor contact lens storage (such as use of tap water, lack of cleansing/regular replacement of case, using homemade solutions for storage)
- Poor ocular surface (such as dry eye disease, blepharitis)

The history of contact lens wear is thus important in any case of corneal abrasion. Bacteria are responsible for almost 90% of contact lens microbial keratitis and Gram-negative bacilli such as Pseudomonas aeruginosa and Serratia marcescens are the most involved group [31, 32].

Another important organism involved with contact lens keratitis is acanthamoeba. Even though uncommon it is a well-known cause of contact lens-related keratitis [33]. Consider acanthamoeba keratitis in contact lens wearers with a history of exposure to soil or contaminated water, especially in patients who go for swimming with the lenses on [33].

5.8.1.2 Clinical Features

In cases of CLMK, a history of severe pain, redness, watering with associated diminution of vision are the common symptoms. Slit lamp findings a ring infiltrate on examination can point towards the diagnosis. At times, sterile inflammatory infiltrates can be seen in patients wearing contact lens, like marginal keratitis or contact lens-related peripheral ulcer (CLPU). These occur due to an inflammatory response to the contact lens and can be differentiated by lesser severity of symptoms and signs which are sectoral and mild.

5.8.1.3 Investigations

Corneal scraping of the infiltrate is done if well-defined corneal ulcer is seen on examination. The contact lens along with its solution can be send for microbiological examination for identification of the organism and better treatment of the same. Culture on non-nutrient agar medium streaked with E. Coli strains should be used whenever acanthamoeba is suspected.

5.8.1.4 Management

Patients with a contact lens-related abrasion should be given treatment similar to other cases of corneal abrasion but not be patched because of the risk of bacterial superinfection [34]. Treatment should include a fourth-generation fluoroquinolone like E/D moxifloxacin for 4 times/day with lubricant drops (E/D CMC 0.5% 6 times/day) and cycloplegic for pain relief in the initial 4–5 days (E/D HA 2% QID). Frequent follow-ups to avoid unwanted complications is advisable. Any epithelial defect with infiltrate should be treated with a high index of suspicion and should be started on broad-spectrum antibiotics and if needed fortified drops covering both Gram-positive and Gram-negative organisms. Further reductions in the incidence of CLMK (contact lens microbial keratitis) will depend on improvements in the composition of lenses, their surface coatings, their solutions and cases, wearing schedules and the education of contact lens wearers.

In cases of CLPU, as the aetiology is inflammatory, treatment is with topical steroid drops (E/D prednisolone acetate 4–6 times/day and tapered) given with proper antibiotic coverage [35].

5.8.2 Neurotrophic Keratitis

A neurotrophic ulcer usually manifests as a well-defined rolled out margin and commonly seen in patients with a history of varicella zoster virus or HSV infection, diabetic neuropathy or in chronic contact lens wearers. Dua et al. [36] defined neurotrophic keratitis as "a disease related to alterations in corneal nerves, leading to impairment in sensory and trophic function with consequent breakdown of the corneal epithelium, affecting the health and integrity of the tear film, epithelium and stroma resulting in a decrease or even absence of corneal sensation."

5.8.2.1 Aetiology

The pathology mainly involves disorders wherein the nerve supply of the cornea is affected such as central nervous system disorders (postsurgical procedures for acoustic neuromas for trigeminal neuralgia, surgical injury to trigeminal nerve), systemic conditions (diabetes, vitamin A deficiency, amyloidosis, multiple sclerosis), genetic disorders (various genetic syndromes as Riley Day syndrome, Goldenhar syndrome, Moebius syndrome) and certain ocular diseases (ocular surface infections especially herpes simplex keratitis and chronic inflammation, post-ocular surgery, contact lenses and corneal dystrophies).

5.8.2.2 Clinical Features

The major manifestation includes inflammation and corneal epithelial keratitis, which can evolve into vision-threatening non-healing epithelial defect (Fig. 5.9) and stromal ulceration which may go on to frank perforation.

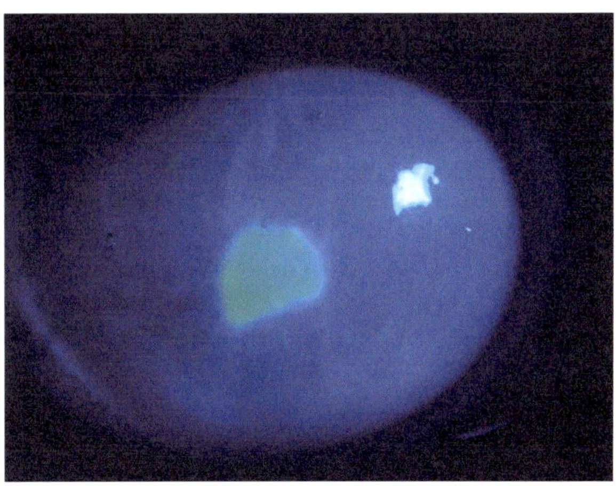

Fig. 5.9 Slit lamp photograph of a patient showing a central neurotrophic ulcer with well-delineated margins, as seen on fluorescein staining under cobalt blue filter

5.8.2.3 Management

Treatment includes withdrawing all toxic medications, application of a bandage contact lens, copious use of preservative-free lubricants and surgical management in the form of tarsorrhaphy, amniotic membrane transplantation or if needed keratoplasty. Novel promising approaches include topical nerve growth factor (cenegermin 0.002% solution) and surgical corneal neurotization [37].

5.8.3 Exposure Keratopathy

In this disease process, damage to the cornea occurs primarily from prolonged exposure of the ocular surface to the outside environment. The exposure results in drying up of the tear film with resultant keratitis, ulceration and even can lead to perforation and scarring leading to permanent vision loss.

5.8.3.1 Aetiology

Patients with seventh cranial nerve palsy and lagophthalmos or Parkinson's disease with infrequent blinking are usually affected. Comatose patients in Intensive Care Units on mechanical ventilation with incomplete eye closure are another group. Rarely, a patient can present following an epi bulbar block with a sudden bleed behind the eye which results in proptosis and inability to close the eyes. In certain situations, following trauma or thermochemical injury, loss of eyelid tissue can occur with resultant exposure of the inferior cornea. Other causes of exposure to keratopathy include thyroid eye disease and other causes of proptosis.

5.8.3.2 Clinical Features

Patients usually present with acute symptoms of foreign body sensation, watering, pain and photophobia due to exposure to keratitis. Dryness of the ocular surface with subsequent decompensation, ulceration and perforation can complicate the situation in many cases [38].

Resultant corneal opacity can lead to long-term ocular disability.

5.8.3.3 Management

Whatever is the aetiology, as uniform distribution of tears is necessary for maintaining a healthy ocular surface, the mainstay of management is the frequent instillation of tear substitutes. Another important strategy is to patch or cover the eye after applying lubricant gel as a temporary measure to avoid exposure. A temporary suture like frost suture or temporary/ permanent tarsorrhaphy might be needed in extreme situations to protect the globe. If there is a retrobulbar bleed with proptosis and inability to close eyes, performing a canthotomy to relieve pressure in itself will suffice [39].

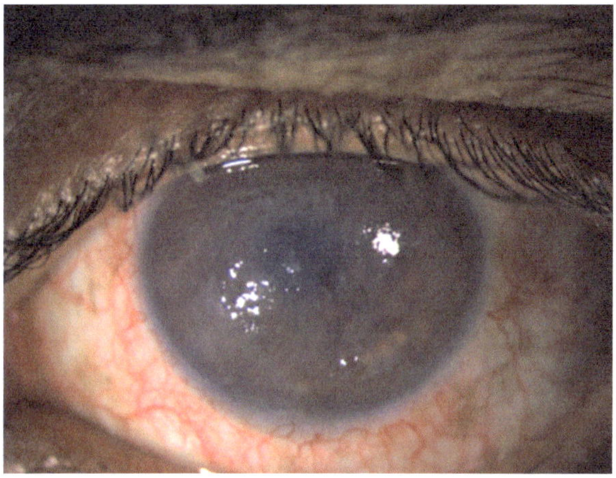

Fig. 5.10 Slit lamp photograph of a patient with bullous keratopathy, demonstrating diffuse corneal edema and multiple bullae. The bulla (yellow arrow) may rupture and cause acute onset of pain and redness

5.8.4 Ruptured Corneal Bulla

Another situation wherein a patient can present to the emergency department with acute onset pain, watering and intolerance to light is a case of ruptured bullae.

5.8.4.1 Aetiology

The aetiology for bullae formation can vary, for example, a patient on treatment for pseudophakic or aphakic bullous keratopathy can have an acute presentation when bulla ruptures and give rise to intolerable symptoms. Similarly, a patient with localised thermal or firecracker injury who was relatively asymptomatic may present acutely following rupture of an associated epithelial bullae (Fig. 5.10) in the area involved. Patients with acute chronic glaucoma, viral keratitis and endothelial dystrophy may present to the emergency with such features.

5.8.4.2 Clinical Features

The symptoms include mild to severe diminution of vision, pain, excessive watering, foreign body sensation and increased sensitivity to light. The pain is typically due to the exposure of subepithelial plexus whenever a bullae rupture.

Signs can vary depending on the severity. The common findings are stromal and epithelial oedema with bullae formation, margins of the ruptured bullae with defect taking up stain on examination after fluorescein staining. In some cases, scarring and opacity of resolved bullous keratopathy may be seen.

5.8.4.3 Management

The diagnosis is usually made from detailed history and clinical examination. The first-line treatment in an emergency situation should be to relieve the patient from pain. Application of a soft bandage contact lens is a useful method to reduce the pain, the patient should be started on antibiotics and IOP lowering medications. Hypertonic saline drops to reduce the stromal oedema can be started as the epithelial defect heals. The patient should be further planned for a posterior lamellar or full thickness keratoplasty and interim procedures like bowman's membrane cautery and anterior stromal puncturing to prevent epithelial bullae formation can be helpful.

5.9 Conclusion

Most of these minor corneal emergency cases present to the general emergency department and can be very well managed by the first contact physician majority of the time without causing any immediate or long-term consequences. A basic knowledge about these situations and their appropriate management is thus crucial for any physician. Appropriate identification of cases that require ophthalmology specialist opinion and unwanted delay in referring should always be kept in mind. Most of these conditions start responding in 2–3 days of starting treatment and if unresponsive should raise suspicion of a wrong diagnosis and should be referred to a higher centre for better timely care.

Key Points

- Corneal abrasions and foreign bodies constitute a frequent presentation to the ophthalmic emergency department.
- Minor corneal emergencies can be effectively managed medically with broad-spectrum antibiotics and lubricant drops.
- Removal of foreign bodies from the corneal surface should be done with extreme caution and under aseptic precautions.
- A proper history coupled with a detailed slit lamp examination can help make the correct diagnosis in cases of recurrent corneal erosions and photokeratitis.
- Any corneal infection should be identified at the earliest and should be referred to a specialist for proper management.
- Neurotrophic keratitis and exposure to keratopathy require careful ophthalmic and systemic evaluation to elicit the primary cause.
- Any delay in treatment of minor corneal emergencies is associated with poor outcomes.

References

1. McGwin G Jr, Xie A, Owsley C. Rate of eye injury in the United States. Arch Ophthalmol. 2005;123(7):970–6.
2. Fraser S. Corneal abrasion. Clin Ophthalmol. 2010;4:387–90.

3. Wipperman JL, Dorsch JN. Evaluation and management of corneal abrasions. Am Fam Physician. 2013;87(2):114–20.
4. Lin YB, Gardiner MF. Fingernail-induced corneal abrasions: case series from an ophthalmology emergency department. Cornea. 2014;33(7):691–5.
5. Harris PM. Bureau of Labor Statistics. Workplace injuries involving the eyes, 2008; 2011.
6. Menghini M, Knecht PB, Kaufmann C, et al. Treatment of traumatic corneal abrasions: a three-arm, prospective, randomized study. Ophthalmic Res. 2013;50:13–8.
7. Lim CHL, Turner A, Lim BX. Patching for corneal abrasion. Cochrane Database Syst Rev. 2016;7:CD004764.
8. Campanile TM, St Clair DA, Benaim M. The evaluation of eye patching in the treatment of traumatic corneal epithelial defects. J Emerg Med. 1997;15:769–74.
9. Agrawal C, Girgis S, Sethi A, Sethi V, Konale M, Lokwani P, et al. Etiological causes and epidemiological characteristics of patients with occupational corneal foreign bodies: A prospective study in a hospital-based setting in India. Indian J Ophthalmol. 2020;68:54–7.
10. Barash D, Goldenberg-Cohen N, Tzadok D, Lifshitz T, Yassur Y, Weinberger D. Ultrasound biomicroscopic detection of anterior ocular segment foreign body after trauma. Am J Ophthalmol. 1998;126:197–202.
11. Jancevski M, Foster CS. Anterior segment optical coherence tomography. Semin Ophthalmol. 2010;25:317–23.
12. Al-Ghadeer HA, Al-Assiri A. Identification and localization of multiple intrastromal foreign bodies with anterior segment optical coherence tomography and ocular Pentacam. Int Ophthalmol. 2014;34:355–8.
13. Guier CP, Stokkermans TJ. Cornea foreign body removal. In: StatPearls. Treasure Island, FL: StatPearls; 2020.
14. Macedo Filho ET, Lago A, Duarte K, Liang SJ, Lima AL, Freitas D. Superficial corneal foreign body: laboratory and epidemiologic aspects. Arq Bras Oftalmol. 2005;68(6):821–3.
15. Hykin PG, Foss AE, Pavesio C, Dart JK. The natural history and management of recurrent corneal erosion: a prospective randomised trial. Eye. 1994;8(Part 1):35–40.
16. Ramamurthi S, Rahman MQ, Dutton GN, Ramaesh K. Pathogenesis, clinical features and management of recurrent corneal erosions. Eye (Lond). 2006;20(6):635–44.
17. Ionides AC, Tuft SJ, Ferguson VM, Matheson MM, Hykin PG. Corneal infiltration after recurrent corneal epithelial erosion. Br J Ophthalmol. 1997;81:537–40.
18. Brown N, Bron A. Recurrent erosion of the cornea. Br J Ophthalmol. 1976;60:84–96.
19. Chandler P. Recurrent corneal erosion of the cornea. Am J Ophthalmol. 1945;28:355–63.
20. Dausch D, Landesz M, Klein R, Schroder E. Phototherapeutic keratectomy in recurrent corneal epithelial erosion. Refract Corneal Surg. 1993;9:419–24.
21. Fagerholm P, Fitzsimmons TD, Orndahl M, Ohman L, Tengroth B. Phototherapeutic keratectomy: long-term results in 166 eyes. Refract Corneal Surg. 1993;9:S76–81.
22. Izadi M, Jonaidi-Jafari N, Pourazizi M, Alemzadeh-Ansari MH, Hoseinpourfard MJ. Photokeratitis induced by ultraviolet radiation in travelers: A major health problem. J Postgrad Med. 2018;64(1):40–6.
23. Clare G, Suleman H, Bunce C, Dua H. Amniotic membrane transplantation for acute ocular burns. Cochrane Database Syst Rev. 2012;9:CD009379.
24. Rathi A, Sinha R, Aron N, Sharma N. Ocular surface injuries & management. Community Eye Health. 2017;30(99):S11–4.
25. Souza PM, Holland EJ, Huang AJ. Bilateral herpetic keratoconjunctivitis. Ophthalmology. 2003;110(3):493–6.
26. Wilhelmus KR. Antiviral treatment and other therapeutic interventions for herpes simplex virus epithelial keratitis. Cochrane Database Syst Rev. 2015;9:CD002898.
27. Lim CHL, Stapleton F, Mehta JS. Review of contact lens-related complications. Eye Contact Lens. 2018;44(Suppl 2):S1–10.
28. Aslam SA, Sheth HG, Vaughan AJ. Emergency management of corneal injuries. Injury. 2007;38:594–7.

29. Dart JKG, Radford CF, Minassian D, Verma S, Stapleton F. Risk factors for microbial keratitis with contemporary contact lenses: a case-control study. Ophthalmology. 2008;115:1647–54.
30. Stapleton F, Edwards K, Keay L, et al. Risk factors for moderate and severe microbial keratitis in daily wear contact lens users. Ophthalmology. 2012;119:1516–21.
31. Sharma S, Gopalakrishnan S, Aasuri MK, et al. Trends in contact lens-associated microbial keratitis in Southern India. Ophthalmology. 2003;110:138–43.
32. Cheung N, Nagra P, Hammersmith K. Emerging trends in contact lens-related infections. Curr Opin Ophthalmol. 2016;27:327–32.
33. Kilvington S, Gray T, Dart J, et al. Acanthamoeba keratitis: The role of domestic tap water contamination in the United Kingdom. Invest Ophthalmol Vis Sci. 2004;45:165–9.
34. Clemons CS, Cohen EJ, Arentsen JJ, Donnenfeld ED, Laibson PR. Pseudomonas ulcers following patching of corneal abrasions associated with contact lens wear. CLAO J. 1987;13(3):161–4.
35. Baum J, Dabezies O. Pathogenesis and treatment of 'sterile' midperipheral infiltrates associated with soft contact lens use. Cornea. 2000;19:777–81.
36. Dua HS, Said DG, Messmer EM, et al. Neurotrophic keratopathy. Prog Retin Eye Res. 2018;66:107–31.
37. Versura P, Giannaccare G, Pellegrini M, Sebastiani S, Campos EC. Neurotrophic keratitis: current challenges and future prospects. Eye Brain. 2018;10:37–45.
38. Mathenge W. Emergency management: exposure keratopathy. Community Eye Health. 2018;31(103):69.
39. Wolkow N, Chodosh J, Freitag SK. Innovations in treatment of lagophthalmos and exposure keratopathy. Int Ophthalmol Clin. 2017;57(4):85–103.

6 Corneal Laceration and Penetrating Injuries

Bharat Patil, M. Vanathi, and Nimmy Raj

Cornea contributes to one sixth of total ocular wall and two thirds of total optical power of eye. Corneal trauma is one of the major reasons for visual disability. If left untreated, may result in permanent blindness. In spite of this, ocular trauma does not get sufficient weightage in National blindness control programme, due to larger share of bilaterally blinding disorders.

6.1 Epidemiology

With most of the epidemiological studies emphasising on ocular trauma in a broader aspect there is limited epidemiological data on corneal laceration, and hence the exact magnitude of problem is not known. Bever Dam Eye study reported that a 20% of population suffers from an ocular trauma in their lifetime [1]. About 5–16% of all admissions in eye hospitals are related to trauma and up to 3% of all visits to emergency department are due to eye trauma [2, 3]. The Baltimore eye survey reported a 14.4% cumulative prevalence of eye injury in the general population [4].

As per data published by World Health Organization (WHO) in 1998, 16 lakh people were blind in both eyes and 19 million people were uniocularly blind due to ocular trauma, and 55 million people had restrict ed activities for more than 1 day a year due to ocular injuries [5]. Andhra Pradesh eye study reported prevalence of

B. Patil
Cataract, Refractive and Glaucoma Services, Sarvadrishti Eye Hospital, Patna, Bihar, India

Ex-Senior Resident, Phaco-Refractive & Glaucoma Services, Dr Rajendra Prasad Centre for Ophthalmic Sciences, AIIMS, New Delhi, India

M. Vanathi (✉) · N. Raj
Cornea, Lens & Refractive Services, Dr R P Centre for Ophthalmic Sciences, All India Institute of Medical Sciences, New Delhi, India

B. Sharma, J. S. Titiyal (eds.), *Corneal Emergencies*,
https://doi.org/10.1007/978-981-16-5876-1_6

7.5% in rural population and 3.9% in urban population [6]. The Aravind Comprehensive Eye Survey reported a prevalence of 4% ocular trauma in rural population [7].

The incidence, prevalence and mode of penetrating ocular injury vary according to many factors like age, sex and socioeconomic background. Mechanical trauma is the most common cause for lacerations and penetrating injuries to the cornea. Blunt trauma can also result in globe rupture resulting in tears involving the corneal tissue.

6.1.1 Age and Sex

Ocular trauma has tri modal age of presentation. Age group of less than 15 years, age 20–44 years and more than 65 years are more susceptible. Mode of injury is different in different age groups. Due to occupational risk factors and more time spent outdoor males have double the risk of eye trauma as compared to females. The manual labourers, farmers are at high risk of ocular trauma due to occupational risk factor. The usual modes of ocular injury in adult population are assault by fist, road traffic accidents, wooden stick, or trauma by branch of tree while working in field.

Worldwide almost 6 million children (less than 15 years) have ocular trauma episodes in a year. The UK Paediatric Trauma Study 2 (POTS2) reported median age of presentation as 7.7 years [8], with boys more than twice as likely to be affected as girls. Since children spend most of their time at home, they have equal or more risk of eye trauma at home than outside, with 25% ocular injuries occurring at school or nursery. Victims may be bystanders. Sharp objects like pen, pencil, toys, etc., or blunt objects like corners of household furniture, ball, gili, wooden stick, etc., are usual cause of eye trauma in children. In Indian scenario, 'Bow and arrow' and firecracker injury are responsible for considerable percentage of eye trauma in children.

A third spike of age occurs at more than 65 years, due to tendency to fall and slowed reflexes. Risk of eye getting injured increases as the age increases. A 50-year-old has 3.6 times more risk of eye trauma than that in 15-year-old [9].

6.1.2 Socioeconomic Background

Socioeconomic background also seems to influence the incidence and mode of eye trauma, with the lower socioeconomic group being at higher risk. Literates have lesser risk of ocular trauma [7]. Injury related to recreational sports like badminton, paint ball gun, etc., is seen in higher socioeconomic class. Rural and industrial population has high risk of ocular trauma due to occupational risk factors. In rural India, ocular trauma incidence correlates with the agricultural activity, more cases reported during crop harvest season and rainy season, most common mode of injury is trauma by thorn or by branch of tree. Eye trauma is an occupational hazard for industrial workers, construction site workers and chemical factory workers. More than half of the accidents involving eye takes place at workplace. Workers at rubber industry, metal industry, refineries, pipe industries, etc., are at high risk. Projectile injury while working with chisel hammer is an important cause in manual labourers. Eye injuries accounts for almost 15% of battlefield injuries worldwide and these injuries usually result in severe visual impairment [10].

Studies have shown that, up to 90% of all ocular injuries are preventable or avoidable by using proper safety eyewear and health education of supervising adults [11–13].

6.2 Betts Classification and Nomenclature

The Birmingham Eye Trauma Terminology System (BETTS) [14] ocular trauma classification system was devised in order to create uniformity, avoid confusion and to promote research (Table 6.1). It mainly classifies ocular trauma either as open globe injury or closed globe injury, depending upon loss of integrity of eye wall. Loss of anatomical continuity of eye wall after trauma is termed as open globe injury (Figs. 6.1 and 6.2). When ocular wall is intact after trauma it is called as close globe injury. For all practical purposes, cornea and sclera are considered as ocular wall or coat. Closed globe injury is further classified into either contusion or lamellar laceration.

Corneal laceration is either full-thickness or partial-thickness injury of cornea which can be due to either direct ocular trauma or by an indirect impact [15]. A direct impact can be cuased by a sharp object like knife, pen or pencil, etc., resulting in either partial/fullthickness laceration or simple abrasion. An indirect impact is caused by eye trauma by blunt object like cricket ball, fist, etc., resulting in inside out trauma to the cornea resulting in full-thickness corneal laceration. In this scenario, it is called ***globe rupture***.

The term ***penetrating injury*** is used when only entry wound is present and when both entry and exit wound are seen it called as ***perforating injury***.

The classification system further divides the open globe injury into three zones (Fig. 6.3).

- Zone I—limited to cornea.
- Zone II—trauma involving limbus and anterior sclera up to 5 mm posterior to limbus.
- Zone III—trauma involving sclera more than 5 mm posterior to limbus.

Table 6.1 Assessment of open globe injuries as per BETTS recommendation

<table>
<tr><th>Type (nature of injury)</th><th>Grade Severity: functional (visual acuity)</th><th>Examination (pupillary reaction)</th><th>Anatomical (zones)</th></tr>
<tr><td>Rupture</td><td>≥20/40</td><td rowspan="5">Positive: RAPD+ in affected eye
Negative: No RAPD in affected eye</td><td rowspan="5">I: isolated to cornea inclusive of corneo-scleral limbus
II: corneo-scleral limbus to a point 5mm into sclera
III: posterior to the anterior 5 mm of sclera</td></tr>
<tr><td>Perforation</td><td><20/40–20/100</td></tr>
<tr><td>Penetration</td><td><20/100–5/200</td></tr>
<tr><td>IOFB</td><td><5/200–PL</td></tr>
<tr><td>Mixed</td><td>No PL</td></tr>
</table>

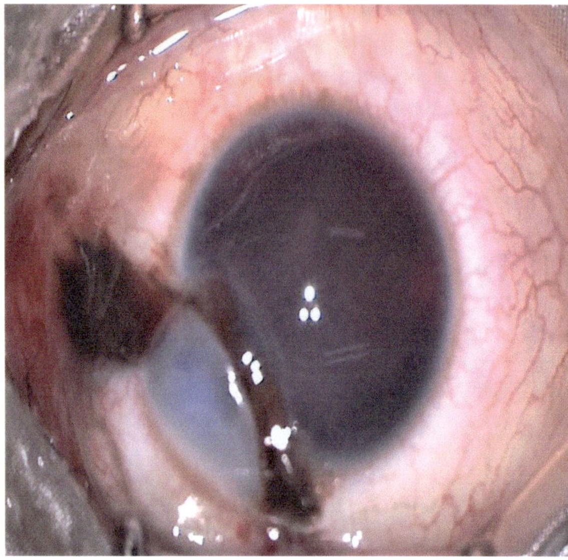

Fig. 6.1 Clinical picture of an open globe injury showing corneo-scleral tear with iris prolapse with turbid aqueous and hyphema

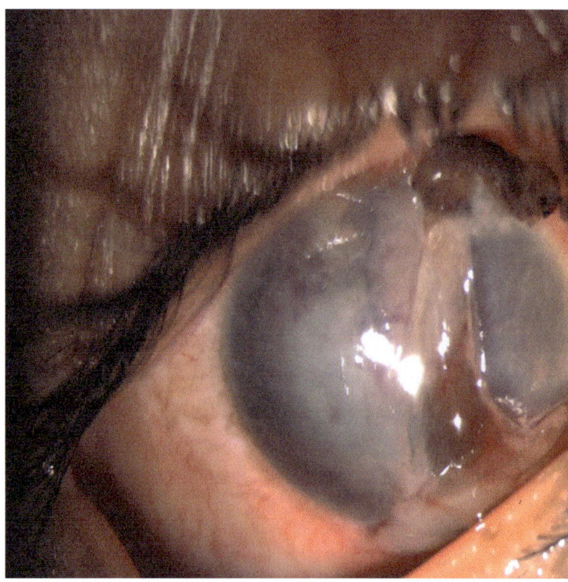

Fig. 6.2 Clinical picture of an open globe injury showing cornea tear with iris incarceration in the wound with corneal edema shallow irregular anterior chamber and cataract

Thus, while documenting the diagnosis of any ocular trauma case, all the above points should be noted, for example, if patient has a full-thickness corneal laceration caused by direct impact of sharp object with only entry wound visible and extent limiting only to the cornea—according to BETTS classification, it should entered into the case record sheet as Open globe Penetrating injury, Zone I Corneal Laceration, preferably aided with a diagrammatic representation or photographic documentation.

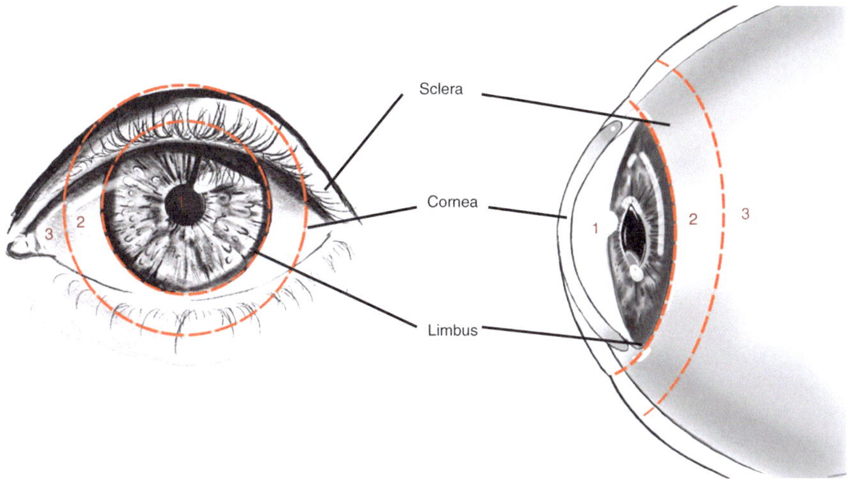

Fig. 6.3 Zones according to BETTS classification system

The ocular trauma score (OTS) was proposed by Kuhn et al. [16] in the early 2000s to provide a simple set of variables which can predict the final visual outcome in an injured eye. This scoring system helps an ophthalmologist in counselling, triage, management and research purposes. The raw score sum which is equal to the sum of raw points is taken to categorise the cases into OTS 1–5 with higher score indicating better visual prognosis (Table 6.2).

As eye trauma in children differs from adults in many ways and as the examination of kids cannot always be relied upon, a similar but slightly different scoring system was proposed by Acar et al. [17] for the paediatric population (paediatric ocular trauma score, POTS), with points assigned for variables considered. The variables that were considered included presenting visual acuity [no light perception (10 points) light perception/hand movements (20 points), counting fingers (30 points), 20/2000–20/40 (40 points) and 20/33–20/20 (50 points)]; age of the child [0–5 years (10 points), 6–10 years (15 points) and 11–15 years (25 points)]; location of the injury [zone 1 (25 points), zone II (15 points) and zone III (10 points)], along with the presence of co-morbidities [iris prolapse, hyphema, endophthalmitis, organic/unclean injury, delay of surgery for >48 h (–5 points each), traumatic cataract (–10 points), vitreous haemorrhage (–20 points), retinal detachment (–20 points) and endophthalmitis (–30 points)]. The POTS gave lesser points for initial visual acuity considering the limitations in obtaining accurate visual acuity measurements from children. The patients were divided into 5 prognostic groups [group 1 (≤45), group 2 (46–64), group 3 (65–79), group 4 (80–89) and group 5 (90–100)] based on the total score obtained with a higher trauma evaluation scores were considered indicative of a better prognosis. The formulae 2 × (age + zone)—corresponding pathologies were used to determine trauma score in children in whom initial visual acuity could not be obtained [17]. Studies have shown that paediatric

Table 6.2 Ocular trauma score (OTS)—variables and method of calculation

Step 1: take raw points based on visual acuity	**Visual acuity**	**Raw points**
	NPL	60
	LP to HM	70
	1/200–19/200	80
	20/200–20/50	90
	>20/40	100
Step 2: take raw points based on other associated injuries	**Ocular injuries**	**Raw points**
	Globe rupture	–23
	Endophthalmitis	–17
	Perforating injury	–14
	Retinal detachment	–11
	Afferent pupillary defect	–10
Step 3: obtain the raw score by adding the points from steps 1 and 2 An OTS is decided based on the raw score	**Raw score**	**OTS**
	0–44	1
	45–65	2
	66–80	3
	81–91	4
	92–100	5

ocular trauma score (POTS) is more sensitive and specific than ocular trauma score in predicting outcomes in children [18].

6.3 History Taking and Clinical Presentation

Mechanism of injury, extent of initial damage and initial visual acuity are the most important factors in predicting visual outcome [19]. Hence evaluation of eye trauma case revolves around these three factors. These factors need to be well documented in history taking at the time of presentation (Table 6.3). The time duration of presentation from the period of injury is also to be noted.

Corneal laceration usually presents as an acute ocular condition with history of sudden diminution of vision. When there is only minimal or local involvement, the vision loss is also not profound. A neglected case can present late with pain and profound vision loss, which can get complicated with infection leading to corneal ulcer, endophthalmitis or panophthalmitis.

All cases of ocular trauma are of medico legal importance, especially in scenarios of road traffic accidents, assaults and workplace related trauma. Hence a detailed and careful history taking and its meticulous documentation is extremely important in every trauma case. During every ophthalmic visit/round, the date and time of patient's presentation and of clinical examination must be documented in every case of ocular trauma. Informant should always be documented in all cases. A sympathetic and compassionate approach to patient is to be adopted while examining and counselling the patient. Obtaining an exact history from post trauma patient is a challenge and more difficult than from non-injured patient. Children may try to hide

Table 6.3 Key points in history and examination

Key points in history	Key points in examination
Rule out life threatening injuries	Projection of rays
Ensure patient is oriented in time, place and person	RAPD and Reverse RAPD
Note down informant, witness and exact time of examination	Rule out canalicular injuries
In cases of associated head injury—ask for h/o loss of consciousness, bleed from mouth, nose/ear	Copious wash before proceeding for any examination in case of chemical injury.
Elicit exact mode of injury	Siedel's Test
General history for anaesthesia fitness	Classify wound according to BETTS classification system
Immunisation history of tetanus In case of animal bite enquire for rabies vaccination of the animal and r/o rabid animal	Look for subtle signs for infection
H/o previous ocular treatment	EUA for uncooperative child Avoid performing forced examination
Ensure Nil Oral	

history due to fear of punishment. History may be fabricated by a victim of assault or by workplace related trauma patient for secondary gains. Hence the clinical findings must always be corroborated with history.

Before proceeding to ophthalmic history and examination, life threatening injuries and non-ophthalmic emergencies threatening life must be ruled out. Orientation of patient to time place and person is to be confirmed. Examiner should try to elicit a detailed history and complete description of presenting complaint. As stated earlier presenting symptoms is typically an acute painful red eye which may or may not be associated with vision loss. Examiner should ask detailed questions to confirm about when, where and how exactly the eye trauma has occurred. Knowing duration is important both for planning treatment and to prognosticate the case. Fresh wounds, if repaired timely will have good prognosis. A risk of wound getting infected increases as the duration increases. Knowing exactly how trauma has occurred and how things have evolved further will help in management and prognosticating the case. A history regarding mode of injury and what exactly caused the trauma should be elicited. History about use of protective eyewear should be asked and the same should be examined for any physical damage. Eye witnesses/family members should also be encouraged to provide details. The most probable agent causing trauma should be traced, for planning the treatment and for prognostication. For example, prognosis and management of a vegetative matter trauma is different from 'chisel hammer' mechanism trauma. History should be asked about any treatment received for eye trauma elsewhere. Past treatment for eye trauma, self-treatment by irritants, antibiotics should be asked. In some part of India, there is a custom of instilling clarified butter, rose water in eye, which may further complicate situation causing secondary infection in wound. A brief history about past medical and surgical history of any pre-existing ophthalmic conditions will help in risk assessment. For example, an operated LASIK patient may present with flap displacement even after trivial eye trauma, an operated corneal transplant patient may present with graft dehiscence. Implants (intra ocular lens, glaucoma drainage devices) or explants (buckle, band) may get displaced or dislocated and will complicate the situation further.

History regarding systemic conditions should be elicited. Besides diabetes mellitus, hypertension and history of cardiovascular accidents a general history to be targeted to rule out conditions which if present may complicate the general anaesthesia. Rule out any bleeding tendency or use of anticoagulant and any drug allergy. History of loss of consciousness, epistaxis, head injury, seizures, etc., should also be looked for and if neurology/neurosurgery, ENT consultation needs to be obtained.

If trauma is secondary to animal bite, attempt must be made to find out whether the animal was rabid or not. Vaccination status of animal if known must be documented.

Fasting status of patient is assessed, and is advisable to inform his/her attendant to ensure that patient is to be placed on nil oral in order to enable an early general anaesthesia administration for surgical repair.

If patient's eye is patched, patch is removed gently under aseptic precautions. Patient is encouraged to open his/her eyes, avoid any forceful eye opening. Best corrected vision with proper documentation of projection of rays must be done. A thorough clinical examination should be carried out. Range of ocular movements, adnexal trauma, RAPD and reverse RAPD if any, should be documented on torch light. Eye lid and punctal-canalicular trauma needs oculo-plasty consultation. Aqueous humour leak from anterior chamber is looked for using fluorescein dye under cobalt blue filter on slit lamp (Seidel's test). If leak is present, Seidel's test is documented as positive. In cases of self-sealed corneal laceration, spontaneous Seidel's test may be negative but leak may be documented on slight pressure on globe (provocative Seidel's test). Extent of corneal wound is noted and is classified according to BETTS system. Condition of iris, depth and contents of anterior chamber (hyphema/hypopyon), lens changes, rupture of anterior capsule, associated zonulopathy if any should be noted. Fornices should be examined thoroughly for presence of foreign body. Meticulous examination of corneal stroma or anterior chamber for foreign body by slit lamp biomicroscopy in cases when possible should be done. Foreign body if freely lying in fornix can be removed in OPD but that impaled in ocular wall or in anterior chamber should better be removed in operation theatre. Signs of infection like corneal infiltrates, exudates in anterior chamber may be seen in cases of eye trauma of longer duration or trauma by vegetative matter. Posterior segment examination is not always possible due to associated hyphema or vitreous haemorrhage and poor visibility. If the perforation is small and media is clear, fundus examination should be done and documented. A gentle preoperative USG might be useful in prognosticating the case in those with poor glow.

Detailed examination may not be possible in children due to poor cooperation. Hence child's further ocular examination is completed during examination under anaesthesia.

Fellow non-traumatic eye of a patient should be examined thoroughly at the time of presentation and especially on follow-up for visual acuity for near and anterior chamber cells, which can be the earliest signs of sympathetic ophthalmia. It is usually seen to occur after a latent period which can vary from as early as 5 days to as long as 50 years. About 70–80% of sympathetic ophthalmia cases occur within 3 months of injury, and 90% occur within 1 year. Others signs to look for are circumciliary congestion, mutton fat keratic precipitates, vitritis or/and exudative retinal detachment.

After assessing the trauma, eye is patched gently. Patient is asked not to press or rub eye. Patient is instructed to avoid straining and blowing nose. A booster dose of 0.5 ml tetanus toxoid is given intramuscularly, if history for vaccination for tetanus is not available or more than 10 years has passed from last injection. Inj. diclofenac 75 mg/1 ml IM can be given for relieving pain. Routine haemoglobin, complete blood counts and any other relevant blood investigation are to be done. Patient is kept fasting in view of general anaesthesia fitness.

6.4 Ocular Investigations

6.4.1 Ultrasonography

In presence of opaque media, ultrasound helps the clinician not only to complete the ocular examination but also to prognosticate and plan the treatment. A-scan is a one-dimensional scan, while B-scan enables two-dimensional cross-sectional imaging. Both scans when used together give maximum information. A gross idea about posterior segment of eye can be obtained. Retinal detachment, vitreous haemorrhage, foreign body in the vitreous cavity may be detected by ultrasonic examination. If lens is not visible, status of anterior and posterior capsule, cataractous changes can also be detected on B-scan. It must be performed carefully in eyes with open globe injury due to potential risk of infection, damage and extrusion of ocular tissues.

B-scan is useful when a foreign body cannot be visualised with a computed tomography scan, e.g. glass, wood or plastic. It is sensitive in detecting foreign bodies with concurrent vitreous haemorrhage and retinal detachment. However, an intra-lenticular foreign body, foreign body lodged in angle and small sized foreign bodies can be missed on USG.

6.4.2 X-Ray

Low radiation exposure, easy availability even in rural areas and low cost are advantages while low resolution is disadvantage. Metallic foreign body, fracture of orbital wall can be detected on X-ray. Both antero-posterior and lateral views are helpful. It has sensitivity of 64–78% for orbital fracture [20]. Hence small orbital fractures can be missed on X-ray. Radiograph is not suitable for detecting soft tissue damage.

6.4.3 CT Scan

CT scan is the imaging modality of choice in open globe injury, orbital trauma and for detecting intraocular foreign bodies specially metallic objects. Lens status and anterior chamber evaluation can also be done on CT scan. CT images can readily show lens position and traumatic displacement/subluxation if any can be easily documented.

CT scan is 71–75% sensitive for detection of occult globe rupture [21]. Signs of globe rupture on CT scan are loss of volume of globe, the ‘flat tire sign’, unusually deep anterior chamber, scleral discontinuity, intraocular air, etc. Retinal and choroidal detachment, vitreous haemorrhage can also be documented on CT scan. CT scan also provides information about the optic nerve status, optic canal fracture, any bony fragment/foreign body pressing over optic nerve, optic nerve avulsion, etc., if present can also be detected by CT scan.

These investigations not only help in planning the treatment but are also of medico legal importance. MRI is contraindicated in ocular trauma due to potential fear of ferromagnetic foreign body.

6.4.4 Special Attention to Be Given to Following Points While Reading Radiograph/CT Scan

- Bony orbit continuity
- Status of Sinuses—look for herniated orbital contents if any
- Orbital apex—a tiny fracture may be an indication of emergency—look for fragment compressing optic nerve
- Evaluate anterior chamber—increased attenuation is s/o hyphema. Shallow chamber may have anteriorly subluxated lens.
- Evaluate position of lens.
- Evaluate posterior chamber for vitreous haemorrhage, choroidal detachment and RD
- Look for retained foreign body. Remember wooden foreign body may mimic air.

6.5 Treatment

6.5.1 Corneal Abrasion

Any surgical intervention needed is best done as early as possible. Majority of corneal abrasions heal spontaneously and treatment is targeted to prevent infection and control pain. Abrasions less than 2 mm usually heal within 24 h.

Indication for Surgical Intervention

The indications for surgical repair include:

- Large corneal laceration
- Complicated corneal laceration
- A positive Seidel’s test
- Retained intraocular (potentially reactive) foreign body

6.5.2 Corneal Laceration Management

6.5.2.1 General Principles

Surgery is usually needed for full-thickness laceration. The primary goal of surgery is to restore the anatomical integrity of eye ball and not the visual gain. Secondary goal is to remove foreign body, manage damaged lens, disrupted vitreous and uveal tissue incarceration/prolapse from the wound.

Patient and his/her attendant should be well informed about the plan of management. A proper, written informed consent must be obtained. For patients less than 18 years of age or poorly oriented unconscious patients, consent is obtained from guardians. A signature of witness must always be taken in all cases of ocular trauma.

6.5.2.2 Simple Corneal Laceration

Full-thickness corneal laceration limited between limbus, without traumatic lens damage and without incarceration of uveal tissue or vitreous or lens in wound is called as simple full-thickness corneal laceration. Management of simple full-thickness laceration varies with the size of laceration, lacerations less than 2 mm and can be managed conservatively while those with more than 2 mm need surgical intervention.

Partial lamellar lacerations which are simple and small without extensive tissue disruption can be managed with topical antibiotic and lubricants along with bandage contact lens/pad and bandage if required. It is imperative to take care to examine the interface thoroughly and during follow-ups to rule out the presence of infection in these cases. Those associated with tissue lift may require suture placement. Majority of simple corneal lacerations tend to heal spontaneously. Goal of therapy is to prevent secondary infection and pain relief. Corneal lacerations are painful due to exposure of nerve endings. In larger corneal lacerations, in order to facilitate healing, and prevent discomfort due to blinking, eye may be patched for 24 h after topical antibiotic instillation. A preservative free ointment preparation maybe preferred. Cycloplegics (2% homatropine/0.75% cyclopentolate) are also instilled to relieve cycloplegia and pain. Patching is contraindicated in vegetative matter trauma and trauma associated with contact lens use. Topical anaesthetics prescription for pain relief is not advisable. On follow-up visit, edges and bed of wound need to be examined for infiltrates. Corneal scraping may be performed if required to identify the infecting microorganisms in order to initiate appropriate therapy. Topical antibiotics in eye drop with broad spectrum coverage (0.5% moxifloxacin) and lubricants (0.5% CMC/1% HPMC) are continued till complete healing of wound.

Simple corneal lacerations heal without leaving corneal scar within 7 days and has good prognosis if not complicated by secondary infection. Patient is advised to avoid eye rubbing and washing eyes with tap water. Dark glasses and cycloplegics can be continued to avoid discomfort. Glare and astigmatism can be a problem with larger laceration scars on healing.

Bandage Contact Lens A soft bandage contact lens (BCL) is an effective alternative of patching for abrasions larger than 2 mm. Bandage contact lens prevents rubbing of lid over epithelial edges, decreases pain and also promotes binocularity. Patient is to be reviewed in 24 h after placement of BCL. Prophylactic topical antibiotics and preservative free lubricants are to be given. Patient is instructed to visit immediately if he/she reports either displacement of lens/pain/photophobia with lens and not to replace lens at home if it is dislodged from eye. Patient is examined after 7 days. On follow-up, status of cornea is examined though BCL specifically for epithelisation status and infiltrates. Examination iperformed after BCL removal enables a detailed evaluation. Epithelium is stained with fluorescein and examined for epithelisation, base and edges are examined for signs of secondary infection (fluorescein is not to be used with BCL in situ as it stains the BCL). Most cases heal within 7 days and reapplication of BCL may not be required. BCL is contraindicated in cases of abrasion associated with—contact lens use/vegetative eye trauma and in the presence of frank infection.

6.5.2.3 Simple Full-Thickness Laceration Less Than 2 mm

Self-sealing simple laceration less than 2 mm, with negative Seidel's test, with well opposed and bevelled edges and formed anterior chamber can be managed conservatively. A soft bandage contact lens (BCL) application and topical medications are sufficient in such cases. Topical antibiotics (0.5% moxifloxacin) QID and cycloplegics (homatropine 2%) QID and lubricant (Carboxy Methyl Cellulose 0.5%) QID are sufficient. Topical steroids (prednisolone acetate 1%) QID is added only in cases not associated with vegetative matter trauma. In cases with vegetative matter trauma, topical steroid is added after a week, after documenting no evidence of secondary infection. Patient is closely followed up with first visit after 24 hours and subsequently, weekly for first month. When wound margins are displaced or not bevelled, a soft bandage contact lens with tissue adhesive is applied.

Tissue Adhesives Two tissue adhesives are available for laceration repair, Cyanoacrylate and fibrin glue.

Cyanoacrylate glue is synthetic while fibrin glue is of animal origin. For cooperative patients BCL with glue application can be done under topical anaesthesia. For non-cooperative patients, it may be done under general anaesthesia (peribulbar/retrobulbar is contraindicated due to risk of prolapse of ocular structures through an open wound, secondary to rise in intra-orbital pressure). Eye is cleaned and draped under aseptic precautions. Anterior chamber is formed either with air/viscoelastic after making a clear corneal stab incision. Area of interest is dried before applying glue. A drop of cyanoacrylate glue is applied over laceration area with the help of 26-gauge needle or cannula (Fig. 6.4). Care is taken to avoid spillage of glue over normal corneal tissue and conjunctiva. If spillage occurs, extra glue is removed by scraping. Glue gets polymerised in 3–5 min, after which BCL

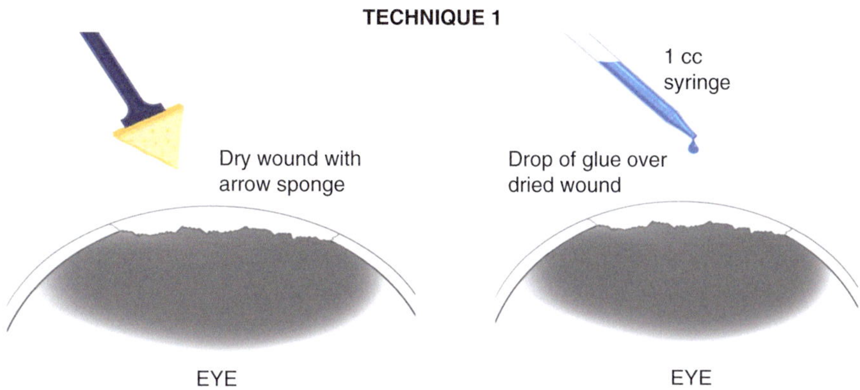

Fig. 6.4 Application of cyanoacrylate glue in corneal laceration

is applied. Do not apply BCL before period of polymerisation, as lens will stick to glue, not allowing movement to enable proper positioning of the BCL over the cornea. It will be prudent to avoid applying glue repeatedly over an area of interest, as after polymerisation glue will form a hump, disallowing optimal BCL fitting and predispose to discomfort and lens dislodgement. Retained viscoelastic is removed. Stab incision is hydrated. Glue usually sheds off after re-epithelisation occurs, and if not, it can be scraped off after 4–6 weeks. Cyanoacrylate glue is a double-edged sword, it helps in sealing the wound, it is bacteriostatic for Gram positive bacteria but as it also prevents penetration of medication to the deeper layers of cornea, vigilance is maintained. Topical medications and follow-up schedule are similar to that of self-sealed full-thickness laceration. Only glue, without a BCL must never be applied as its surface is extremely rough and will cause constant irritation and severe discomfort to the patient. Common complications of cyanoacrylate glue application are giant papillary conjunctivitis, excessive deep stromal corneal vascularisation. Inadvertent leakage of glue into the anterior chamber can cause severe iritis, iridocorneal synechia, posterior synechia, and endothelial damage.

Another tissue adhesive option is fibrin glue. Fibrin glue is FDA approved for haemostasis and is widely used in ophthalmology in suture less pterygium surgery, amniotic membrane grafting, etc. Commercially it comes in four components in four different colours coded vials (Fig. 6.5). Fibrin glue needs to be constituted just before application.

The four components are:

1. Sealer protein
2. Concentrate
3. Fibrinolysis inhibitor solution
4. Thrombin

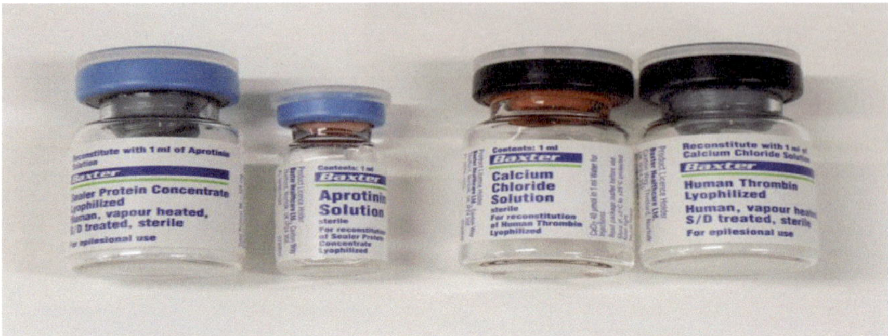

Fig. 6.5 Components of fibrin glue

First two components are heated and mixed to form the sealer protein solution, and the third and fourth components are heated and mixed to form thrombin solution. The heating is done in special machine called the fibrinotherm at 37 °C. The whole process takes 20 min and the two components, i.e. sealer protein solution and thrombin solution are aspirated in two syringes and mounted on to the duploject assemble. On injecting through the duploject assemble, when these two solutions are combined fibrin glue will set in 30 s. BCL is applied over it after few minutes after confirming that there is no wound leak.

Application of cyanoacrylate glue with BCL in laceration less than 3 mm was noted to have faster healing in comparison to application of fibrin glue with BCL with lesser corneal vascularization [22]. Overall rate of healing is however similar with both types of glues application [22]. Cyanoacrylate is a cheaper and easily available option without the requirement of special equipment for reconstitution which makes it preferred choice for most of the ophthalmic surgeon, especially in ocular emergency scenarios.

6.5.2.4 Simple Full-Thickness Laceration More Than 2 mm

Simple full-thickness laceration greater than 2 mm in length constitutes an open globe injury and must always be repaired under general anaesthesia (GA) unless contraindicated. Facial block is an effective alternative when GA is contraindicated. Surgical field is cleaned and draped under aseptic precaution. Wire speculum is used to open eyelids. When laceration is associated with eye lid trauma a retraction suture with 4-0 silk retraction suture may be used. A clear corneal stab incision is given at 90° away from area of corneal laceration, or at the most comfortable location for surgeon with the help of 15° blade or Micro-Vitreoretinal (MVR) blade. While making a stab incision, undue pressure on globe is avoided by lifting limbus with Lim's forceps by other hand. Surgeon must keep blade parallel to underlying iris tissue, to avoid damage to iris or lens. Anterior chamber is formed with viscoelastic (2% HPMC). If anterior chamber is extremely shallow and corneal stab entry is not possible, viscoelastic can be flush injected through wound, taking care not to touch the edges by cannula. But once side port incision is made, it is advisable not to use the wound entry for injection of substances into the anterior chamber, as it may damage the edges of wound, which will further complicate the suturing and results. 10-0 nylon monofilament suture on fine spatulated microsurgical needle is material of choice for corneal laceration suturing. Basic principles of corneal laceration suturing are covered later in the chapter. After complete suturing, all knots are buried away from visual axis. Viscoelastic is removed. Stab incision is hydrated. In children less than 6 years of age, it is recommended to suture all incisions. A subconjunctival injection (gentamycin 0.5 ml with dexamethasone 0.5 ml) is given. Dexamethasone is not given in cases of suspected vegetative matter trauma or presence of infection. Subconjunctival injection of atropine sulphate (0.6 mg/ml) can be given if not contraindicated. It relieves pain and ciliary spasm, reduces postoperative inflammation. Eye is patched at the end of the surgery. In children, application of Cartella shield is also preferred. Patch is removed after 24 h during the postoperative evaluation.

6.6 Basic Principles of Corneal Laceration Suturing

6.6.1 Preferred Anaesthesia

General anaesthesia is the anaesthesia of choice. Absolute no to retrobulbar or peribulbar block.

6.6.2 Preferred Suture Material

10-0 nylon monofilament suture on fine spatula design microsurgical needle is optimal for repair of corneal tear. While repairing corneo-scleral tears, the scleral part of the wound is best repaired with vicryl sutures.

The components of effects of suturing include compression, torque, tissue eversion, tissue inversion and splinting. Single interrupted sutures are best for corneal tear repair and work by the effect of the overlapping zone of compression.

Zone of Compression The zone of compression (Fig. 6.6a, b) is a square shaped area defined around the suture, within which, the suture exhibits a compression effect. The diagonal of this square is formed by suture and corneal laceration/tear segment.

Simple opposition of wound edges is not sufficient, as due to intraocular pressure and elasticity of tissue, wound may gap subsequently. To achieve a watertight closure of wound, the zone of compression of neighbouring sutures should overlap.

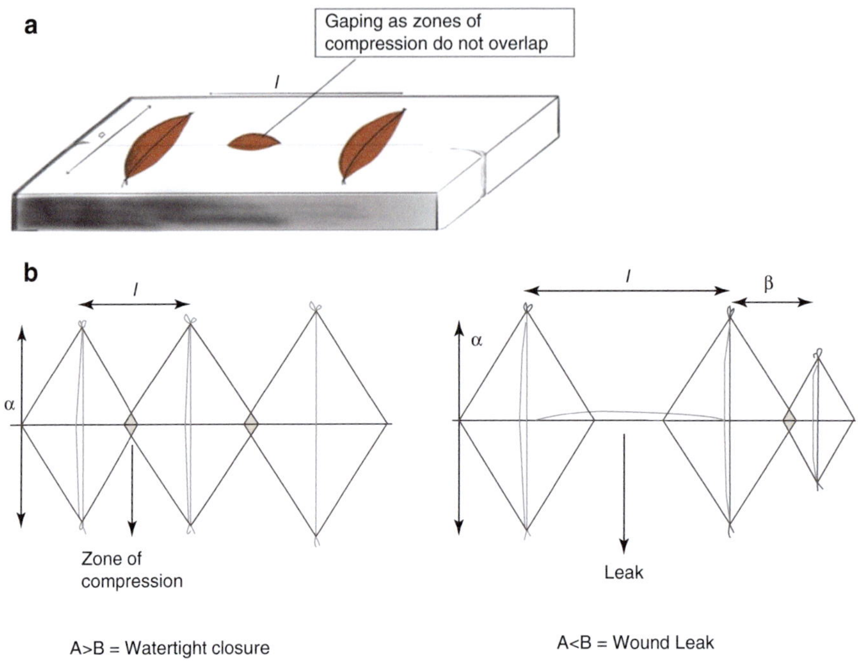

Fig. 6.6 (**a**) Diagrammatic depiction of zone of compression in corneal suturing. (**b**) Diagrammatic representation depicting adequate and inadequate zone of compression in corneal tear repair suturing

6.6.3 'No Touch' Technique

In this technique, suturing is done without holding the edges of the wound. As wound edges are never manipulated, there is minimal damage and water tight closure is possible. Globe is stabilised by holding it at area away from laceration; corneal wound edges are not held with forceps. Undue pressure over globe is avoided. After forming anterior chamber with a viscoelastic or air, the needle tip is placed perpendicular to corneal surface and is rotated through the tissue following curvature of a needle. To pass a needle though tissue, surgeon should rotate his/her wrist while keeping his/her elbow constant and steady. Tissue override is avoided by passing needle up to 80–90% depth of corneal tissue, keeping entry and exit of needle perpendicular to surface of cornea, opposing the internal edge of wound rather than the external edge and taking a suture bite equidistant from internal edge of wound rather than external edge. A 2-1-1 knot locking may be preferred over 3-1-1 as this would enable suture tension adjustment in accordance to optimal wound apposition during the second throw tie of the suturing. Suture knots are to be buried after completion of suturing. It is desirable to repair corneal tear by placing long, tight sutures in the corneal periphery and the subsequent shorter sutures towards the centre (Fig. 6.7) in an effort to conserving steepened central cornea (Rowsey-Hays

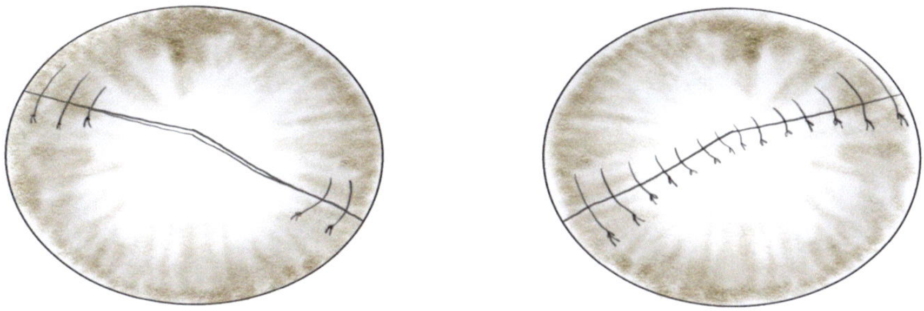

Fig. 6.7 Rowsey-Hay technique of corneal tear suturing

technique) [23]. For corneal tears involving the limbus, the first suture is placed at the limbus ensuring optimal apposition, with care to avoid misalignment. The sutures closer to the limbus are longest with the size decreasing with approach towards the centre. The suture spacing should be taken care of to enable optimal overlap of adjacent zones of compression. Longer sutures closer to the visual axis lead to greater tissue distortion and more astigmatism.

Scar formation and astigmatism can be minimised by burying knot away from visual axis. After knot is buried, the orientation of knot is reversed to facilitate subsequent suture removal. Suture bite is kept smaller for laceration near the visual axis as compared to peripheral laceration. Interrupted sutures are preferred over continuous suture technique as continuous suturing technique may induce a torque effect with difficulty in titrating tightening. Selective suture removal is also not possible in continuous suturing technique.

6.6.4 Astigmatism and Suturing

A tight suture causes localised flattening of cornea but induces steepening along its axis. Incision or laceration in cornea causes flattening along the axis of area of incision/laceration. Larger the incision or laceration more flattening is induced. Location of laceration is also important; lacerations nearer to the visual axis induce more flattening along its axis than lacerations away from visual axis. If laceration is crossing the visual axis; to minimise induced astigmatism, it is sutured with smaller bites, suture is not passed through central area of visual axis and knots are buried away from visual axis

6.6.5 Suturing Large Wound with Stellate or Branching Pattern

In corneal tears which are stellate or branching, each branch of stellate tear/laceration is treated as individual laceration and sutured accordingly. Perpendicular rather than bevelled segments of wound are sutured first; irregular segments are divided into relatively straight segments and sutured with the usual technique. To achieve

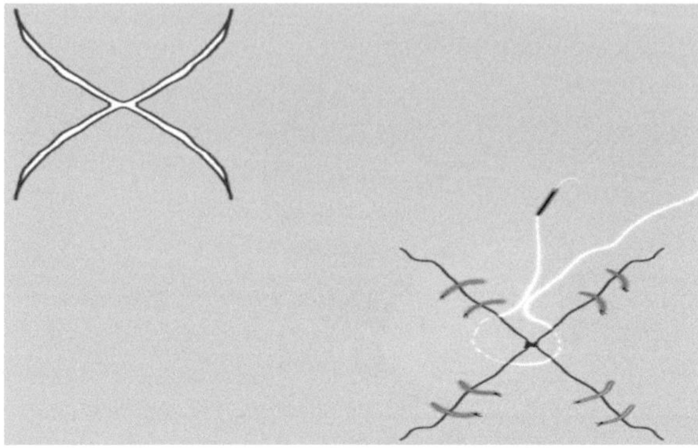

Fig. 6.8 Purse-string suturing in stellate corneal tear repair

water tight closure at the centre a purse-string suture(Fig. 6.8), bridge suture may be used. Glue-BCL is also a good option for good closure of central arc.

6.7 Complicated Corneal Lacerations

6.7.1 Corneal Laceration with Uveal Incarceration or Prolapse

Large corneal lacerations secondary to globe rupture are usually associated with uveal tissue prolapse, incarceration in wound and iris tear. If left unattended, it may lead to dreaded complications like endophthalmitis, panophthalmitis or sympathetic ophthalmia. The decision on management of the prolapsed uveal tissue in corneal/corneo-scleral repair is important and should be carefully examined for signs of infection and epithelialisation. Exposure to external environment for more than 24 h increases risk of infection. Reposting back the dead and necrotic tissue which has been lying exposed in the tear is avoided, as reposition will lead to transfer of infection to anterior chamber. If epithelised, tissue must be removed to prevent epithelial seeding in anterior chamber. The two forms of management of prolapsed uveal tissue in the wound in corneal/corneo-scleral wound repair include prolapsed iris tissue abscission and excision. Abscission is preferred over excision. In ***abscission***, tissue is gently pulled outside though wound and cut flush with cornea, taking out a rim of healthy iris tissue along with dead devitalised tissue. This minimises the risk of anterior chamber seeding by infectious tissue. In ***excision***, tissue is cut flush without pulling it out. While removing the tissue, all attempts should be made to save as much tissue as one can, but not at the cost of increasing risk of infection. Large areas of tissue damage not amenable to suturing should be managed with Corneal patch graft. Thus back up tissue should be available while repairing cases with significant tissue defect

Incarcerated tissue if healthy, with exposure lesser than 24 h, may be reposited back in the anterior chamber. A blunt iris spatula/simple visco cannula can be used. Cannula is introduced through the side port incision and tissue is reposited by gentle sweeping movements, followed by suturing of wound in usual way. Surgeon must double check before closing the surgery for any inadvertent or residual uveal tissue incarceration in suture/wound, as uveal tissue in wound is potential risk factor for sympathetic ophthalmia. Uveal tissue in wound can lead to anterior synechia formation and adherent leucoma subsequently, which may complicate course of treatment by causing astigmatic changes and secondary glaucoma.

Owing to handling of uveal tissue and broken blood aqueous barrier, excessive anterior chamber reaction may be expected in the postoperative period. To minimise this, subconjunctival injection of atropine sulphate (0.6 mg/ml) along with dexamethasone is given. Strong cycloplegic (like atropine sulphate 1%), frequent topical steroids (prednisolone acetate 1%) with or without oral steroids (prednisolone 1 mg/kg/day) are added to the postop regimen along with topical antibiotics. Starting of postoperative topical steroids is withheld for 48–72 h or used more cautiously post repair in setting of infection to rule out wound infection. Fellow eye must be examined for signs of sympathetic ophthalmia at each visit.

6.7.2 Corneal Laceration Along with Limbus or Scleral Involvement

Limbal or scleral involvement is commonly seen in globe rupture. Usually, corneal laceration if associated with scleral tear is usually continuous. Scleral tear with healthy area in between it and corneal laceration is extremely rare. All cases of a full-thickness corneal laceration which are extending up to limbus, a limited peritomy must be done at the area adjacent to corneal laceration to find out extent of damage. If scleral involvement is present, a limbal area is secured first by 10-0 nylon suture. Then an area of laceration just posterior to limbus is sutured using 7-0 vicryl suture. Theses sutures are cut long, ends of the suture can used as an anchoring suture for mobilising globe to maximise surgeons view during scleral wound suturing. Posterior most extent of scleral tear is to be looked for by globe exploration at time of surgery to identify it in extensive tears. For this a surgeon should dissect as posterior as he/she can. In rare cases if tear is extending up to unreachable posterior part of globe, surgeon should suture the globe up to the maximum extent of wound. If needed, planned disinsertion of recti can be done, which can be restored at place after scleral tear repair. Care must be taken to cut the incarcerated vitreous and uveal tissue at wound. A mechanical vitrectomy cutter is preferred to remove the vitreous from wound. After suturing scleral tear, corneal tear is sutured in usual way. Conjunctival peritomy is sutured with 8-0 vicryl suture. These cases need postoperative regimen targeted to tackle expected reaction and inflammation. Life time follow-up for sympathetic ophthalmia and retinal detachment is needed.

6.7.3 Corneal Laceration with Traumatic Cataract

Traumatic cataract is encountered in 27–65% of the ocular trauma cases [24–26]. In certain cases, traumatic cataract may be visually significant and needs concurrent management at the time of repair surgery. Cases with minor injury and with minimal or localised lens opacity, can be observed and the lens opacification can be dealt with later (Fig. 6.9a, b) [27]. The common question encountered is to whether simultaneous cataract surgery is also to be done in the same setting as tear repair or to operate cataract later on once eye is quiet (Fig. 6.10). Ruptured anterior capsule with lens matter in anterior chamber, if not removed will cause intense inflammatory reaction, endothelial touch, secondary glaucoma, etc.; hence needs to be tackled at the time of primary laceration repair. Besides inflammation and visual disturbances, a significant cataract also precludes fundus view in postoperative period. In the absence of significant cataract, anterior capsular rupture, it is better to plan cataract surgery at a later date. This approach gives advantage of better IOL power calculation after suture removal after confirming visual potential.

6.7.3.1 Simultaneous Corneal Tear Repair with Cataract Extraction

After routine corneal laceration repair, two clear corneal side port incisions are made 180° apart, with the help of MVR blade, (3' o clock and 9' o clock, if the

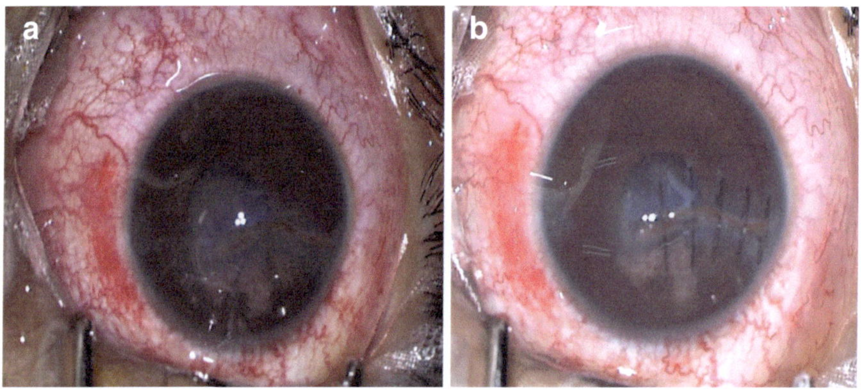

Fig. 6.9 Preoperative clinical picture of an open globe injury showing tear with iris incarceration in wound (**a**) and postoperative picture after corneal tear repair (**b**)

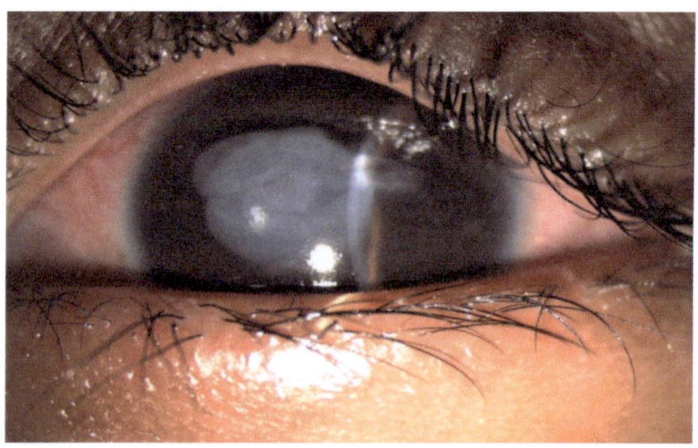

Fig. 6.10 Corneal tear with traumatic cataract with ruptured anterior capsule and lens matter in anterior chamber

surgeon is seated superiorly; locations can be changed according to visibility and site of laceration, but must be 180° apart). Anterior chamber is filled with viscoelastic, preferably high molecular weight cohesive viscoelastics like Helon/HelonGv, if not available HPMC 2% can also be used. Staining anterior capsule by Trypan blue dye (0.06%) increases the visibility. A tangential cut is given at the edge of torn capsule with the help of angled Vannas scissors if the anterior capsule is damaged and the rhexis is completed with the help of forceps. If intra-lenticular pressure is high, the lens is decompressed by aspirating lens material either with bimanual/Simcoe aspiration cannula through the traumatic anterior capsular opening, if posterior vitreous pressure is significant, IV mannitol (5–7 ml/kg) intraoperatively can be given. Low flow parameters are used and bottle height is kept low, else laceration may extend to periphery. Rarely nucleus is hard due to age related changes, in such cases nucleus is delivered with the help of wire vectis though sclera tunnel. Patient is left aphakic. Every attempt is made to salvage 'bag complex'. Secondary IOL may be planed later on after suture removal, after complete healing of corneal wound. Owing to difficulty in IOL power calculation and change in corneal curvature after wound healing; lens aspiration with primary IOL implantation along with corneal laceration repair is not advised.

If posterior capsular rupture noted, a good anterior vitrectomy is done. To aspirate a retained lens matter, instead of automated bimanual/Simcoe aspiration, vitrectomy cutter on 'IA-CUT' mode may be safely used.

Zonules are usually intact in cases of penetrating injuries as compared to non-penetrating injuries. Very rarely, a sharp object/projectile can damage the zonules by direct impact. In such cases when posterior capsule intact and anterior rhexis is not radially torn capsular support devices can be used (Table 6.4).

IOL implantation in traumatic cataracts associated with penetrating injuries:

- Two stage approach: In traumatic cataracts with fresh corneal laceration, two stage approach is used. In first surgery laceration is repaired and lens is aspirated. In second stage of surgery a secondary IOL is planned. Cases where corneal wound is self-sealed and completely healed, primary IOL implantation can be planed.
- Timing of secondary IOL: After 4–6 weeks of primary surgery, after complete removal of corneal sutures—whichever is later

Table 6.4 Extent of Zonular loss and preferred surgical approach

Extent of zonular loss	Preferred surgical approach
Zonular loss 1–3 clock hours	Orientation of haptic of IOL in area of weakness (IOL either PMMA or Multipiece) with or without Capsular tension ring (CTR)
Zonular loss 3–6 clock hours	Modified CTR (Cionni ring) or CTR with Capsular tension segment (CTS)
Zonular loss >6 clock hours but <9 clock hours	Double eyelet Cionni ring with or without CTS
Zonular loss >9 clock hours	ICCE done with secondary IOL

- IOL type and material: Multipiece IOL is preferred. PMMA IOL can also be used. Foldable single piece IOLs are avoided. Acrylic hydrophobic is a preferred IOL material.
- Preferred Location of IOL implantation: Sulcus>Scleral fixation >anterior chamber IOL

6.7.4 Corneal Laceration with Endophthalmitis

Endophthalmitis is potentially devastating complication of ocular trauma, the incidence being 1 in 100 open globe injuries [27]. Compared to postoperative endophthalmitis, posttraumatic endophthalmitis usually has worse prognosis visually. Potential risk factors include trauma by vegetative matter, retained intraocular foreign body, disruption of crystalline lens and delay in primary repair. Ruptured lens is a potential risk factor because it gives microorganisms a direct access to the posterior segment. Penetrating trauma in rural setting has higher risk than that urban setting; owing to higher incidence of soil contamination [28]. Non-metallic foreign body has higher risk as compared to metallic ones. Prophylactic intravitreal and or intracameral antibiotics are recommended for high-risk cases. Organisms isolated are usually Bacillus species, Staphylococcus epidermidis and Streptococcus species, and polymicrobial infections are not uncommon. Bacillus species are common in wounds contaminated by soil. Patient presents with rapid onset severe pain and inflammation, hypopyon, chemosis, ring infiltrates in cornea and even panopthalmitis [29]. Pseudomonas is another cause for rapidly progressing endophthalmitis. Fungal infections are common with vegetative matter injury, particularly aspergillus species while candida species are common in hospitalised patients [30, 31].

Treatment of endophthalmitis with corneal laceration starts with repair of the corneal laceration in the usual fashion. Anterior chamber wash is given with vancomycin 1 mg/0.1 ml and Ceftazidime 2.25 mg/0.1 ml. Use of dexamethasone is controversial. Anterior chamber exudates/vitreous sample is taken by intravitreal tap aspirate for culture and sensitivity before instillation of intravitreal antibiotics injection, subsequent to completion of tear repair. Intravitreal injection and/or anterior chamber wash with Amphotericin B 5 μg/0.1 ml is given in cases with vegetative matter trauma. Fortified topical antibiotics are given along with intravitreal antibiotics from day 1 postoperative period. Similarly, intravitreal injection is to be given if RD is not present on B-scan. For non-responding patients pars plana vitrectomy (PPV) is planned subsequently, after media gets clear providing enabling better visibility. A silicone oil injection is considered in most cases, because it not only supports retina but it also slows down the microbial growth [32–34].

6.7.5 Treatment of Associated Cyclodialysis

Cyclodialysis usually occurs in blunt ocular trauma, though perforating injuries can also have component of cyclodialysis. Cyclodialysis repair is planned after corneal laceration repair. Management of cyclodialysis clefts requires step wise approach, primary corneal laceration repair followed by cyclodialysis repair on subsequent visits. Patient may have more than one cyclodialysis cleft, hence it is necessary to identify the full extent and location of cleft. There is no standardised management for cyclodialysis. Direct cyclopexy remains the most common treatment, followed by vitrectomy with internal tamponade [35, 36]. Diagnosis of cleft is challenging, non-invasive modalities like UBM and AS-OCT can be used along with gonioscopy.

6.8 Postoperative Management

Eye patch is opened after 24 h. On day 1 of postoperative period, sutured wound is examined for leak using fluorescein dye strips. Anterior chamber depth and presence of inflammatory reaction are noted. If fundus is visible, it is examined for any sign of vitritis and retained foreign body. Routine postoperative regimen recommended is e/d moxifloxacin 0.5% QID, e/d homatropine 2% BD and oral analgesic ibuprofen/paracetamol. In case of vegetative material trauma, topical steroids are generally prescribed after 1 week of antibiotic therapy; if wound is clean topical steroids (e/d prednisolone acetate 1%) 2 hourly can be started from day 1. Topical steroids are tapered during subsequent visits. Topical carboxy methyl cellulose 0.5% or hydroxy propyl methyl cellulose 1% drops can be given to minimise foreign body sensation. No proven role of prophylactic oral antibiotics has been noted to prevent traumatic endophthalmitis. If anterior chamber reaction is anticipated (which is usually seen when iridectomy/lensectomy/vitrectomy is done), oral prednisolone once a day 1 mg/kg is given for a week. Subsequent follow-up is done after 7 days, then twice weekly for a month, monthly for first 6 months and then once in a year. More frequent follow-ups may be required in cases with significant inflammation. Besides routine eye evaluation, eye is examined for any loose suture, suture infiltrates or any sign of late endophthalmitis. Suture removal is done after 6–8 weeks upon ensuring optimal wound healing. All sutures are preferably not removed in a single setting; instead an alternate suture removal is done. Sutures at steeper axis are removed first. Other healthy eye should be examined for signs of sympathetic ophthalmia. Patient is also educated for early symptoms of sympathetic ophthalmia, i.e. loss of near vision, photophobia in healthy eye.

6.9 Management of Astigmatism After Corneal Laceration Repair

Addressing postoperative astigmatism after corneal laceration repair is difficult. Hence every attempt is made to reduce it by using simple steps, which are highlighted above, in operation section, to reduce it. Treatment of astigmatism in trauma cases begins after 6 weeks of surgery, after healing of wound. Usually, these cases tend to have irregular astigmatism. Classically it can be managed in step wise manner, first by selective removal of tight sutures. Suture removal is started after 6 weeks of surgery, as stated earlier. If significant astigmatisms remain after complete suture removal which is not amenable to correction by glasses, rigid gas permeable (RGP) contact lenses can be tried. RGP contact lenses provide significant visual improvement by providing smooth refractive surfaces negating the irregular astigmatism secondary to scar. If astigmatism is regular and patient has significant cataract, toric IOL implantation is a viable option.

Key Points

- Traumatic corneal injuries can result in permanent vision loss if inadequately treated.
- Both children and adults are equally susceptible and public awareness to avoid such accidental injuries should be reinforced.
- BETTS classification and OTSS can help in appropriately classifying and prognosticating each case of ocular injury.
- Small lacerations can be managed with tissue adhesives and contact lens alone, whereas larger lacerations will require suturing.
- Appropriate management of corneal/corneo-scleral tears with optimal suturing and postoperative medical care will help in effective visual rehabilitation and decrease ocular morbidity.
- Associated complications need special considerations as explained in the chapter and needs to be managed on a case to case basis.

References

1. Wong TY, Klein BE, Klein R. The prevalence and 5 year incidence of ocular trauma. The Beaver Dam Eye Study. Ophthalmology. 2000;107(12):2196–202.
2. Negrel AD. Magnitude of eye injuries worldwide. Community Eye Health. 1997;10(24):49–53.
3. Willmann D, Moshirfar M, Melanson SW. Corneal injury [updated 2020 Apr 29]. In: StatPearls [Internet]. Treasure Island, FL: StatPearls; 2020. Available from https://www.ncbi.nlm.nih.gov/books/NBK459283/
4. Katz J, Tielsch JM. Lifetime prevalence of ocular injuries from the Baltimore Eye Survey. Arch Ophthalmol. 1993;111(11):1564–8.
5. Negrel AD, Thylefors B. The global impact of eye injuries. Ophthalmic Epidemiol. 1998;5:143–69.
6. Dandona L, et al. Ocular trauma in an urban population in southern India: the Andhra Pradesh Eye Disease Study. Clin Exp Ophthalmol. 2000;28(5):350–6.
7. Praveen KN, et al. Ocular Trauma in a Rural South Indian Population The Aravind Comprehensive Eye Survey. Ophthalmology. 2004;111:1778–81.
8. Sii F, et al. The UK Paediatric Ocular Trauma Study 2 (POTS2): demographics and mechanisms of injuries. Clin Ophthalmol. 2018;12:105–11.
9. Thylefors B. Epidemiological patterns of ocular trauma. Aust N Z J Ophthalmol. 1992;20(2):95–8.

10. Coats B, Shedd DF. Biomechanics of eye injury in the military. In: Gefen A, Epstein Y, editors. The mechanobiology and mechanophysiology of military-related injuries. Studies in mechanobiology, tissue engineering and biomaterials, vol. 19. Cham: Springer; 2015.
11. Pizzarello LD. Ocular trauma: time for action. Ophthalmic Epidemiol. 1998;5(3):115–6.
12. Philip SS, Hoskin AK. Children's protective eyewear: the challenges and the way forward. Med J Aust. 2014;201(2):87–8.
13. Shah A, Blackhall K, Ker K, Patel D. Educational interventions for the prevention of eye injuries. Cochrane Database Sys Rev. 2009;4:CD006527.
14. Kuhn F, Morris R, Witherspoon CD. Birmingham Eye Trauma Terminology (BETT): Terminology and classification of mechanical eye injuries. Ophthalmol Clin N Am. 2002;15:139–43.
15. Saka ES, Monsudi KF, Olatuji V. Traumatic corneal laceration in Northwestern Nigeria. J West Afr Coll Surg. 2017;7(4):72–84.
16. Kuhn F, Maisiak R, Mann L, Mester V, Morris R, Witherspoon CD. The ocular trauma score (OTS). Ophthalmol Clin North Am. 2002;15(2):163–vi. https://doi.org/10.1016/s0896-1549(02)00007-x.
17. Acar U, Tok OY, Acar DE, Burcu A, Ornek F. A new ocular trauma score in pediatric penetrating eye injuries. Eye (Lond). 2011;25(3):370–4. https://doi.org/10.1038/eye.2010.211.
18. Shah MA, Agrawal R, Teoh R, et al. Pediatric ocular trauma score as a prognostic tool in the management of pediatric traumatic cataracts. Graefes Arch Clin Exp Ophthalmol. 2017;255(5):1027–36. https://doi.org/10.1007/s00417-017-3616-y.
19. Ainbinder DJ, Mazzoli RA, Raymond WR, Hansen EA, Sanford EG. Ophthalmic care of the combat casualty, Ocular trauma scores. Section 2, Chapter 6.
20. Chaithanyaa N, Devireddy SK, Kishore Kumar RV, Gali RS, Aneja V. Sympathetic ophthalmia: a review of literature. Oral Surg Oral Med Oral Pathol Oral Radiol. 2012;113(2):172–6. https://doi.org/10.1016/j.tripleo.2011.01.036.
21. Kubal WS. Imaging of orbital trauma. Radiographics. 2008;28(6):1729–39.
22. Sharma A, Kaur R, Kumar S, et al. Fibrin glue versus N-butyl-2-cyanocrylate 9n corneal perforations. Ophthalmology. 2003;119(20):291–8.
23. Rowsey JJ, Hays JC. Refractive reconstruction for acute eye injuries. Ophthalmic Surg. 1984;15(7):569–74.
24. Dannenberg AL, Parver LM, Brechner RJ, Khoo L. Penetration eye injuries in the workplace. The national Eye Trauma System Registry. Arch Ophthalmol. 1992;110(6):843–8.
25. Slusher MM, Greven CM, Yu DD. Posterior chamber intraocular lens implantation combined with lensectomy-vitrectomy and intraretinal foreign body removal. Arch Ophthalmol. 1992;110(1):127–9.
26. Pieramici DJ, Sternberg P Jr, Aaberg TM Sr, et al. A system for classifying mechanical injuries of the eye (globe). The Ocular Trauma Classification Group. Am J Ophthalmol. 1997;123(6):820–31.
27. Mosseiev J, Segev F, Harizman N, et al. Primary cataract extraction and intraocular lens implantation in penetrating ocular trauma. Ophthalmology. 2001;108(6):1099–103.
28. Ahmed Y, Schimel AM, Pathengay A, Colyer MH, Flynn HW Jr. Endophthalmitis following open globe injuries. Eye (Lond). 2012;16(2):212–7.
29. Boldt HC, Pulido JS, Blodi CF, Folk JC, Weingeist TA. Rural endophthalmitis. Ophthalmology. 1989;96(12):1722–6.
30. Gupta A, Srinivasan R, Kaliaperumal S, et al. Post-traumatic fungal endophthalmitis—a prospective study. Eye. 2008;22:13–7.
31. Durand ML. Endophthalmitis. Clin Microbiol Infect. 2013;19(3):227–34.
32. Azad R, Ravi K, Talwar D, Rajpal, Kumar N. Pars plana vitrectomy with or without silicone oil tamponade in posttraumatic endophthalmitis. Graefes Arch Clin Exp Ophthalmol. 2003;241(6):478–83.

33. Yan H, Lu Y, Yu J, et al. Silicone oil in the surgical treatment of traumatic endophthalmitis. Eur J Ophthalmol. 2008;18(5):680–4.
34. Dave VP, Joseph J, Jayabhasker P, et al. Does ophthalmic-grade silicone oil possess antimicrobial properties? J Ophthal Inflamm Infect. 2019;9:20.
35. Morin A, Delbarre M, Friang C, Marechal M, Froussart-Maille F. Cyclodialyse : un challenge thérapeutique, revue de la littérature sur les pratiquesactuelles [Cyclodialysis, a therapeutic challenge: Review of the literature on current practices]. J Fr Ophtalmol. 2019;42(8):852–63.
36. Ioannidis AS, Barton K. Cyclodialysis cleft: causes and repair. Curr Opin Ophthalmol. 2010;21(2):150–4. https://doi.org/10.1097/ICU.0b013e3283366a4.

Emergencies in Microbial Keratitis

7

Bhavana Sharma, Samendra Karkhur, and Deepak Soni

7.1 Introduction

Microbial keratitis frequently presents as corneal emergency in clinical practice. It necessitates well-timed appropriate therapeutic interventions to salvage visual function and structural integrity. Small-sized corneal ulcers are amenable to treatment by broad-spectrum antibiotics. Whereas, while dealing with a large-sized corneal ulcer ophthalmologists are faced with dilemma of mixed microbial aetiology as a result of long duration, already instated cocktail of treatment and rapidly progressing damage. In such a case despite initiation of treatment, ulcer may show suboptimal response with progressive damage. Visual and structural loss can be devastating in such cases. This chapter intends to discuss clinical features, diagnostic differentiators, investigations and treatment, of microbial keratitis (MK) most likely to require emergent care.

7.2 Incidence

The incidence and type of MK largely vary with factors related to geography, ethnicity and trends in antibiotic usage [1]. Bacterial keratitis is reported to be more prevalent in developed countries as opposed to mycotic keratitis in the developing world. This variation is largely attributed to the organic matter-related ocular trauma as one of the most common risk factors for mycotic keratitis in the developing

B. Sharma (✉)
Department of Ophthalmology, All India Institute of Medical Sciences, Bhopal, Madhya Pradesh, India
e-mail: head.ophtho@aiimsbhopal.edu.in

S. Karkhur · D. Soni
All India Institute of Medical Sciences, Bhopal, Madhya Pradesh, India

B. Sharma, J. S. Titiyal (eds.), *Corneal Emergencies*,
https://doi.org/10.1007/978-981-16-5876-1_7

world. The incidence of MK varies from 10/lakh persons/year in the United States to 799/lakh persons/year in developing countries [2, 3]. Moreover, bacterial keratitis is the most common form of MK, accounting for 90–95% cases with highest reported cases in temperate climate regions [1].

Fungal keratitis is a common cause of corneal infection in developing nations owing to tropical climate with higher temperature and humidity. In sub-Saharan Africa and Asia, filamentous fungi account for more than 40% of cases of MK. In the United States, *Candida* and *Aspergillus* are regarded as most common cause of fungal keratitis while *Fusarium species* is predominant in the southern United States [4]. However, *Aspergillus* remains the most common cause of mycotic ulcers all over the world including India [4].

7.3 Aetiology

The variable aetiological agents in different types of MK are an important determinant of severity of lesion and corneal emergencies associated with it. In bacterial keratitis, the most common causative pathogen has been reported to be Gram-positive cocci which include *Staphylococcus aureus and Streptococcus pneumonia* [5, 6]. Gram-negative bacilli like *Pseudomonas aeruginosa*, *Haemophilus influenzae and Serratia* species are other less common causative agents [7]. *Staphylococcus epidermidis and Fusarium species* are the most common organisms seen in polymicrobial keratitis. Among viral keratitis, Herpes simplex virus (HSV) is one of the leading and emerging causes of corneal blindness worldwide. Stromal necrotising HSV keratitis may lead to severe stromal necrosis and neurotrophic ulcer but rarely perforates. Rare pathogens causing microbial keratitis includes the protists, *Acanthamoeba* spp., *Pythium* and *Microsporidia*.

The aetiology of fungal keratitis varies depending on geographical region, climatic condition and socio-economic status [6]. The common fungal agents associated with infectious keratitis include filamentous as well as yeast variants. Filamentous fungi are responsible for more than 70% of cases [6]. Mycotic keratitis carries a significantly higher potential for corneal perforation in comparison to other infective aetiologies [8]. *Aspergillus* keratitis shows a higher tendency for descemetocele formation and perforation in comparison to *Candida* and *Fusarium* keratitis. In addition, up to 20% cases of mycotic keratitis (mainly candidiasis) are complicated by bacterial coinfection [9].

Pseudomonas is the commonest pathogen identified in contact lens-associated bacterial keratitis and subsequent sloughing in such cases. It is also the most common bacterial organism detected in cases with corneal perforation [1]. While *Staphylococcus aureus* also exhibits considerable propensity towards corneal abscess, sloughing and perforation [10]. Incidence of secondary glaucoma is observed to be more in cases of *Pneumococcal*, mycotic and advanced stage of *Acanthamoeba* keratitis. *Acanthamoeba* keratitis may lead to corneal perforation in advanced cases, especially when initially misdiagnosed and inappropriately managed.

7.4 Approach to Diagnosis

7.4.1 History

The relevant history together with the evaluation of clinical features is an important step towards formulating a clinical diagnosis. Identification of predisposing factors along with characteristic onset of symptoms can be indicative of causative organism (Table 7.1). Important predisposing factors that should be elicited during pre-treatment workup should comprise ocular trauma, conjunctivitis and subsequent use of over-the-counter medications, contact lens wear (including type and duration of lens used, time since last change to a new pair of lenses, cleaning regimen and frequency of use) and whether the patient was engaged in activities such as sleeping or swimming with contact lenses in place, tear film abnormalities, use of topical steroids, ocular surgery, neurotrophic keratopathy, systemic diseases and immune compromised states.

7.4.2 Clinical Examination

A meticulous clinical examination is an important step towards further management of the case. Patients presenting with microbial keratitis-related corneal emergencies should be first assessed for visual acuity in the involved eye. The extent of deterioration in visual acuity is indicative of severity of the lesion and provides a useful guide to the prognosis and potential response to treatment. Careful slit lamp aided ocular examination is important for presumptive diagnosis of the causative pathogen by determining the morphology of lesion, growth pattern within the cornea and other unique clinical signs (Table 7.2).

Slit lamp photography is a useful tool to monitor the clinical progress and is a strong aid in counselling the patient for improved compliance. Ultrasound B-scan (USG B-scan) should be employed to assess the posterior segment in severe cases where endophthalmitis is suspected and visualisation of fundus is not possible. Clinical grading of ulcer is indicative of extent and severity of disease and is further helpful in treatment and prognosis of the case. Corneal ulcer can be graded into mild moderate and severe depending on the extent of involvement [11] (Table 7.3). Documenting the clinical features as a colour-coded diagram and/or a clinical photograph can serve as an important guide for prognosis and follow-up (Fig. 7.1).

7.4.3 Microbiological Evaluation

Microbiological evaluation for identification of causal organism is undoubtedly the most important step towards proper management of corneal ulcer. Cultures are helpful to guide in modification of therapy in patients with a poor clinical response and to decrease toxicity by eliminating unnecessary medications (Table 7.4). Obtaining a corneal culture is a means of identifying the causative organism(s) and the only

Table 7.1 Pre-disposing factors and corneal emergencies associated with various pathogens

Sr. no.	Predisposing factor	Indolence	Perforation	Sloughing	Descemetocele	Secondary glaucoma	Toxic epitheliopathy	Neurotrophic ulcer	Corneal abscess	Corneal fistula
Bacterial										
Staphylococcus	Diseased corneas like PBK, DED, viral keratitis, exposure keratopathy	Common	In advanced cases and in suboptimal treatment	In advanced cases an in suboptimal treatment	Progressive corneal thinning leads to descemetocele formation	Common	Common with long term treatment	Common with long-standing cases	Hallmark feature	Associate with central perforation
Pseudomonas	Corneal trauma	–	Most common cause of corneal perforation in microbial keratitis	Rapidly progressing	Severe ulceration leads to descemetocele formation	Longstanding severe inflammation leads to rubeotic glaucoma	–	–	Suppuration and abscess are very common	Rare
Pneumococcal	Corneal trauma; Coexistent dacryocystitis, persistent epithelial defects consequent to lid abnormalities	Common	Common with 'Ulcus Serpens'	Seen in advanced inadequately treated cases	Common	Can be seen with a long duration	Common	–	Common	Associate with central perforation
Herpes simplex virus (HSV)										
Epithelial	Active viral replication	Untreated and recurrent cases are commonly associated with PED	Uncommon	Not seen	Chronic recurrent cases may lead to descemetocele	Not seen	Seen commonly	Chronic recurrent cases may lead to neurotrophic ulcer	Uncommon	Not seen
Stromal necrotising	Active viral replication; when topical steroids are given without antiviral cover	Common	Perforation in advanced cases	Sloughing in advanced cases	Common	Common	Seen commonly	Necrosis with decreased corneal innervation leads to neurotrophic ulcer	Uncommon	Associate with central perforation

Immune stromal	Type III hypersensitivity to viral antigen	Rare	Very rare	Not seen	Rare	Secondary trabeculitis may lead to secondary glaucoma	Common with chronic cases	Common with chronic cases	Not seen	Rare
Disciform	Type IV hypersensitivity to viral antigen	Rare	Rare	Not seen	Rare	Secondary trabeculitis may lead to secondary glaucoma	May be seen in chronic cases	Common with chronic cases	Rare	Rare
Mycotic										
Aspergillus	Trauma with vegetative matter; contact lens wear; prolonged topical steroids/antibiotic usage	Very common, especially in steroid-treated cases	Very common	In advanced cases	Progressive thinning leading to descemetocele	In long-standing and steroid-treated cases	Common		Suppuration and abscess	Associate with central perforation
Fusarium	Contact lens wear; trauma with vegetative matter	Common	Very common		Progressive thinning leading to descemetocele	In long-standing and steroid-treated cases	Common		Suppuration and abscess	Associate with central perforation
Candida	Diseased cornea like DED, chronic HSV keratitis; Immunosuppression; contact lens wear	Common	Very common	Uncommon	In advanced cases	In long-standing and steroid-treated cases	Common		Common	Rare
Acanthamoeba										
	Contact lens wear; trauma with agricultural matter; contaminated water bodies	Commonly seen	Common	Common		Very common		Radial keratoneuritis and neurotrophic ulcer	Common	Associate with central perforation
Pythium										
	Exposure to aquatic flora and soil, especially in rainy season	Common; Response to medical treatment is poor	Common	Common	Causes rapid perforation	Common		Common		

Table 7.2 Morphological pattern of different pathogens causing microbial keratitis

Sr. no.	Pathogen	Subtype	Morphology	Associated findings	Corneal emergency
1	Bacterial		Greyish white infiltrates at epithelium and stromal level with associated stromal oedema and overlying epithelial defect	Papillary and ciliary congestion with conjunctival chemosis Anterior chamber reaction with or without hypopyon	Descemetocele; Perforation Sloughing Fistula
		Staphylococcus	Centrally located oval greyish white opaque ulcer with distinct margins and mild oedema of surrounding cornea	Mild AC reaction Long-standing cases Stromal abscess	Corneal abscess Hallmark is 'suppuration' Secondary glaucoma
		Pseudomonas	Spreads concentrically and symmetrically to involve increasing depth of cornea forming 'Ring ulcer' with greenish-yellow discharge. Marked surrounding stromal oedema	Severe AC reaction; Hypopyon Rapidly progressing ulcer; secondary glaucoma	Stromal necrosis and corneal liquefaction progressing to descemetocele; perforation and sloughing
		Pneumococcal	Greyish white or yellowish disc-shaped ulcer near centre of the cornea Starts at periphery and spreads towards centre	Hypopyon Severe AC reaction and anterior uveitis Tendency to creep over the cornea in serpiginous manner	'Ulcus Serpens' leading to corneal perforation

Table 7.2 (continued)

Sr. no.	Pathogen	Subtype	Morphology	Associated findings	Corneal emergency
2	Mycotic		Elevated branching ulcers with feathery irregular margins; associated overlying epithelial defect and satellite lesions Advanced stage might be associated with ring infiltrates, endothelial plaques and corneal perforation	Hypopyon in advanced cases Secondary glaucoma	Persistent epithelial defect Perforation; sloughing ulcer
		Filamentous fungi	Dry looking ulcer with irregular feathery extensions into normal cornea	Fixed hypopyon	Perforation and sloughing. *Fusarium* species typically have a severe course with rapid perforation
		Candida	Elevated yellowish-white plaque-like lesion with surrounding infiltration and oedema	Fixed hypopyon	Perforation in advanced cases or immunocompromised subjects

(continued)

Table 7.2 (continued)

Sr. no.	Pathogen	Subtype	Morphology	Associated findings	Corneal emergency
3	Acanthamoeba	Early phase	Punctate lesions, pseudo-dendrites, subepithelial and perineural infiltrates	Ring infiltrates Symptoms disproportionate to clinical signs	Radial keratoneuritis Secondary glaucoma
		Advanced phase	Advanced stages show multiple large stromal infiltrates associated with thinning of stroma and corneal melting	Hypopyon Anterior Uveitis	Corneal perforation
4	Viral	Epithelial	Superficial punctate keratitis which coalesce to form dendritic ulcer, terminal bulbs and swollen borders	Loss of corneal sensations Symptoms may be less than clinical signs	Persistent epithelial defect Dendritic ulcer Neurotrophic ulcer
		Stromal Non-necrotising	White opaque stromal infiltration, without ulceration	Anterior Uveitis Secondary glaucoma	Neurotrophic ulcer
		Necrotising	Grey-white stromal infiltration with ulceration and necrosis	Anterior Uveitis; Secondary glaucoma	Corneal thinning leading to corneal perforation, necrosis Neurotrophic ulcer
		Disciform	'Ground glass appearance' Stromal oedema not associated with infiltration or vascularization Thickening of all layers of the affected cornea with Descemet's folds	Keratic precipitate (KPs) just behind the involved area	Secondary trabeculitis leading to secondary glaucoma

Table 7.3 Grade of ulcer and stage-wise treatment

S. No	Grade of ulcer	Size (mm)	Depth of involvement (%)	Features	Treatment	Regimen
1	Mild	<2	< 20	Superficial involvement No scleral involvement	Monotherapy • Ciprofloxacin 0.3% • Gatifloxacin 0.3% • Moxifloxacin 0.5%	• 4–6 times • Asses the response • Improvement—continue for 7 days and taper over another 7 days
	Moderate	2–5	20–50	Mid-stromal infiltrates No scleral involvement	Combination therapy • Fortified Cefazolin5% +Tobramycin 1.3% Or • Fortified Cefazolin 5%+Gatifloxacin 0.3%or Moxifloxacin 0.5% Cephalosporin for Gram +ve cocci and AG/FQ for Gram –ve bacilli	• 2 hourly day time, 4 hourly night time for 2 days • Taper over next 1 week, later 4 times for another 1 week
	Severe	>5	>50	Deep stromal, scleral involvement	Combination therapy • Fortified Cefazolin5% +Tobramycin 1.3% OR • Fortified Cefazolin 5%+Gatifloxacin 0.3% or Moxifloxacin 0.5% Cephalosporin for Gram +ve cocci and AG/FQ for Gram –ve bacilli Systemic antibiotics	• Loading dose Every 5 min for half-hour; every 15 min for 2 h; every half to 1 h for 24 h • Assess the clinical response • Improvement: 2 hourly day time 4 hourly night time for 2 days and taper over next 1 week; 4 times for another 1 week
2	Perforated ulcers or Impending perforation				Systemic antibiotic—oral or intravenous Ciprofloxacillin 500–1000 mg BD Tab Doxycycline 100 mg BD along with topical therapy as described	1–2 weeks

(continued)

Table 7.3 (continued)

S. No	Grade of ulcer	Size (mm)	Depth of involvement (%)	Features	Treatment	Regimen
3	Scleral involvement *Neisseria, Corynebacterium* and *Haemophilus* infection				Systemic antibiotic—oral or intravenous Ciprofloxacillin 500–1000 mg BD	1–2 weeks
4	Descemetocele				BCL; Tissue glue; AMT	
5	Perforation <2 mm				BCL; tissue glue; AMT	
6	Perforation >2 mm				Patch graft Therapeutic keratoplasty	
7	Sloughing				Therapeutic keratoplasty	
8	Corneal Fistula				Patch graft	
9	Endophthalmitis				I/V antibiotics	

AG/FQ: Aminoglycosides/Fluroquinolones
BCL: Bandage contact lens
AMT: Amniotic membrane transplantation

method to determine antibiotic sensitivity. However, with the advent of broad-spectrum antibiotics many ophthalmologists tend not to culture the microbe. Small peripheral ulcers may not require culture but central ulcers and ulcers more than 2 mm, should be cultured prior to initiating therapy to prevent progression, indolence and relapse. If access to the culture media is not available, valuable information can still be achieved from Gram stain. The site should be cultured even in patients already on antibiotics as, there always remains a possibility to get conclusive result. In event of inconclusive microbiological report of non-responding ulcers, patients should be evaluated for non-bacterial aetiology. Samples of the eyelids/conjunctiva, topical eye medications and contact lens solutions should also be cultured wherever deemed necessary.

Indications for Culture Sensitivity

- A corneal infiltrate which is central, more than 2 mm and/or associated with significant stromal involvement or melting.
- Infection is chronic in nature or unresponsive to broad-spectrum antibiotic therapy.
- History of corneal surgeries.
- Atypical clinical features suggestive of fungal, amoebic, or mycobacterial keratitis.
- Infiltrates in multiple locations over the cornea.

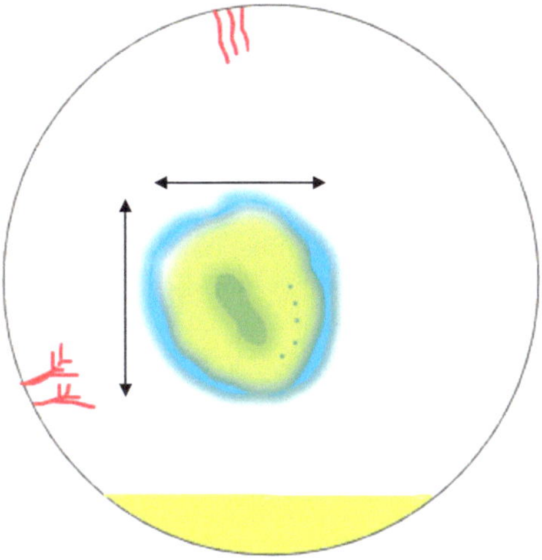

Fig. 7.1 Colour-coded diagram for documentation

Table 7.4 Microscopy and microbial culture in microbial keratitis

	Microscopy (smear)	Culture media
Bacterial	Gram's stain Giemsa stain	Chocolate agar (*Haemophilus* and *Neisseria* spp.) Blood agar (aerobes) Thioglycollate broth Roberson cooked meat media (anaerobes)
Fungal	KOH mount (10%) Calcofluor white Gram's stain Periodic acid-Schiff (PAS)	Sabouraud dextrose agar without chlorhexidine Brain heart infusion agar with chloromycetin
HSV keratitis	–	Tube culture isolation—traditional gold standard Cell culture (cell lines—human foreskin fibroblasts, MRC-5)
Acanthamoeba	Calcofluor white	Non-nutrient agar with seeded *Escherichia coli*
Mycobacteria/ Acid-fast bacilli	Ziehl-Neelsen (ZN) stain	Lowenstein-Jensen (LJ) media Middlebrook media
Pythium	Acridine orange hydrochloride, Lactophenol blue	Potato dextrose agar Sabouraud dextrose agar, and Chocolate agar

7.4.4 Response to Treatment

Response to treatment should be assessed after 24 and 48 h. Stable clinical features after initiation of treatment without any worsening, even if not showing any improvement on clinical parameters is indicative of resolving infection. Subsequently, the ulcer should start consolidating with progressive healing of epithelial defect, decrease in infiltration and stromal oedema. Other clinical signs also, should noticeably be decreasing. However, the visual acuity is the last to improve in majority of cases. Consequent to signs of healing, gradually reduce the frequency of topical treatment and follow up over 2 weeks. If morphological looking and culture-proven bacterial ulcers fail to show any improvement even after 7 days it is reasonable to consider methicillin-resistant *Staphylococcus aureus* (MRSA).

7.4.5 When to Refer?

Referral guidelines largely depend on the level of health care delivery system, where the patient reports for the first time. Decision to refer the patient for further management is dependent on multiple factors like onset and duration of symptoms, severity of disease and associated complications if any.

At Primary Centre
With limited resources and lack of skilled care at primary centre urgent referral to higher centre is mandatory along with prescription of broad-spectrum antibiotic eye drops for hourly instillation, until they are seen at the referral centre.

At Secondary Centre
Management of mild-to-moderate grades and uncomplicated corneal ulcers can be effectively done at secondary eye care centres. In cases of severe grades and complicated variants, the decision to refer the case can be taken as per the guidelines (Fig. 7.2).

At Tertiary Centre
Different tertiary eye care centres have their own protocols for management of corneal ulcer. However, the WHO recommended guidelines to be followed at eye care facilities are as follows [12]:

- Careful history, background examination findings and treatment history.
- Meticulous corneal scraping.
- Hospitalisation to ensure adequate treatment and regular follow-up.
- Documentation.

If the keratitis responds to treatment, instituted therapy should be continued for 1–2 weeks in a bacterial aetiology and at least 2–3 weeks in fungal. In cases with

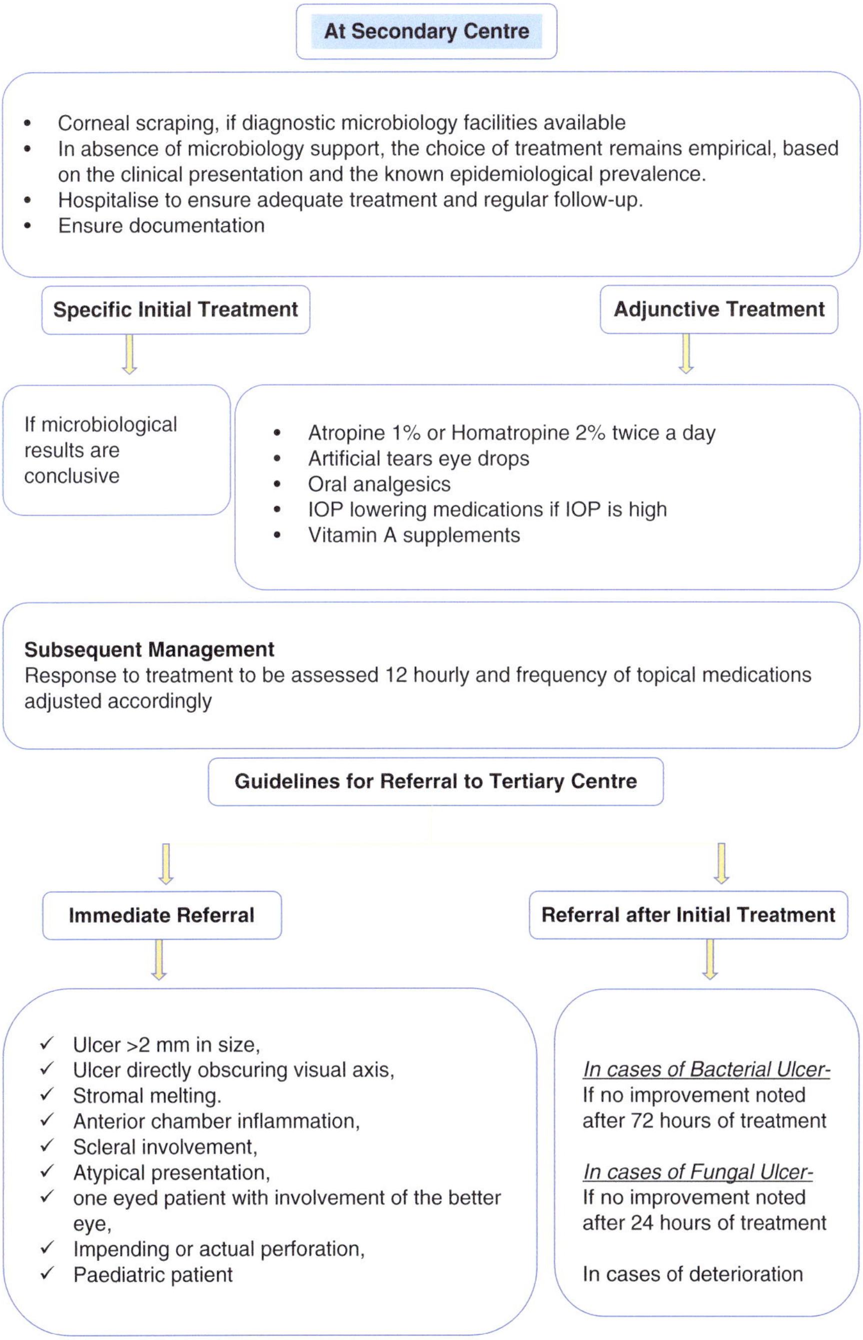

Fig. 7.2 Management and referral guidelines for secondary centre

poor response manifested as increase in size of epithelial defect, increase in infiltrations, AC reaction and hypopyon, progressive thinning and perforation, it is prudent to re-evaluate the case for possible cause of indolence.

7.5 Bacterial Keratitis

Bacterial keratitis is the most common cause of microbial keratitis and accounts for more than 85% of all microbial keratitis cases [12]. It is a corneal emergency which if not managed properly, can lead to vision threatening complications such as perforation, sloughing, endophthalmitis and/or corneal scarring/opacification [12]. Since it is characterised by rapidly progressing clinical course, an early diagnosis and treatment are paramount to minimising visual deterioration. The clinical features and morphological appearance of important causes of bacterial keratitis are described below.

7.5.1 Diagnostic Differentiators

Patients presenting with bacterial keratitis exhibit distinct morphological patterns amenable to be correlated to particular pathogen which is immensely helpful in initiating an appropriate and timely treatment. However, in advanced cases the morphological distinction is not discernible. Lid oedema, conjunctival and circumciliary congestion, epithelial defect, stromal infiltration, surrounding oedema and endotheliitis associated with anterior chamber reaction with or without hypopyon are some of the important clinical signs that help differentiate bacterial corneal ulcer from other aetiologies.

7.5.1.1 Staphylococci

Staphylococcus being a commensal of conjunctival flora is seen to be a cause of keratitis more frequently in compromised corneal surface (Table 7.1). Corneal lesions are usually pale white, round or oval disc-shaped ulcer with dense deep surrounding infiltration. Presence of stromal oedema, folds in Descemet's membrane along with moderate-to-severe AC reaction and hypopyon are indicative of deeper involvement. Abscess formation may be seen in long standing cases with suboptimal treatment (Fig. 7.3).

7.5.1.2 Streptococci

Streptococcus pneumoniae usually presents with rapidly progressing lesion with severe mucopurulent discharge. Typical morphology being round or oval central or paracentral ulcer with formation of deep stromal abscess. It is accompanied by severe fibrinous AC reaction and hypopyon formation. Rest of the cornea is usually clear (Fig. 7.4).

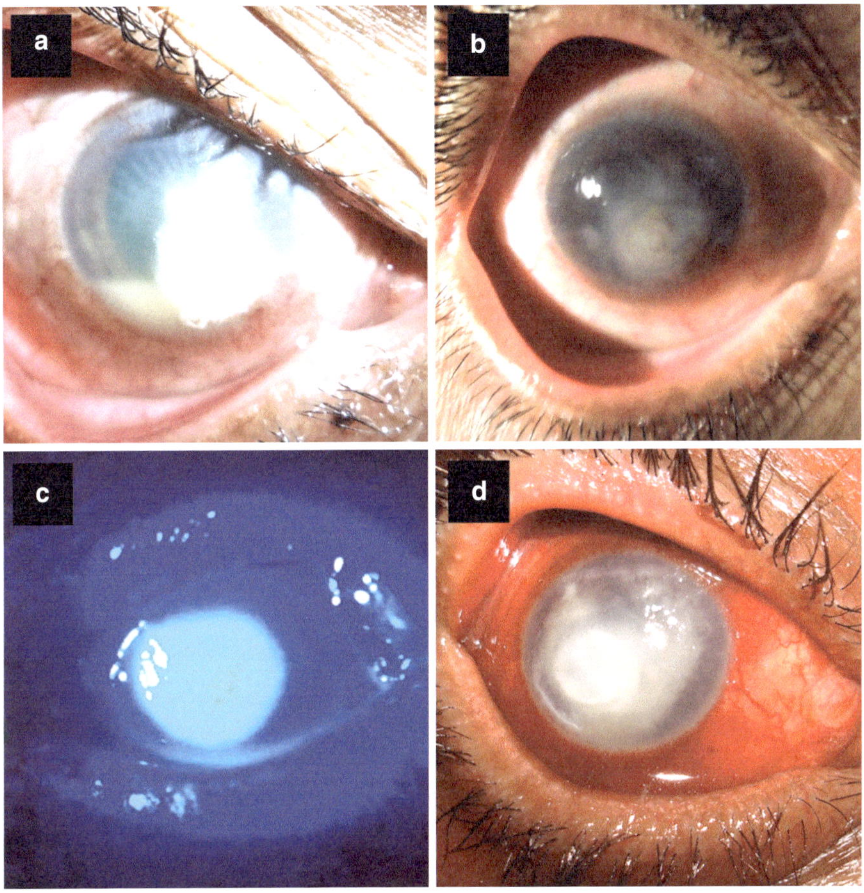

Fig. 7.3 (**a**) Pale white disc-shaped ulcer with dense deep surrounding infiltration, stromal oedema, folds in Descemet's membrane and hypopyon indicative of *Staphylococcus*. (**b**) Status post healing with the formation of leucomatous corneal opacity. (**c**, **d**) Larger pale white Staphylococcal central ulcer with surrounding infiltration

7.5.1.3 Pseudomonas

Pseudomonas aeruginosa typically presents with rapidly progressing ulcer both in size and in depth with dense deep stromal infiltrate and oedema, intense necrosis and greenish-yellow mucopurulent discharge (Fig. 7.5). Rest of the cornea has steamy inflamed ground glass appearance. In event of suboptimal treatment, the aggressive pathological course of *Pseudomonas* causes rapid descemetocele formation and subsequent corneal perforation or sloughing. Immune ring may be seen in a slowly progressing lesion.

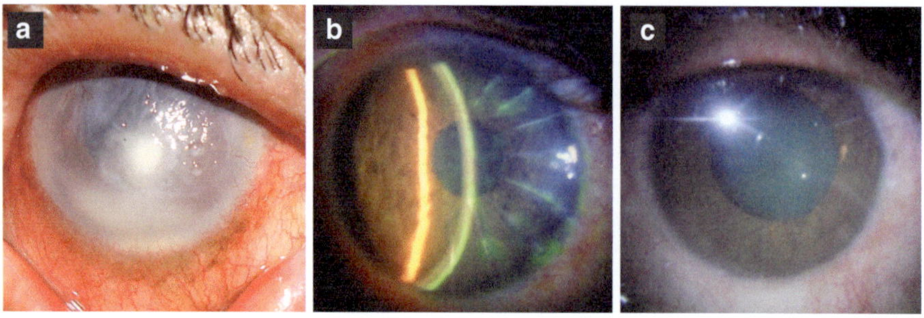

Fig. 7.4 (**a**) Round paracentral ulcer with formation of deep stromal abscess with hypopyon (**b**) *Streptococcus* keratitis status post radial keratotomy, and (**c**) Healed keratitis at follow up of 7 days

Fig. 7.5 Slit lamp picture showing Grade III corneal ulcer with dense stromal infiltrates, liquefactive necrosis and intense yellow exudates, causative organism being *Pseudomonas*. Note the marked thinning with peripheral gutter formation (arrow) and perforation sized 2 × 3 mm (arrowhead)

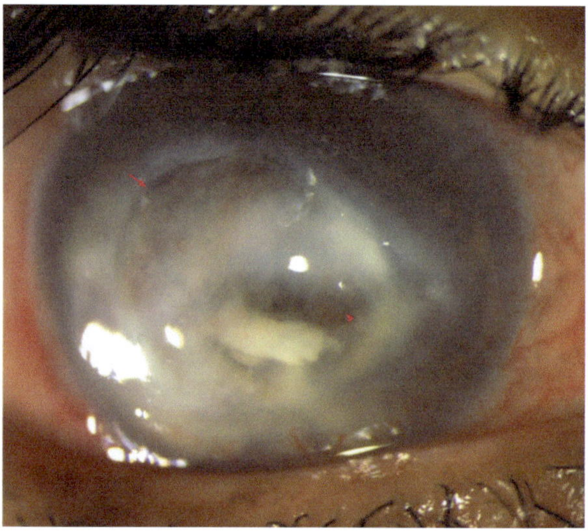

7.5.2 Management

Empirical therapy should be started in cases of mild keratitis, obviating the need for corneal scraping, especially in centres where laboratory facilities may not be readily available for plating and inoculation. However, in moderate and severe grades of ulcers microbiological workup and antibiotic sensitivity should necessarily be done. Subsequently, empirical treatment should be started with broad-spectrum antibiotics in accordance with the sensitivity report (Table 7.5) [12]. Corneal biopsy could be considered in cases with deep stromal infiltrates, particularly in setting of negative culture and poor clinical improvement.

Bacterial keratitis is effectively managed (including severe cases) using fortified antibiotics, tobramycin (14 mg/mL) one hourly alternating with cefazolin or vancomycin (50 mg/mL). General guidelines for antibiotic usage in the management of

Table 7.5 Antimicrobial therapy for the management of bacterial keratitis

Organism	Antibiotic	Topical concentration	Subconjunctival dose
No organism identified or multiple types of organisms	Cefazolin or vancomycin with Tobramycin or gentamicin or Fluoroquinolones[a]	50 mg/mL 9–14 mg/mL Various[b]	100 mg in 0.5 mL 20 mg in 0.5 mL
Gram-positive cocci	Cefazolin Vancomycin[c] Bacitracin[c] Fluoroquinolones[a]	50 mg/mL 15–50 mg/mL 10,000 IU Various[b]	100 mg in 0.5 mL 25 mg in 0.5 mL
Gram-negative rods	Tobramycin or gentamicin Ceftazidime Fluoroquinolones	9–14 mg/mL 50 mg/mL Various[b]	20 mg in 0.5 mL 100 mg in 0.5 mL
Gram-negative cocci[d]	Ceftriaxone Ceftazidime Fluoroquinolones	50 mg/mL 50 mg/mL Various[b]	100 mg in 0.5 mL 100 mg in 0.5 mL
Nontuberculous mycobacteria	Amikacin Clarithromycin Azithromycin Fluoroquinolones	20–40 mg/mL 10 mg/mL 10 mg/mL Various[b]	20 mg in 0.5 mL
Nocardia	Sulfacetamide Amikacin Trimethoprim/ sulfamethoxazole: Trimethoprim Sulfamethoxazole	100 mg/mL 20–40 mg/mL 16 mg/mL 80 mg/mL	20 mg in 0.5 mL

Reprinted with permission from: Lin A, Rhee MK, Akpek EK, Amescua G, Farid M, Garcia-Ferrer FJ, Varu DM, Musch DC, Dunn SP, Mah FS. Bacterial Keratitis Preferred Practice Pattern®. Ophthalmology. 2019 Jan;126(1):P1

[a]Fewer Gram-positive cocci are resistant to gatifloxacin, moxifloxacin and besifloxacin than other fluoroquinolones

[b]Besifloxacin 6 mg/mL; ciprofloxacin 3 mg/mL; gatifloxacin 3 mg/mL; levofloxacin 15 mg/mL; moxifloxacin 5 mg/mL; ofloxacin 3 mg/mL, all commercially available at these concentrations

[c]For resistant *Enterococcus* and *Staphylococcus* species and penicillin allergy. Vancomycin and bacitracin have no Gram-negative activity and should not be used as a single agent in empirically treating bacterial keratitis

[d]Systemic therapy is necessary for suspected gonococcal infection

bacterial keratitis are illustrated in Table 7.5. Adjunctive treatment of cycloplegics, tear supplements and antiglaucoma medication should be instituted along with antibiotics. Less-severe forms of keratitis can be effectively managed by monotherapy with fourth-generation fluoroquinolones such as moxifloxacin or Gatifloxacin. MRSA should be considered in a culture-proven bacterial ulcer, if it fails to show any improvement in 24–48 h [13]. Ocular surface disease should be ruled out in such cases. Figure 7.6 summarises the treatment approach to bacterial keratitis at a tertiary level facility.

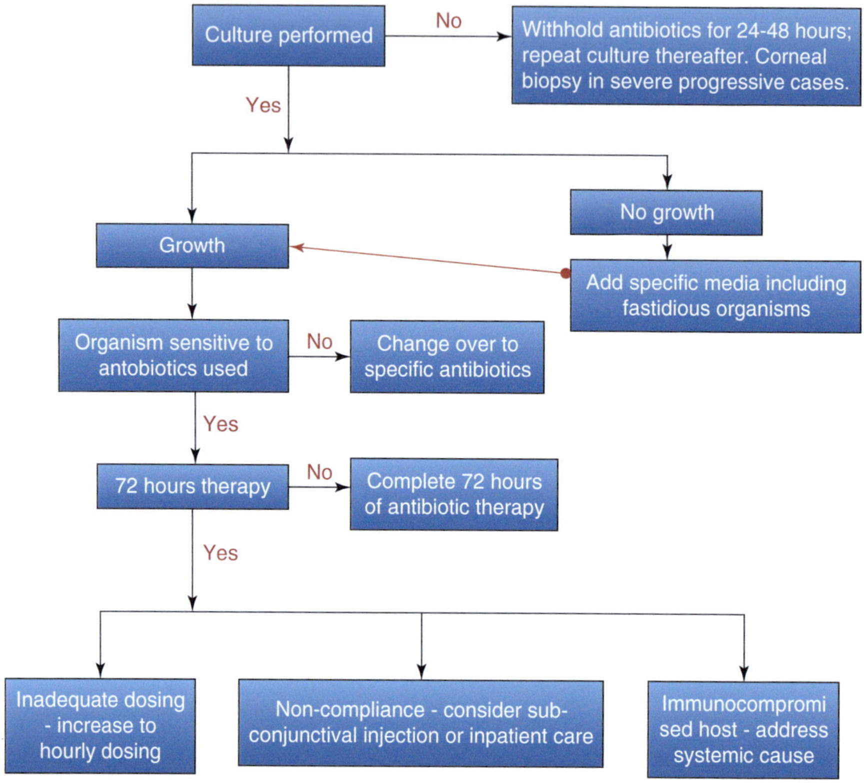

Fig. 7.6 Treatment approach to bacterial keratitis at a tertiary level facility

7.6 HSV Keratitis

HSV keratitis is by far the most underdiagnosed and an equally challenging entity in clinical practice both from diagnostic and from therapeutic perspective. It can affect all the layers of cornea individually or as mixed variants. The diagnostic dilemma and therapeutic concerns can be challenging for the ophthalmologist, because HSV keratitis often masquerades as *Acanthamoeba* keratitis, mixed microbial keratitis, toxic epitheliopathy and neurotrophic keratitis [14]. Thus, it warrants an emergent intervention to alleviate symptoms minimise visual loss and prevent complications. As opposed to other types of microbial keratitis, HSV keratitis can have clinical manifestations ranging from infectious to immunological variants requiring varied treatment in diverse circumstances.

It can be broadly categorised as epithelial disease, caused by active virus replication, stromal disease, usually caused by immunologic mechanisms in addition to active viral replication and endotheliitis (Table 7.6). The commonest cause of corneal emergency in HSV keratitis which necessitates emergent intervention is

Table 7.6 HSV keratitis

	Morphology	Corneal emergencies	Symptoms	Complications	Treatment	Outcomes	Etiopathogenesis
Epithelial infective	Superficial punctate keratitis: branching epithelial dendrites	Persistent epithelial defect Toxic epitheliopathy	Pain, photophobia, redness, watering	Epithelial and faint anterior stromal opacities	Topical antiviral; Surface debridement	Self-limiting in immune-competent hosts; Ghost scarring; footprints	Active virus replication in epithelial cells, causing cell destruction
Stromal necrotising	Grey-white stromal infiltration with ulceration and necrosis	Persistent epithelial defect Corneal thinning and perforation	Pain, photophobia, redness, watering diminution of vision	Anterior chamber inflammation; Iritis; Thinning and Progressive corneal scarring	Topical and systemic anti-viral followed by topical corticosteroid therapy	Stromal opacity and neovascularisation; thinning and scarring leading to visual impairment	Active Virus proliferation within the stroma
Immune stromal	Stromal infiltration with intact epithelium Punctate Stromal opacities and haze Immune ring	Stromal oedema	Pain, photophobia, diminution of vision	Anterior chamber inflammation; iritis; Mid-to-deep stromal neovascularisation Corneal scarring	Topical /systemic corticosteroids with systemic anti-virals	Stromal opacity and neovascularisation; ghost vessels; lipid keratopathy leading to visual impairment	Antibody complement cascade against retained herpes antigens in stroma

(continued)

Table 7.6 (continued)

	Morphology	Corneal emergencies	Symptoms	Complications	Treatment	Outcomes	Etiopathogenesis
Endotheliitis	Stromal oedema not associated with infiltration or vascularisation epithelial microcysts; keratic precipitate, Descemet's folds	Stromal oedema; endothelial decompensation	Pain, photophobia, decreased vision	Anterior chamber inflammation; Iritis	Topical and or systemic corticosteroids	Corneal decompensation in severe cases and in absence of treatment	Cell-mediated immune reaction to stromal tissue
Neurotrophic ulcer	Greyish white oval ulcer with rolled and smooth borders; Inter-palpebral location	Corneal perforation	Non-specific	Corneal thinning Neovascularisation	Discontinuation of potentially toxic eye drops; Artificial tear supplements soft corticosteroid eye drops; Bandage contact lens		Decreased tear secretion consequent to impaired corneal innervation; toxic epitheliopathy

necrotising stromal keratitis. However, it is imperative to have knowledge of all types of clinical presentations, their morphology and treatment.

7.6.1 Diagnostic Differentiators

7.6.1.1 HSV Epithelial Keratitis

Infective epithelial keratitis is the most common manifestation and generally presents as dendritic and geographic ulcers in addition to marginal keratitis in infrequent cases [15]. Raised clear epithelial vesicles which later coalesce to form the typical dendritic or geographical ulcers are the hallmark of disease (Fig. 7.7a). The patient presents with symptoms of photophobia, pain, foreign body sensation and serous discharge. Blurring and diminution of vision may be seen in cases of central involvement.

The typical dendritic ulcer is a central or paracentral branching, linear lesion with terminal bulbs and swollen epithelial borders containing live viruses. However, immune compromised subjects may fail to show a typical dendrite and may have only vesicles.

The fluorescein-stained lesion is an important differentiator from other branching lesions of the corneal epithelium often regarded as pseudo dendrites particularly of varicella-zoster virus (VZV). Psuedodendrites are raised lesions usually peripherally located and arranged in cluster of cells without break in surface epithelium and hence do not stain with fluorescein. Coalescent and enlarged dendrites with scalloped borders are referred to as geographic ulcer (Fig. 7.7b). It has swollen epithelial borders that contain live viruses while staining brightly with fluorescein. If treatment is not initiated promptly the disease can progress to stromal necrotising keratitis, immune stromal keratitis or neurotrophic keratopathy [15].

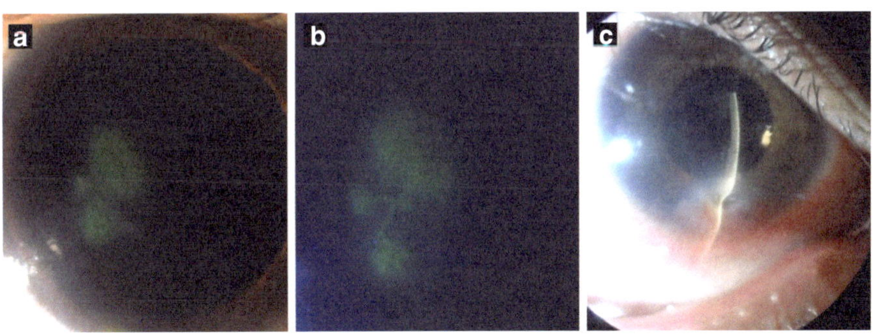

Fig. 7.7 (**a**) Slit lamp picture showing herpetic dendritic ulcer. (**b**) Slit lamp picture showing herpetic dendritic ulcer with dichotomous branching as visualised on cobalt blue filter with fluorescein staining. Broad terminal end pattern is indicative of progression to geographical ulcer. (**c**) Corneal thinning consequent to marginal keratitis of HSV associated with superficial and deep vascularisation extending up to the lesion

Treatment

Epithelial keratitis is a self-limiting disease with resolution in more than 50% of cases within 2 weeks [15, 16]. However, it is prudent to initiate timely treatment to promote healing, prevent progression and subsequent subepithelial scarring. It is advisable to do debridement of ulcer by a cotton-tipped blunt applicator which facilitates shedding of virus thereby decreasing the viral load. This is to be followed by topical antiviral agents in adequate doses.

Recommended treatment agents comprise of ganciclovir gel 0.15%, trifluridine 1% ophthalmic suspension, every 2–4 h [17]. Acyclovir 3% or vidarabine 3% ointment five times a day can also be used. To prevent drug-induced epithelial toxicity dosing frequency can be reduced over the next 2 weeks. Ganciclovir/ trifluridine can be reduced to 4–6 times and acyclovir/ vidarabine to 3 times per day and can be discontinued completely by 3 weeks. There is no role of topical corticosteroids in management of HSV epithelial keratitis. Supportive treatment in the form of topical cycloplegics (homatropine acetate 1%/ cyclopentolate 2%), broad-spectrum antibiotic (ofloxacin 0.3%/ moxifloxacin 0.5%) and preservative-free tear substitutes (HPMC 0.3%/ CMC 0.5%) are initiated to prevent iritis, ciliary spasm and superimposed secondary infection. Systemic antivirals are indicated in infants, immunocompromised patients, and patients not responsive or not compliant to topical therapy. They can shorten the course of disease, reduce the chances of complications and recurrences.

7.6.1.2 Marginal Ulcer of HSV

Marginal ulcer of HSV is a frequently misdiagnosed entity which is characterised by severe inflammation, anterior stromal infiltrates and accompanying vascularisation as a sequel to active viral replication and resultant immune response (Fig. 7.7c). It has to be differentiated from marginal keratitis of bacterial origin which is purely an immune response to bacterial antigen and presents with an intact overlying epithelium with a clear zone between the lesion and corresponding limbus. The HSV lesion rarely progresses centrally even in advanced stage. In event of confounded diagnosis of bacterial marginal keratitis with initiation of topical corticosteroids without antiviral cover, the lesion can rapidly progress to larger size and central extension [15]. Treatment involves topical antiviral agents followed by topical corticosteroids once the infiltrates start to decrease and epithelial lesion is healed.

7.6.1.3 Stromal Keratitis

Is representative of true corneal emergency in HSV keratitis and presents either as primary or secondary affection (Table 7.6). Secondary involvement may occur as a complication of endotheliitis, epithelial keratitis or neurotrophic keratopathy. Stromal keratitis manifests as two major entities:

- *Necrotising stromal keratitis*—which involves active viral replication in stroma
- *Immune stromal keratitis*—sequel of an immune reaction to viral antigen within the stroma

Necrotising Stromal Keratitis

Necrotising stromal keratitis occurs as a result of direct viral invasion of the corneal stroma. Clinical features include intense infiltration of the stroma, stromal necrosis and ulceration with an overlying breached epithelium (Fig. 7.8). If untreated it rapidly progresses to thinning and perforation. The condition needs to be differentiated from other types of microbial keratitis mainly bacterial and mycotic (Fig 7.9).

Treatment

Treatment is more complex in necrotising keratitis, in which both live virus and immune response are present and depend on severity of disease. For mild-to-moderate cases prednisolone 1% ophthalmic suspension 4 times and in severe grades 2 hourly dosing is started which can be tapered over a period of 8–10 weeks

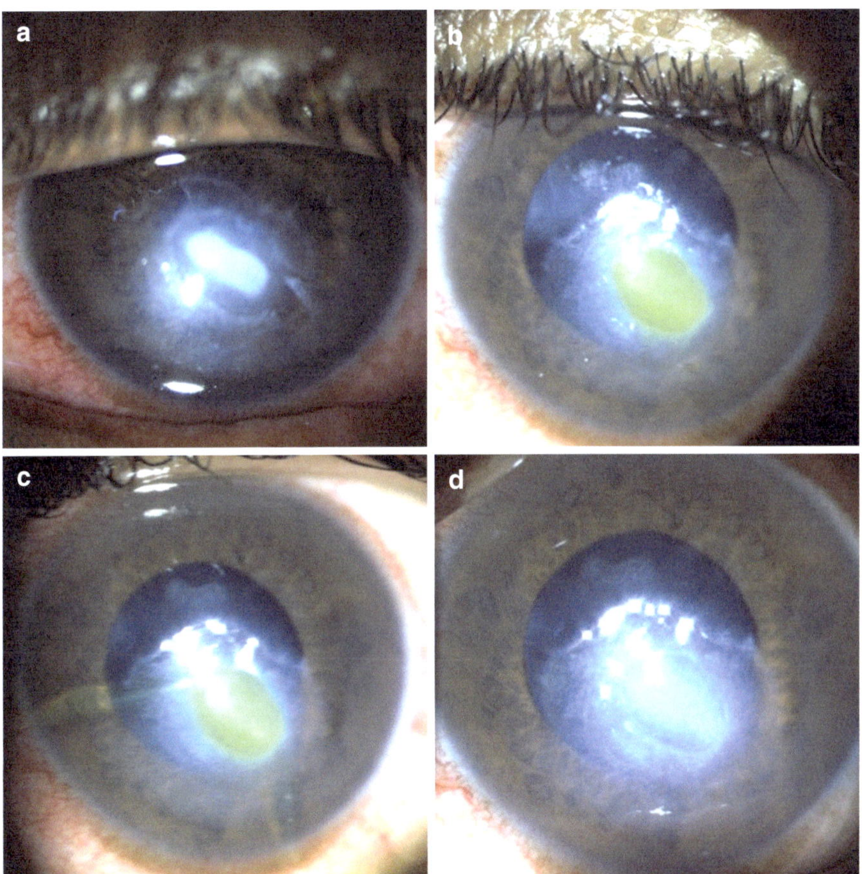

Fig. 7.8 (**a**) Stromal necrotising keratitis as visualised with fluorescein stain showing dense stromal infiltrates and epithelial defect sized 4 × 4 mm. (**b**, **c**) Subsequent pictures show progressive healing with decrease in size of ulcer, infiltrates and healing epithelial margins

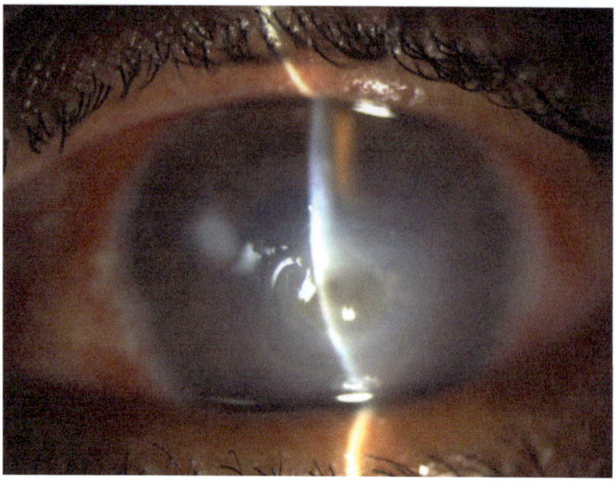

Fig. 7.9 Slit lamp picture showing necrotising viral keratitis with super-added bacterial infection (image courtesy—Prof. Namrata Sharma; Dr. R. P. Centre for Ophthalmic Sciences, All India institute of Medical Sciences, New Delhi)

[17]. It should always be supplemented with topical and systemic antiviral agents, cycloplegics and surface lubricants (Table 7.6).

Immune Stromal (Interstitial) Keratitis

It involves immune-mediated inflammation to retained viral antigen within the stroma. The viral antigen is thought to trigger an antigen-antibody-complement (AAC) cascade that results in intrastromal inflammation [18]. Stromal involvement occurs in the form of infiltration and stromal oedema with an intact overlying epithelium accompanied with anterior chamber inflammation. The lesion heals by varying grades of stromal opacification depending on virulence of organism and host immune response. Wessely immune ring is seen as a consequence of AAC precipitate in mid stroma of central or paracentral cornea.

Immune stromal keratitis may lead to stromal neovascularisation and intense inflammation as a response to ongoing inflammation. The neovascularization may range from sectoral in less inflamed cases to complete involvement in severe inflammation. It can be a cause of visual impedance if not managed timely. Emergent treatment of inflammation can result in resolution of blood vessels. Visual deprivation may occur consequent to stromal scarring, lipid keratopathy, corneal neovascularisation and ghost vessels. Such lesions may show reactivation after a period of quiescence which may range from weeks to months necessitating long-term topical corticosteroids to suppress the ongoing inflammatory reaction.

Treatment

Topical corticosteroids used in conjunction with systemic and topical antivirals are the mainstay of treatment in HSV immune stromal keratitis [19]. Dosing schedule largely depends on severity at the time of presentation. For mild-to-moderate disease prednisolone acetate 1% ophthalmic suspension four times a day and for severe cases 2 hourly regimen is to be instated. Topical antiviral agents should always be supplemented with topical steroids. Acyclovir 3% ointment, trifluridine 1%

suspension or ganciclovir 0.15% gel 3–5 times a day should be started. Mydriatic cycloplegic drops of HA 2% /cyclopentolate 1% 2–3 times a day are to be given for ensuing iritis. Additionally, systemic antivirals like oral acyclovir 400 mg five times for 1 week and then three times for 1 week should be started. They shorten the course of the disease and reduce the chances of complications and recurrences.

Topical steroids work by reducing inflammation, scarring and neovascularisation. However, injudicious use of topical steroids can be a cause of perforation, secondary infection and secondary glaucoma. Systemic corticosteroids are to be reserved for severe stromal keratitis with endotheliitis and iritis. They should be given for long term up to 6 months till complete resolution occurs, otherwise, there is a risk of continuing inflammation and sequel.

7.6.1.4 HSV Endotheliitis

HSV endothelitis is characterised by immune-mediated inflammation of corneal endothelium manifesting as moderate to severe stromal oedema associated with keratic precipitates (KP) and overlying epithelial oedema in severe cases. Oedema is clearly demarcated from surrounding uninvolved cornea with or without presence of immune ring. Ongoing inflammation can be a cause of moderate-to-severe iritis. Characteristically the KP's are always present along the line of endothelial, stromal and epithelial oedema and absent over the rest of cornea. Initiation of timely treatment results in complete resolution of lesion. However, if untreated stromal oedema may persist leading to bullous keratopathy, scarring and secondary neovascularisation. Most agreed upon aetiology is immune mediated, however, some studies have demonstrated live virus in the lesion [20]. HSV endotheliitis can be classified as disciform, diffuse, and linear based on their morphology. Disciform endotheliitis is by far the most common variant present in central or paracentral area and typically with round configuration (Fig. 7.10). Patient presents with photophobia foreign body sensation with mild-to-moderate ocular discomfort. Clinical signs composed

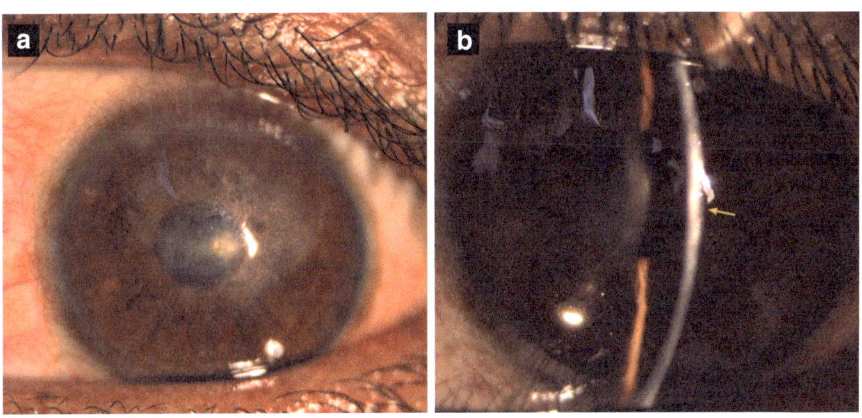

Fig. 7.10 Slit lamp picture showing disciform keratitis of HSV. Note the central circular 3 × 3 mm lesion (**a**) with stromal oedema (arrow) seen on slit beam (**b**)

of varying grades of visual acuity impairment, circumciliary congestion and the typical morphological lesion (as described above) with or without iritis. Secondary open-angle glaucoma may be seen in advanced cases and in severe involvement.

Diffuse endotheliitis is a rare form of HSV endotheliitis. Lesion typically is of diffuse distribution with diffuse stromal oedema and KP over the entire cornea. Severe cases may show epithelial bullae and hypopyon due to intense inflammation. Linear endotheliitis typically presents as a line of stomal oedema with KP and secondary iritis that progresses centripetally from the limbus [21–23].

Treatment

It necessitates aggressive treatment with both corticosteroids and antiviral agents. Oral acyclovir may have a beneficial role and should be considered in all cases. Adjuvant therapy with hyperosmotic agents, anti-glaucoma medication and lubricating eye drops are to be given as per the clinical requirement.

7.6.1.5 Neurotrophic Ulcers

Neurotrophic ulcers are oval ulcers with smooth scalloped borders accompanied by lack of corneal lustre and decreased corneal sensations. They are formed consequent to piling up of epithelial cells over the margin of ulcer mainly as a sequel to corneal nerve involvement, toxic epitheliopathy due to overtreatment with topical antiviral drugs and resultant decreased tear secretion. Neurotrophic ulcers can complicate stromal ulceration and resultant perforation in absence of appropriate treatment [24].

Treatment

Treatment aims to promote epithelial regeneration thereby healing the ocular surface. All topical antivirals, antibacterial and cycloplegic agents should be discontinued. Soft bandage contact lens can be supplemented to prevent shedding of regenerating epithelium. Frequent use of preservative-free artificial tears promotes epithelial healing. In non-responsive cases debridement of the epithelium from the margin of ulcer is advisable to facilitate migration of new epithelial cells thereby facilitate healing. Temporary tarsorrhaphy or eyelid stay suture can be employed as temporary measures to promote epithelisation and healing.

7.7 Fungal Keratitis

The incidence of fungal keratitis has increased over the years owing to frequent use of corticosteroids and antibiotics. Corticosteroids suppress the host immune response and antibiotics provide a non-competitive environment for the fungi to grow. Of the several agents known to cause fungal keratitis, two are important, namely—yeast (*Candida* spp.) and filamentous fungi (septate and aseptate). Former causes secondary fungal keratitis in already compromised corneas following use of topical steroids or preexistent ocular surface disease while the latter overall, constitutes the most common cause of fungal corneal ulcer. Few if any, fungi can penetrate intact corneal tissue. Risk factors for invasion and infection have been summarised in Table 7.1.

7.7.1 Diagnostic Differentiators

The clinical picture combined with relevant history makes for a good diagnostic differentiator in isolating fungal aetiology among other causes of infectious keratitis. Although the most frequently presented signs of fungal keratitis are similar to other microbial keratitis, an intact epithelium over deep stromal infiltrate should alert the examiner in favour of fungal aetiology. Certain characteristic findings such as greyish white elevated ulcer with hyphate or branching edges, dry rough texture, satellite lesions, immune ring, endotheliitis/ endothelial plaque and fixed hypopyon with convex upper edge can be helpful in narrowing down the cause of keratitis to filamentous fungi (Fig 7.11). *Fusarium* species show a more aggressive course with deeper involvement and rapid perforation (Fig. 7.12). Corneal ulcer caused by yeast is a cheesy white elevated plaque-like lesion with small central ulcer and wider deep stromal infiltrates in a collar stud configuration. Dematiaceous fungi, such as *Curvularia lunata* are identified by the presence of gross brown pigmentation in the region of keratitis.

7.7.2 Treatment

Topical antifungal therapy is the mainstay of treatment of fungal keratitis. However, topical antifungal agents have poor corneal penetration; hence it is advisable to perform epithelial debridement at the time of initiating treatment. Topical 5% Natamycin eye drop being a wide-spectrum antifungal agent, is the drug of choice for most cases of mycotic keratitis. It is given in hourly dosing at daytime, and 2 hourly at bedtime with tapering over 4–7 days if improvement is seen. The treatment should be continued preferably for a period of 3–4 weeks or until complete resolution. Adjunctive treatment in the form of topical fluoroquinolone, Gatifloxacin, cycloplegics, tear supplements and antiglaucoma medication should be continues as per the clinical condition. In event of worsening of clinical features, it is advisable to introduce 0.15% Amphotericin B or 2 % Voriconazole eye drops. Systemic treatment with oral Fluconazole 100–150 mg BD, oral Voriconazole 200 mg BD or oral Itraconazole 200 mg BD for 1–2 weeks is indicated in large-sized ulcers >5 mm, deep keratitis with more than 2/3rd involvement, scleritis, post-PK and in impending endophthalmitis.

Targeted therapy with intracameral or intrastromal antifungal agents can be given in severe cases which are non-responsive to medical therapy, have endothelial

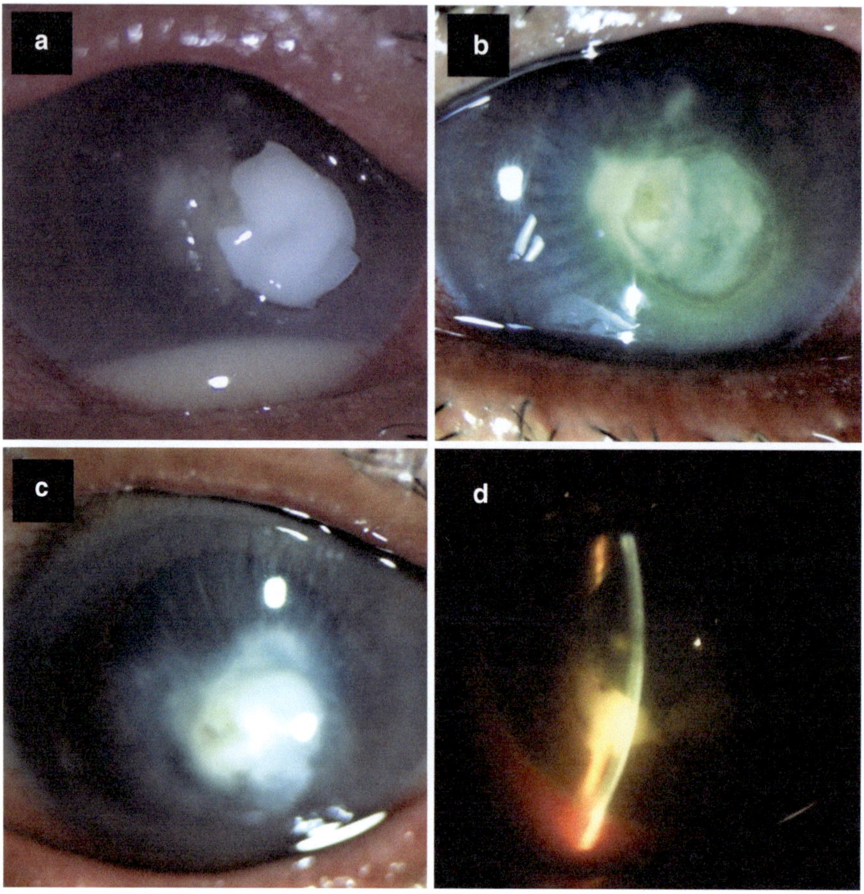

Fig. 7.11 (**a**–**d**) Mycotic corneal ulcer with deep stromal abscess, endothelial plaque formation and fixed hypopyon. Large-sized corneal ulcer with satellite lesion and endothelial plaque is seen after removal of epithelial debris

exudates and severe AC reaction. Amphotericin B 5–7.5 μgm/0.1 mL of 5% dextrose or Voriconazole 50–100 μgm/0.1 mL of 5% dextrose can be given. Repeat dose can be given after 1 week. In severe cases such as deep infections, associated scleritis, anterior chamber infiltration—systemic therapy combined with intracameral or intrastromal injections should be considered. Collagen cross-linking and cryotherapy have also been proposed as a useful adjunct to medical therapy [25].

Advanced cases involving the stroma often require prolonged and intensive topical and systemic antifungal therapy [26, 27]. Failure with medical management alone is common. Surgical interventions (therapeutic keratoplasty (TKP), penetrating keratoplasty (PK), conjunctival flap, lamellar keratoplasty or cryotherapy) are required for visual rehabilitation and control [28, 29].

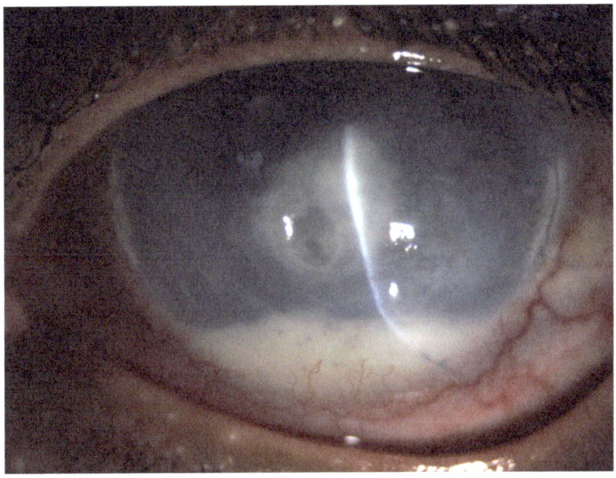

Fig. 7.12 Slit lamp picture of mycotic corneal ulcer with hypopyon, surrounding dense infiltration, marked thinning in centre and impending perforation

7.8 Acanthamoeba Keratitis

It is a fairly uncommon cause of infective keratitis caused by a protozoa—*Acanthamoeba* which is found ubiquitously in water and soil. The patient typically presents as a chronic case of contact lens wear with history suggestive of improper hygiene, exposure to contaminated water bodies or an organic matter-related trauma [30]. In patients with indolent features, leading history of previous use of topical steroids should be elicited. Predominant symptoms of severe pain, photophobia, watering, foreign body sensation even in milder looking lesions should alert the ophthalmologist about *Acanthamoeba* as a possible causative agent.

7.8.1 Diagnostic Differentiators

It primarily presents as ulcer with features similar to herpes simplex. Morphological features consist of epithelial microcysts and erosions, pseudo dendrites, stromal infiltrates and ulceration, radial keratoneuritis and immune ring formation [31] (Fig. 7.13). The pseudo dendrites are raised above the surface with symptoms disproportionate to signs. Presence of satellite lesion is indicative of replicating trophozoites. In advanced case with stromal ulceration disease may be indistinguishable from HSV.

Confocal microscopy is a useful, non-invasive imaging technique for diagnosis, and treatment of *Acanthamoeba* keratitis. *Acanthamoeba* cysts are identified as high contrast round configuration with double-walled structure of the ectocyst surrounding the endocyst, while trophozoites as more irregular structures. Radial keratoneuritis can be demonstrated, as irregularly swollen nerve fibres. Identification and subsequent resolution of these lesions are important to evaluate the response to treatment and can serve as prognosis indicators.

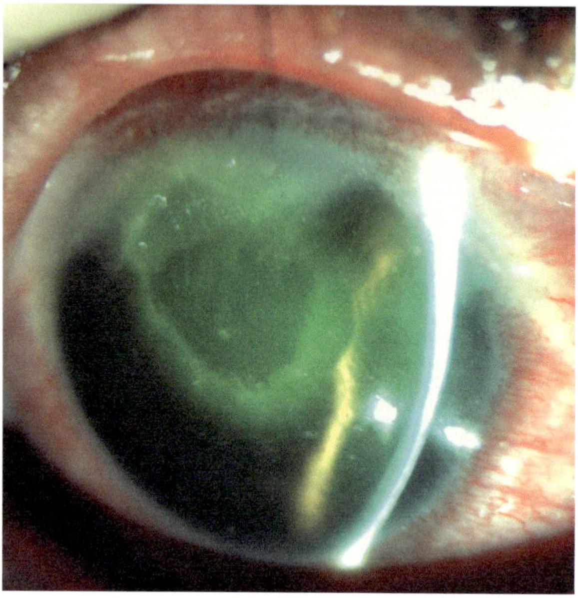

Fig. 7.13 Corneal ulcer sized 5 × 5 mm with deep stromal infiltrates and immune ring formation caused by *Acanthamoeba*

It should be differentiated from mycotic keratitis when a similar history of trauma with vegetative matter is present. However, clinical signs of radial keratoneuritis, pseudo dendrites and epithelial erosions are important differentiating features. Advanced cases present as deep stromal infiltrate and abscesses which can progress to descemetocele and perforation. Uncontrolled infection can be a cause of scleritis, iridocyclitis, secondary glaucoma and complicated cataract.

7.8.2 Treatment

Microbial keratitis due to *Acanthamoeba* is difficult to treat requiring treatment for longer duration up to 6–12 months. Combination therapy includes cytocidal drugs like Propamidine isethionate 0.1%, Chlorhexidine 0.02%, polyhexamethylene biguanide 0.02%, hexamidine and miltefosine (65.12 μg/mL) are effective when given for prolonged period [30]. Chlorhexidine 0.02% is given 1–2 hourly for 2–4 weeks, which can later be tapered to 4–6 times for 6–12 months. Adjuvants like mydriatic cycloplegic agents, surface lubricants and broad-spectrum antibiotics can be supplemented. Recommended dosing frequency varies, but they are initially used hourly for the first several days and tapered slowly over 4–6 weeks to four times a day. The maintenance therapy is tapered more slowly to ensure complete eradication of cyst, lasting 3–6 months, even up to a year or more in resistant cases.

Systemic drugs found to be useful in *Acanthamoeba* keratitis are Voriconazole and Miltefosine. Oral Voriconazole in a dose of 200 mg twice daily for 4–6 weeks can be started. Miltefosine is an alkyl phosphocholine that has demonstrated efficacy in other protozoal infections such as visceral leishmaniasis, *Trichomonas vaginalis* and *Entamoeba histolytica*. Oral Miltefosine in the dose of 50 mg three times for 4–6 weeks has shown to be efficacious. Gastrointestinal symptoms after prolonged treatment have been of concern in some patients. However, the dosing frequency can be reduced to 50 mg once or twice daily in such cases

Mechanical debridement of the ulcer helps to remove organism and also to improve drug penetration. Patients requiring therapeutic corneal transplantation should be evaluated carefully to identify the healthy margins free from infection in host cornea. However, recurrence of infection in the graft has been commonly reported by various authors [30, 32].

7.9 Pythium Keratitis

Microbial keratitis caused by *Pythium insidiosum* has garnered much interest over the last decade. It is an oomycete that causes a devastating infection of the cornea and can cause severe visual loss owing to its aggressive course refractory to standard treatment. Incidence is found to be more in tropical and subtropical climates. Clinical, microbiological, histopathological and confocal microscopy features of *Pythium insidiosum* closely resembles that of fungus, increasing the difficulty in diagnosis and resulting in an under diagnosis of *Pythium* keratitis (Fig. 7.14). Major reports have identified it to be refractory to both medical and surgical treatment

7.9.1 Diagnostic Differentiators

Morphological features on clinical presentation comprise mainly of cotton wool or dot-like infiltrates in early stage which later progress to larger size ulcer with hyphate edges extending into surrounding cornea resembling that of filamentous fungi [33]. Additionally, tentacle-like lesions and peripheral furrowing may be seen. Pythium

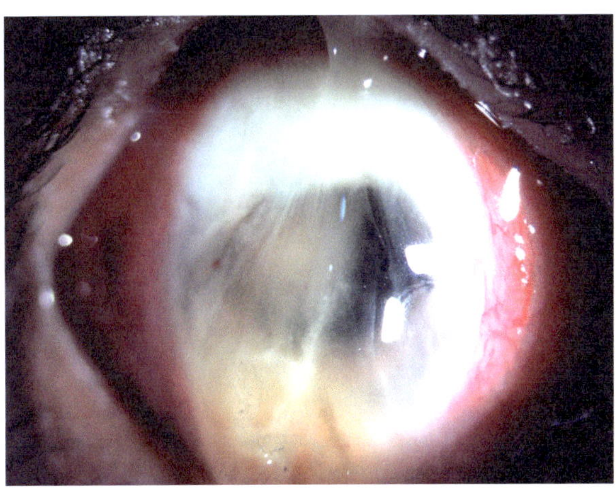

Fig. 7.14 Rapidly sloughing corneal ulcer due to *Pythium Insidiosum*

keratitis has an aggressive course that can lead to descemetocele formation, perforation and sloughing within a week (Fig 7.14). At times the lesions mimic the radial keratoneuritis of *Acanthamoeba* keratitis misleading the diagnosis and management.

7.9.2 Diagnosis

Electron microscopy of Pythium filaments on cursory look mimic filaments of hyphate fungi, however, important differentiating feature being a sparse or complete absence of septae in filaments. They are broad ribbon shaped with right angle branching. The growth on SDA/blood agar is characterised by flat, colourless or light brown glabrous colonies. Identification is best confirmed by demonstrating zoospore formation or PCR DNA sequencing [33, 34].

7.9.3 Treatment

Various treatment options have been suggested for treatment of *Pythium* keratitis. In vitro sensitivity of antibiotics such as azithromycin, minocycline and tigecycline have been tested and found to be effective. Topical azithromycin 1% and linezolid 0.2% eyedrop every hour along with oral azithromycin 500 mg once per day or linezolid 1200 mg/day has been found to be effective [33]. Treatment needs to be continued for 2–4 weeks. Additionally, Tetracycline ointment four times a day, Chloramphenicol eye drops hourly and Caspofungin 200 mg twice a day has been shown to be effective. However, despite the initiation of medical treatment the aggressive course of pathogen warrants surgical intervention in majority of cases. Therapeutic keratoplasty is the treatment of choice in such cases. Recurrence of disease in grafted tissue remains an important impedance to visual and structural improvement.

7.10 Surgical Management

Occasionally, adjuvant surgical therapy is indicated in the treatment of microbial keratitis composed of therapeutic contact lenses, collagenase inhibitors, tarsorrhaphy, conjunctival flap [35], cyanoacrylate glue [36] and lamellar or penetrating keratoplasty [37].

Impaired healing manifesting as persistent epithelial defect that fails to respond to conventional therapy of lubricating eye drops, necessitates the use of soft bandage contact lens, amniotic membrane transplantation and temporary tarsorrhaphy. Gundersen conjunctival flap can be advanced over the defect for surface healing and control of inflammation. Nevertheless, such eyes may need a penetrating keratoplasty at a later date.

Small perforations less than the size of 3 mm are amenable for closure by cyanoacrylate glue. Larger perforations more than 3 mm in size will require penetrating keratoplasty [38]. The size of the graft in such cases should be compatible with size of the defect by oversising of 0.25–0.5 mm.

Corneal transplantation done for HSV keratitis are likely to have stronger post-operative inflammation causing a risk of graft rejection in addition to recurrence of infection in the graft. Post-operative treatment regimen in such cases should include topical and systemic antivirals and corticosteroids in tapering doses for a period of 6 months. Patients with deep stromal opacity may be benefitted from DALK which has the advantage of a low rejection rate.

7.11 Corneal Emergencies Associated with Microbial Keratitis and Their Management (Table 7.1)

7.11.1 Penetrating Trauma with/Without Foreign Body

In microbial keratitis associated with penetrating trauma primary management is directed towards repair of the corneal tear followed by treatment of keratitis as described above. Foreign body if present must be removed during primary repair. Special attention should be given to clinical signs indicative of endophthalmitis. Cautious use of steroids must be exercised.

7.11.2 Descemetocele and Corneal Melt or Perforation

Severe ulceration may lead to descemetocele formation which may progress to perforation or sloughing particularly in *Pseudomonas, Pythium* and necrotising stromal mycotic keratitis. This can further be complicated with the onset of endophthalmitis or expulsion of the contents of eyeball leading to an irreversible visual and structural damage. Depending on the extent of involvement treatment can be initiated by following procedures:

- Tissue adhesives—cyanoacrylate glue, fibrin glue [39]
- Conjunctival flaps—Gundersen or Cies's racquet conjunctival flap [35, 40]
- Amniotic membrane transplantation—especially for central lesions [41]
- Tenon's patch graft
- Keratoplasty—lamellar or penetrating keratoplasty
- Superficial keratectomy and/or tectonic epikeratoplasty

7.11.3 Scleritis

Peripheral corneal and perilimbal infections can be complicated with scleritis. Various predisposing factors include trauma, systemic infection with or without immunocompromised state, use of corticosteroids and immunomodulators, or previous ocular surgery [42, 43]. If not addressed timely and adequately infectious scleritis follows a more rapid and aggressive course, requiring evisceration to address the disease course [44]. Hence, infectious keratitis associated with scleritis usually evolves into a poorer visual and anatomical outcome in comparison to that without scleritis.

The management often presents a greater challenge due to lack of consensus on therapeutic intervention. Early microbiological analysis, institution of specific antimicrobial therapy and complete cessation of all forms of corticosteroids combined with surgical debridement if needed, especially in deeper scleral involvement remain standard treatment approaches in cases of keratitis associated with infectious scleritis especially fungal. Simultaneously the underlying predisposing factor must be addressed while the infection is being managed.

7.11.4 Endophthalmitis

Microbial keratitis associated endophthalmitis carries a dismal prognosis and requires extensive surgical management. A major challenge in such a condition is the inability to visualise posterior segments to carry out complex vitreoretinal procedures, due to corneal opacification. Often surgeons' resort to using combined penetrating keratoplasty and pars plana vitrectomy and lensectomy assisted by temporary keratoprosthesis. Long-term silicone oil tamponade is required and the procedure remains globe salvaging more often than vision restoring.

7.12 Conclusion

Microbial keratitis is a frequent cause of corneal emergency requiring well-timed appropriate intervention to salvage visual and structural integrity. Last two decades have witnessed a sea change in the treatment of corneal ulcers with excellent visual and structural outcomes. Nevertheless, diagnosing and treating corneal ulcers should not be regarded as a simple task. Optimal treatment aims at maximising the chances of complete recovery by identifying the exact aetiology and then instituting a tailored treatment.

Key Points

- Microbial keratitis is a frequent cause of corneal emergency. Appropriate and timely intervention can salvage visual and structural integrity.
- The incidence of microbial keratitis varies according to geographical location, climatic conditions and socio-economic status.
- Meticulous history, clinical examination, microbiological evaluation and knowledge of pre-disposing factors, are crucial in management.
- Knowledge about morphological patterns is an important diagnostic differentiator in arriving at a provisional diagnosis of probable pathogen.
- Bacterial keratitis is the most common form of microbial keratitis accounting for more than 90% of cases, while fungal keratitis contributes maximally to the burden of corneal perforations.

- HSV keratitis is by far the most under diagnosed and an equally challenging entity, both from diagnostic and therapeutic perspectives.
- *Acanthamoeba keratitis* is commonly associated with contact lens wear and is particularly difficult to treat. It may mimic HSV keratitis and demands a high degree of suspicion for timely diagnosis.
- *Pythium insidiosum* keratitis is usually associated with poor response to medical treatment. Therapeutic keratoplasty is indicated early, however, recurrence of infection in graft is not uncommon.
- Descemetocele, corneal perforation, sloughing, toxic epitheliopathy, neurotrophic ulcer, corneal abscess and corneal fistula are commonly encountered corneal emergencies associated with microbial keratitis.

References

1. Al-Mujaini A, Al-Kharusi N, Thakral A, Wali UK. Bacterial keratitis: perspective on epidemiology, clinico-pathogenesis, diagnosis and treatment. Sultan Qaboos Univ Med J. 2009;9(2):184.
2. Erie JC, Nevitt MP, Hodge DO, et al. Incidence of ulcerative keratitis in a defined population from 1950 through 1988. Arch Ophthalmol. 1993;111:1665–71.
3. Upadhyay MP, Karmacharya PC, Koirala S, et al. The Bhaktapur eye study: ocular trauma and antibiotic prophylaxis for the prevention of corneal ulceration in Nepal. Br J Ophthalmol. 2001;85:388–92.
4. Manikandan P, Abdel-Hadi A, Randhir Babu Singh Y, Revathi R, Anita R, Banawas S, Bin Dukhyil AA, Alshehri B, Shobana CS, Panneer Selvam K, Narendran V. Fungal keratitis: epidemiology, rapid detection, and antifungal susceptibilities of Fusarium and Aspergillus isolates from corneal scrapings. BioMed Res Int. 2019; https://doi.org/10.1155/2019/6395840.
5. Bourcier T, Thomas F, Borderie V, et al. Bacterial keratitis: predisposing factors, clinical and microbiological review of 300 cases. Br J Ophthalmol. 2003;87:834–8.
6. Bharathi MJ, Ramakrishnan R, Meenakshi R, Padmavathy S, Shivakumar C, Srinivasan M. Microbial keratitis in South India: influence of risk factors, climate, and geographical variation. Ophthalmic Epidemiol. 2007;14(2):61–9.
7. Teweldemedhin M, Gebreyesus H, Atsbaha AH, Asgedom SW, Saravanan M. Bacterial profile of ocular infections: a systematic review. BMC Ophthalmol. 2017;17(1):212.
8. Titiyal JS, Negi S, Anand A, Tandon R, Sharma N, Vajpayee RB. Risk factors for perforation in microbial corneal ulcers in north India. Br J Ophthalmol. 2006;90(6):686–9.
9. Pate JC, Jones DB, Wilhelmus KR. Prevalence and spectrum of bacterial co-infection during fungal keratitis. Br J Ophthalmol. 2006;90(3):289–92.
10. Prajna VN, Prajna L, Muthiah S. Fungal keratitis: the Aravind experience. Indian J Ophthalmol. 2017;65(10):912.
11. Harrison SM. Grading corneal ulcers. Ann Ophthalmol. 1975;7(4):537–9, 541–2. PMID: 1147498
12. Lin A, Rhee MK, Akpek EK, Amescua G, Farid M, Garcia-Ferrer FJ, Varu DM, Musch DC, Dunn SP, Mah FS. Bacterial keratitis preferred practice pattern®. Ophthalmology. 2019;126(1):1.
13. Lee KM, Lee HS, Kim MS. Two cases of corneal ulcer due to methicillin-resistant Staphylococcus aureus in high risk groups. Korean J Ophthalmol. 2010;24(4):240–4.
14. Szentmáry N, Daas L, Shi L, Laurik KL, Lepper S, Milioti G, Seitz B. Acanthamoeba keratitis—clinical signs, differential diagnosis and treatment. J Curr Ophthalmol. 2019;31(1):16–23.
15. Wilhelmus KR. Antiviral treatment and other therapeutic interventions for herpes simplex virus epithelial keratitis. Cochrane Database Syst Rev. 2015;1

16. Ahmad B, Patel BC. Herpes simplex keratitis. In: StatPearls. Treasure Island, FL: StatPearls; 2020.
17. White ML, Chodosh J. Herpes simplex virus keratitis: a treatment guideline. Hoskins Centers Compendium of Evidence-Based Eye Care. http://www.aao.org/clinical-statement/herpes-simplex-virus-keratitis-treatment-guideline. 2014.
18. Rowe AM, St Leger AJ, Jeon S, Dhaliwal DK, Knickelbein JE, Hendricks RL. Herpes keratitis. Prog Retin Eye Res. 2013;32:88–101.
19. Wilhelmus KR, Gee L, Hauck WW, Kurinij N, Dawson CR, Jones DB, Barron BA, Kaufman HE, Sugar J, Hyndiuk RA, Laibson PR. Herpetic Eye Disease Study: a controlled trial of topical corticosteroids for herpes simplex stromal keratitis. Ophthalmology. 1994;101(12):1883–96.
20. Kaufman HE, Kanai A, Ellison ED. Herpetic iritis: demonstration of virus in the anterior chamber by fluorescent antibody techniques and electron microscopy. Am J Ophthalmol. 1971;71(2):465–9.
21. Robin JB, Steigner JB, Kaufman HE. Progressive herpetic corneal endotheliitis. Am J Ophthalmol. 1985;100:336.
22. Sugar A, Smith T. Presumed autoimmune corneal endotheliopathy. Am J Ophthalmol. 1982;94:689.
23. Khodadoust AA, Attarzadeh A. Presumed autoimmune corneal endotheliopathy. Am J Ophthalmol. 1982;93(6):718–22.
24. Sacchetti M, Lambiase A. Diagnosis and management of neurotrophic keratitis. Clin Ophthalmol. 2014;8:571–9. https://doi.org/10.2147/OPTH.S45921. PMID: 24672223; PMCID: PMC3964170.
25. Zamani M, Panahi-Bazaz M, Assadi M. Corneal collagen cross-linking for treatment of non-healing corneal ulcers. J Ophthalmic Vis Res. 2015;10(1):16–20. https://doi.org/10.4103/2008-322X.156087. PMID: 26005547; PMCID: PMC4424712.
26. Miller D, Alfonso EC. Management of fungal keratitis: Topical or Systemic therapy? Vis Pan Am Pan Am J Ophthalmol. 2014;13(3):73–7.
27. Lai J, Pandya V, McDonald R, Sutton G. Management of Fusarium keratitis and its associated fungal iris nodule with intracameral voriconazole and amphotericin B. Clin Exp Optom. 2014;97(2):181–3.
28. Ansari Z, Miller D, Galor A. Current thoughts in fungal keratitis: diagnosis and treatment. Curr Fungal Infect Rep. 2013;7(3):209–18.
29. Rogers GM, Goins KM, Sutphin JE, Kitzmann AS, Wagoner MD. Outcomes of treatment of fungal keratitis at the University of Iowa Hospitals and Clinics: a 10-year retrospective analysis. Cornea. 2013;32(8):1131–6.
30. Lorenzo-Morales J, Khan NA, Walochnik J. An update on Acanthamoeba keratitis: diagnosis, pathogenesis and treatment. Parasite. 2015;22:10. https://doi.org/10.1051/parasite/2015010. Epub 2015 Feb 18. PMID: 25687209; PMCID: PMC4330640.
31. Lorenzo-Morales J, Martín-Navarro CM, López-Arencibia A, Arnalich-Montiel F, Piñero JE, Valladares B. Acanthamoeba keratitis: an emerging disease gathering importance worldwide? Trends Parasitol. 2013;29(4):181–7.
32. Rama P, Matuska S, Viganò M, Spinelli A, Paganoni G, Brancato R. Bilateral Acanthamoeba keratitis with late recurrence of the infection in a corneal graft: a case report. Eur J Ophthalmol. 2003;13(3):311–4.
33. Hasika R, Lalitha P, Radhakrishnan N, Rameshkumar G, Prajna NV, Srinivasan M. Pythium keratitis in South India: Incidence, clinical profile, management, and treatment recommendation. Indian J Ophthalmol. 2019;67:42–7.
34. He H, Liu H, Chen X, Wu J, He M, Zhong X. Diagnosis and treatment of Pythium insidiosum corneal ulcer in a Chinese child: a case report and literature review. Am J Case Rep. 2016;17:982–8.
35. Gundersen T. Conjunctival flaps in the treatment of corneal disease with reference to a new technique of application. AMA Arch Ophthalmol. 1958;60(5):880–8.

36. Moorthy S, Jhanji V, Constantinou M, et al. Clinical experience with N-butyl cyanoacrylate tissue adhesive in corneal perforations secondary to herpetic keratitis. Cornea. 2010;29(9):971–5.
37. Brik D, Dunkel E, Pavan-Langston D. Persistent herpes simplex virus in the corneal stroma despite topical and systemic antiviral therapy. Arch Ophthalmol. 1994;111:522–7.
38. Deshmukh R, Stevenson LJ, Vajpayee R. Management of corneal perforations: An update. Indian J Ophthalmol. 2020;68(1):7.
39. Weiss JL, Williams P, Lindstrom RL, Doughman DJ. The use of tissue adhesive in corneal perforations. Ophthalmology. 1983;90(6):610–5.
40. Sandinha T, Zaher SS, Roberts F, Devlin HC, Dhillon B, Ramaesh K. Superior forniceal conjunctival advancement pedicles (SFCAP) in the management of acute and impending corneal perforations. Eye. 2006;20(1):84–9.
41. Sheha H, Liang L, Li J, Tseng SC. Sutureless amniotic membrane transplantation for severe bacterial keratitis. Cornea. 2009;28(10):1118.
42. Albini TA, Rao NA, Smith RE. The diagnosis and management of anterior scleritis. Int Ophthalmol Clin. 2005;45(2):191–204.
43. Jain V, Garg P, Sharma S. Microbial scleritis—experience from a developing country. Eye. 2009;23(2):255–61.
44. Ramenaden ER, Raiji VR. Clinical characteristics and visual outcomes in infectious scleritis: a review. Clin Ophthalmol (Auckland, NZ). 2013;7:2113.

8 Corneal Perforations

Amar Bhat and Vishal Jhanji

8.1 Introduction

Corneal perforations are emergencies that require prompt diagnosis and treatment. Corneal perforation is a full-thickness defect of the cornea that can arise from myriad causes. Corneal perforations can lead to significant ocular morbidity and prevention of perforation in at-risk eyes is of utmost importance. Corneal perforations can be broadly grouped into two categories: traumatic and non-traumatic. Traumatic causes of corneal perforation include penetrating trauma, chemical burns, surgical complications, and thermal injury. Traumatic corneal perforations are often amenable to surgical repair. Non-traumatic causes are varied and will be the focus of this chapter. Etiologies of non-traumatic corneal perforation can further be categorized into infectious and non-infectious causes. Non-infectious perforations can be secondary to autoimmune or inflammatory conditions, corneal degenerations or ectasia, ocular surface disease, neurotrophic keratopathy, or toxic causes.

8.2 Pathophysiology of Corneal Perforations

Most corneal perforations require epithelial defects to begin the process of corneal melting, or keratolysis. The process of keratolysis usually involves proteolytic enzymes such as matrix metalloproteinases that lead to the breakdown of the corneal stroma [1]. Occasionally, significant stromal lysis will lead to a *descemetocele*, where the remaining Descemet's membrane and endothelium begin to bulge forward. Descemetoceles can easily rupture with minimal trauma or straining, so

A. Bhat · V. Jhanji (✉)
University of Pittsburgh School of Medicine, Pittsburgh, PA, USA
e-mail: jhanjiv@upmc.edu

B. Sharma, J. S. Titiyal (eds.), *Corneal Emergencies*,
https://doi.org/10.1007/978-981-16-5876-1_8

counseling and prophylactic treatment are important if descemetoceles are noted on examination.

Owing to a multitude of natural defense mechanisms, the ocular surface is generally resistant to infection. The combination of the innate plus adaptive immune system and the anatomically protective ocular surface contribute to the eye's natural resilience [2]. Tears flush the eye of pathogens and contain protective components like immunoglobulins, lysozyme, and lactoferrin [3, 4]. The normal flora of the ocular surface may serve a protective role by secreting antibiotic-like substances or acidic metabolic waste products [5]. Eyes with a deficient corneal environment are at higher risk to develop microbial keratitis and hence, corneal perforation [6]. Ocular surface pathology in general also may contribute to collagenase activity that may lead to stromal melting [7].

8.3 Clinical History

Eliciting a good history from a patient is of paramount importance, as the clinical history may suggest a diagnosis that can guide treatment. In addition to determining the patient's symptoms (as discussed below), the provider should also discuss key aspects of the patient's medical and ocular history. Specifically, one should inquire about contact lens use, ocular trauma, prior eye surgery, eye drop use, prior herpetic infections, and dry eyes. Additionally, systemic history discussion should be tailored to the patient. For autoimmune corneal perforations, this may include history of joint pain, rashes, cold sores, dry mouth, immunosuppression, and family history of rheumatologic conditions. Diabetes is important systemic comorbidity to inquire about; not only may it contribute to neurotrophic keratopathy, but their blood sugar control may be affected if starting systemic steroids in autoimmune keratitis.

8.4 Symptoms

Patients with a corneal perforation most commonly report symptoms of pain, vision loss, redness, and tearing. Vision loss is the most often reported symptom. Typically, the "tearing" is an egress of aqueous fluid that the patient interprets as excessive tearing. Symptoms vary from patient to patient as the location and type of pathology may prevent the development of some symptoms. For example, a patient with a slow leak, a small peripheral perforation, and a deep chamber may be relatively asymptomatic. Additionally, patients with neurotrophic keratopathy may lack the pain that patients with normally innervated corneas may feel.

8.5 Signs

Corneal perforations often will display the same telltale signs in many eyes, but the entire anterior segment examination may help differentiate from the multitude of causes of corneal perforation. Prior to perforation, a cornea may display progressive

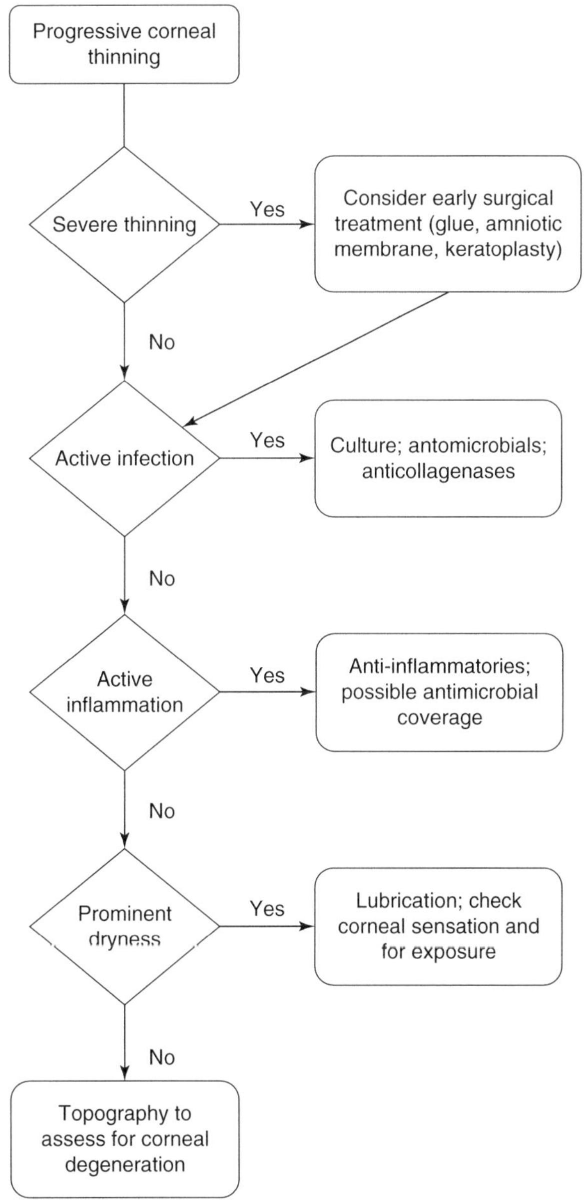

Fig. 8.1 Management of progressive corneal thinning

corneal thinning. Understanding the potential causes of progressive corneal thinning may help guide treatment, so the examiner should assess for severity of thinning, active infection, inflammation, or prominent dryness (Fig. 8.1). The presence of an infiltrate and hypopyon could suggest an infectious cause (or less likely an inflammatory cause) (Fig. 8.2). Peripheral thinning and perforation can suggest an autoimmune etiology, especially if the contralateral eye has signs of peripheral corneal thinning. Lid function is important to assess, as exposure to keratopathy from

Fig. 8.2 Slit lamp picture of paracentral bacterial corneal ulcer with 2 × 2 mm perforation in centre

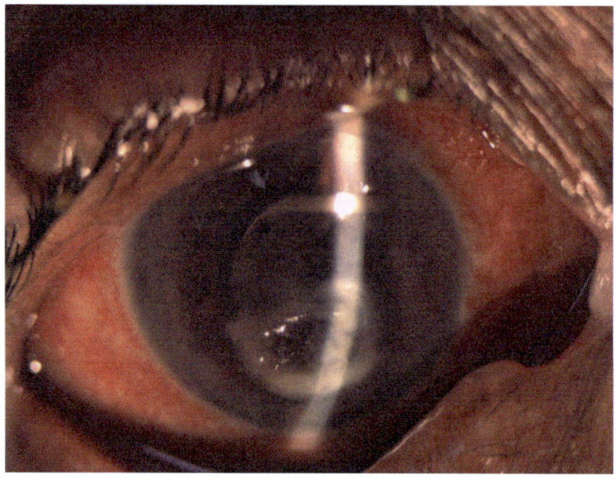

lagophthalmos can put a desiccated cornea at risk of perforation. Corneal hypoesthesia in addition to dryness would suggest neurotrophic keratopathy as a contributing factor.

A corneal perforation itself is best observed with a Seidel's test, the suspected area has fluorescein applied and is subsequently observed under the cobalt blue filter of a slit lamp for a leak. A positive Seidel test will appear as blue fluid moving down the cornea through the green-appearing tear film. Some corneal perforations may not have an obviously positive Seidel test. In cases where the perforation is suspected but the initial Seidel test is not conclusive, one can apply gentle pressure to the globe to see if a fluid egress can be elicited.

Other common signs in corneal perforation can include low intraocular pressure (IOP), a shallow or flat anterior chamber, and pigmentation at the wound. In practice, measurement of intraocular pressure is often deferred to prevent excessive pressure on the globe that could result in further outflow of aqueous fluid. If performed, rebound tonometry may be a safer option of IOP measurement compared to applanation tonometry since less pressure is exerted onto the globe. Pigmentation at the suspected area of the cornea is also suggestive of corneal perforation, as it indicates that iris likely made contact with that area of the cornea at some point. The presence of iris incarceration would be a more obvious sign of corneal perforation, and an iris plug may also result in a negative Seidel test.

8.6 Workup

The workup for any corneal perforation will depend on the constellation of history, signs, and symptoms. In a patient with concurrent infectious keratitis, gentle scraping and culture of the lesion should be performed to determine the infectious agent. The provider should submit to microbiology slides for Gram and Giemsa stains, plates of blood, chocolate, and Sabouraud dextrose agar for cultures, and thioglycolate broth. Drug sensitivities should be checked in the case of recalcitrant infectious keratitis and due to the increasing prevalence of methicillin-resistant *Staphylococcus aureus*. Calcofluor white can also be used to test for both fungi and *Acanthamoeba*. Plating on non-nutrient agar with *E. coli* overlay should be considered if the pre-test probability of *Acanthamoeba* is high. Suspected cases of herpes simplex or herpes zoster keratitis can have swabs taken for polymerase chain reaction (PCR), though clinical diagnosis alone may be sufficient for these. In contact lens wearers, contact lenses and cases should also be submitted to microbiology if available. Empiric therapy should be started prior to getting any culture results back.

Systemic workup (and later, treatment) can be co-managed by the patient's primary medical doctor or other specialists (most often a rheumatologist). Workup can be initiated when clinical suspicion of systemic autoimmune disease is high; this may include rheumatoid factor, SS-A and SS-B, ANA, ANCA, chest X-ray, ACE, RPR/FTA-ABS, or tuberculosis screening.

8.7 Causes of Corneal Perforations

8.7.1 Infectious Corneal Perforations

Bacterial, fungal, and viral keratitis have all been observed to cause corneal perforations. Severe infectious keratitis that is slow to or fails to respond to medical therapy is a common cause of corneal perforation. Infectious keratitis often results in stromal destruction of proteolytic enzymes, though direct destruction of infected keratocytes by cytotoxic T cells has also been reported in mice with herpetic keratitis [8–10].

8.7.1.1 Bacterial Keratitis

Bacteria is a common cause of infectious corneal perforations [11]. Although most bacteria require an epithelial defect to trigger the inflammatory cascade, some bacteria are reported to invade intact epithelium: *Neisseria gonorrheae* and *meningitidis*, *Haemophilus aegyptius*, *Shigella* species, *Corynebacterium diphtheriae* and *Listeria* species (mnemonic: *N*o *H*ard or *S*oft *C*ontact *L*enses). Once bacteria have bypassed the epithelium, pro-inflammatory cytokines lead to increased polymorphonuclear cell (PMN), macrophage, and T cell activity. Even with the appropriate treatment of bacteria, the abundance of cytokines can lead to progressive corneal thinning, melting, and perforation. Proteolytic activity from collagenases can be increased during infection from certain bacteria, most notably *Pseudomonas*.

8.7.1.2 Fungal Keratitis

Fungal keratitis can be a potentially devasting condition, but its incidence has fortunately decreased over recent decades [12]. Fungal keratitis is more common in the developing world; climate and location play a role in fungal keratitis risk. Ocular trauma, especially with the vegetative matter, is another important risk factor in the development of fungal keratitis. While most fungal keratitis is secondary to filamentous fungi, immunocompromised patients may be more prone to yeast keratitis. Fungal keratitis often develops slower than bacterial keratitis, and low ocular penetration of antifungal therapy makes fungal keratitis more difficult to treat. Treatment failure rate is significantly high in fungal keratitis, with approximately a third of primary treatments failing [13]. The high rate of treatment failure leads to a high perforation rate and hence, the need for surgical intervention. *Fusarium* species was classically considered to cause fulminant keratitis that is high risk for perforation, though recent studies in India have demonstrated a higher risk with *Aspergillus* keratitis [14].

8.7.1.3 Viral Keratitis

Corneal perforations from viruses primarily are attributed to herpetic eye disease, classically herpes simplex virus (HSV) and varicella zoster virus (VZV) keratitis. Perforation may occur as a result of stromal destruction from activated lymphocytes, and active viral replication need not be present [9, 15]. Recurrent infections will prompt additional immune responses that can lead to further stromal destruction and corneal thinning, putting the eye at increased risk for perforation [16]. Neurotrophic keratopathy and persistent epithelial defects are additional risk factors for perforation that can be seen after HSV and VZV keratitis.

8.7.2 Non-Infectious Corneal Perforations

Non-infectious corneal perforations can be secondary to myriad causes and can be difficult to treat depending on the etiology. Causes include autoimmune or inflammatory conditions, corneal degenerations or ectasia, ocular surface disease, neurotrophic keratopathy, or toxic injury.

8.7.2.1 Autoimmune Conditions

Multiple autoimmune conditions that affect the cornea can predispose a cornea to perforation by way of causing corneal melting and/or peripheral ulcerative keratitis (PUK). These conditions include (but are not limited to): rheumatoid arthritis, granulomatosis with polyangiitis (GPA), temporal arteritis, polyarteritis nodosa, inflammatory bowel disease, systemic lupus erythematosus, Churg Strauss syndrome, relapsing polychondritis, and sarcoidosis [17]. Rheumatoid arthritis has been the most frequently reported cause of PUK, a rare inflammatory condition involving the juxta limbal cornea and sclera. Keratolysis in PUK may be due to the elevated matrix metalloproteinase-1 (MMP-1) to tissue inhibitor (TIMP-1) ratio [18]. A similar condition exists called Mooren'sulcer; Mooren's ulcer is considered idiopathic (though helminth and hepatitis C associations have been reported), and sclera is usually not involved. The presence of a non-infectious corneal melt with a suspected autoimmune cause should always prompt systemic workup, as an untreated systemic disease may be a cause for patient mortality.

8.7.2.2 Ocular Surface Disease

Conditions that disrupt the natural protective barriers of the ocular surface will predispose the cornea to keratolysis, thinning, and potentially perforation. Dry eye syndrome can contribute to poor healing of the ocular surface and hence increase the probability of corneal perforation. The cause of dryness should be investigated, as exposure to keratopathy or toxic surface disease from eye drops (medicamentosa) may be quickly treatable. Corneal melts have been seen with both topical nonsteroidal anti-inflammatory drug (NSAID) use and topical anesthetic abuse.

Neurotrophic keratopathy is another cause of ocular surface disease, as the change in neuromodulator levels on the ocular surface results in abnormal epithelial healing and metabolism [19]. Early recognition of neurotrophic keratopathy is important, as protective responses of the eye (blinking and reactive ptosis) may be blunted, leading to desiccation of the cornea and accelerated keratolysis. If corneal hypoesthesia is noted, one should inquire about prior herpetic infection, prior eye surgery, topical medication use, and history of diabetes.

8.7.2.3 Corneal Degenerations or Ectasias

Corneal degenerations and ectasias may result in profound corneal thinning that increases the risk of corneal perforation with minimal trauma. Keratoconus, pellucid marginal degeneration, post-LASIK ectasia, and Terrien's marginal degeneration have all been seen in conjunction with corneal perforations. When severe thinning is noted in patients with these conditions, patients should be discouraged from rubbing their eyes and to generally be cautious with their eyes to prevent a corneal perforation.

8.8 Management of Corneal Perforations

Treatment of corneal perforations is varied and depends on multiple factors, including the cause and size of perforation (Fig. 8.3). The management can be broadly categorized into non surgical and surgical treatment. Non surgical treatment varies

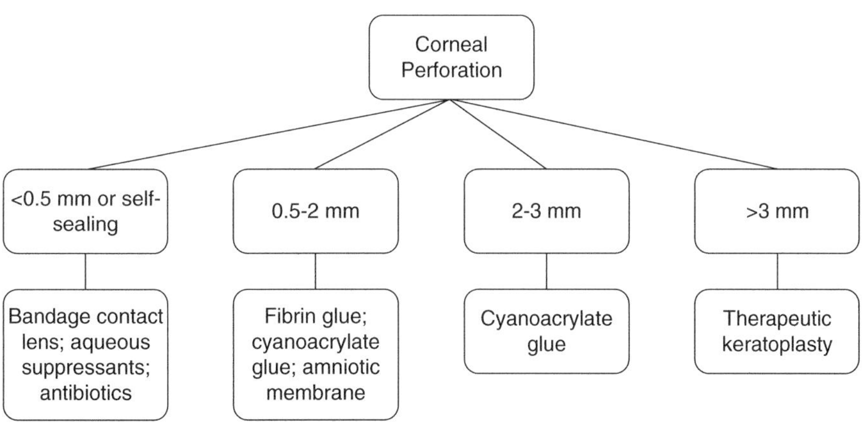

Fig. 8.3 Management of corneal perforations with regards to size of defect

from medical treatment such as antibiotics and antivirals to placement of bandage contact lenses. Surgical treatment includes placement of amniotic membranes, corneal gluing, conjunctival flaps, and corneal transplantation. Many of the non-surgical treatments discussed below are to help decrease the chance of perforation in patients at risk. Often times, the surgical and non-surgical treatments described may be useful in delaying, but not preventing, future keratoplasty.

8.8.1 Non-surgical Treatment

Non-surgical treatment of corneal perforations is primarily directed at treating the underlying cause of the perforation. Infectious keratitis requires timely medical treatment prior to surgical intervention, as surgical intervention will be more successful in an eye with a fully treated infection.

8.8.1.1 Lubricating Treatments

Indication

Aggressive lubrication is often required to prevent a perforation in cases where corneal desiccation is the primary driving force behind keratolysis. Maintenance of a consistent tear film is important in corneal healing. In exposure keratopathy and neurotrophic keratopathy, where corneas may not receive adequate coverage and lubrication from the eyelid, aggressive lubrication is an important step in preventing further corneal thinning. Therapies to lubricate the cornea can work via three different routes: increase the body's production of tears, decrease the outflow of tears, or supply lubrication from an external source (artificial tears, for example).

Technique

The most common first treatment involves supplying topical lubrication through artificial tears, gels, or ointments. Patients with good vision in the affected eye may prefer eye drops to gels or ointments but must be counseled that drops have to be used much more often. Drops should be used every 1–2 h, and hence should be preservative free to prevent secondary toxicity from preservatives. In contrast, gels can be used once every 2–4 h, and ointments can be used every 2–12 h depending on the severity of the disease. Gel or ointment should be used at night time to prevent overnight dryness, especially in cases with lagophthalmos or floppy eyelid syndrome. Autologous serum tears are another great option for providing lubrication as well as nutrients to the cornea that may accelerate healing—autologous tears are often started every 2–4 h initially, and preservative-free tears can be used as needed between serum drop administration.

Decreasing tear outflow is primarily accomplished with punctal plugs and punctal cautery. Temporary or dissolvable punctal plugs are usually a fair first option for treatment, though patients with very severe disease may prompt the physician to start with permanent plugs. Punctal cautery or surgical closure of puncta are other options in severe disease but may also be used when patients cannot receive plugs due to unique anatomical considerations or from adverse effects from plugs such as canaliculitis.

Increasing tear production in the short term is difficult to accomplish as topical formulations of cyclosporine A and lifitegrast take may take months to increase tear production. However, cyclosporine is also a steroid-sparing anti-inflammatory medication that may help prevent a perforation in certain inflammatory conditions by immunosuppressive mechanisms.

8.8.1.2 Antimicrobials

Indication

The presence of significant thinning in the setting of bacterial keratitis should prompt early and aggressive antibiotic therapy to decrease the bacterial load. Proliferation of bacteria can allow further collagenase and hence keratolytic activity.

Technique

Topical fourth-generation fluoroquinolone monotherapy (moxifloxacin 0.5%, frequency may vary between hourly around the clock to four times a day) is often sufficient for many cases of bacterial keratitis, including methicillin-resistant *Staphylococcal aureus* (MRSA) keratitis; however, escalation to fortified antibiotics should not be delayed if there is a poor clinical response to the fluoroquinolone [20]. Drug sensitivities from corneal cultures are of great importance if the ulcer is recalcitrant so that therapy can be adjusted as needed.

Antiviral treatment is primarily used in cases where herpetic stromal keratitis is suspected. Acyclovir (400–800 mg five times daily) and valacyclovir (500–1000 mg three times daily) are commonly used oral antivirals to treat active herpetic infection and decrease recurrences of herpes simplex keratitis. Topical antiviral formulations include trifluridine eye drops and ganciclovir gel (ganciclovir gel 0.15% five times daily); the primary limitations of these are toxicity of trifluridine and cost or availability of ganciclovir gel. More aggressive antiviral treatment should be considered in cases of necrotizing herpetic stromal keratitis. In necrotizing herpetic stromal keratitis, active viral replication is suspected to be present, and hence suppression of viral replication with antivirals is critical to minimize the risk of perforation. Antifungal and antiparasitic treatments are typically not empirically initiated unless there is a very high index of suspicion or if previous antimicrobial treatment has failed.

8.8.1.3 Anti-collagenases

Indication

Progressive keratolysis is often secondary to activated collagenases, so retarding or halting collagenase activity could help prevent a perforation in some patients.

Technique

Oral doxycycline (100 mg twice daily) is the most commonly prescribed medication that has anti-collagenase activity by exerting its effect on matrix metalloproteinases by chelating metal ions [21]. Some success has been seen using oral doxycycline to stabilize epithelial breakdown and prevent subsequent perforation [22]. Although not commonly used, topical acetylcysteine and ethyl enediamine tetraacetic acid (EDTA) have also been found to inhibit collagenase activity and may have some role in delaying or preventing corneal perforation [23, 24].

8.8.1.4 Aqueous Suppressants

Indication

Aqueous suppressants should be reserved for small (<0.5 mm) or self-sealing corneal perforations where re-epithelialization and closure of the perforation can occur quicker.

Technique

In patients with a formed anterior chamber, the combination of a bandage soft contact lens and a topical or systemic aqueous suppressant may promote wound healing and decrease efflux of intraocular contents through the perforation. Commonly used topical aqueous suppressants for corneal perforation include: timolol 0.5% twice daily, or once daily if gel-forming solution; brinzolamide 1% twice daily; dorzolamide 2% twice daily.

Systemic aqueous suppression can be achieved using acetazolamide extended-release capsules (500 mg twice daily) or, if not extended release, acetazolamide tablets (250–500 mg four times daily). If using systemic aqueous suppression with acetazolamide, additional topical carbonic anhydrase inhibitors (brinzolamide and dorzolamide) are unlikely to help further.

8.8.1.5 Anti-Inflammatories

Indication

Primary inflammation of the cornea or inflammation in the cornea secondary to the original insult contributes to keratolysis and the risk of perforation.

Technique

In bacterial keratitis, it is appropriate to start topical corticosteroids if the cultures were done and the organism and its drug sensitivities have been identified. Typically, corticosteroids should only be started at least 2 days after the appropriate antimicrobial has been started. Choice of steroid may vary depending on concurrent risk factors and severity of inflammation. Fluorometholone (0.1% or 0.25%) or loteprednol (0.38% or 0.5%) may be used when there is a history of steroid-induced ocular hypertension and the inflammation is not aggressive. Prednisolone acetate 1% used four times daily is a common first-line therapy. More frequent use of prednisolone (i.e., every 2 h) or more potent steroids such as Difluprednate 0.05% (4–6 times daily) can be considered when inflammation is severe or recalcitrant. Steroids should be tapered when inflammation has subsided; a weekly taper is commonly done, though slower tapers may be necessary if inflammation recurs.

Active herpes simplex epithelial keratitis is a contraindication to starting topical corticosteroids; however, topical corticosteroids in herpes simplex stromal keratitis helps shorten the duration and slows the progression of keratitis [25]. Contact lens wear or trauma with the vegetative matter may hint at potential fungal keratitis where topical corticosteroids should be avoided.

In contrast, primary inflammatory conditions of the cornea may prompt early anti-inflammatory therapy. Conditions such as Mooren ulcer and peripheral ulcerative keratitis may benefit from early steroid treatment even in the presence of an epithelial defect. Antibiotic coverage is often prescribed simultaneously as a safety measure to prevent subsequent infection. Systemic steroids may also be necessary for some recalcitrant noninfectious inflammatory conditions.

Systemic immunosuppression in the form of steroid-sparing agents is warranted in patients that require maintenance therapy to prevent "flare-ups." Oral cyclosporine A has also been used with success in peripheral ulcerative keratitis [26]. Topical cyclosporine A 2% and 0.5% has been reported in some studies to help stop keratolysis with corneal inflammation in collagen vascular diseases [27].

8.8.1.6 Bandage Contact Lens

Bandage contact lenses play an important role in both the prevention and treatment of many types of corneal perforations. They may be placed when there is an impending perforation, as a safeguard while the primary pathology is being treated. They may also supplement therapies such as amniotic membranes or gluing. Finally, for small perforations (<0.5 mm), the combination of a bandage contact lens with aqueous suppressants may be sufficient to treat the perforation.

8.8.2 Surgical Treatment

Other than keratoplasty, most of the below surgical treatments are aimed at delaying corneal transplantation or preventing a perforation. Surgical treatment includes corneal gluing, amniotic membranes, conjunctival flaps, tarsorrhaphy, tenon's patch graft, and keratoplasty.

8.8.2.1 Corneal Gluing

Indication

The primary benefit of corneal gluing is its ability to delay the need for corneal transplantation in perforations <3 mm in size. (Fig. 8.4) Delaying corneal transplantation allows surgery to be performed on an eye that is less inflamed or with a lower infectious burden on the cornea. Differences between the two most common types of corneal glue (cyanoacrylate and fibrin) are discussed below.

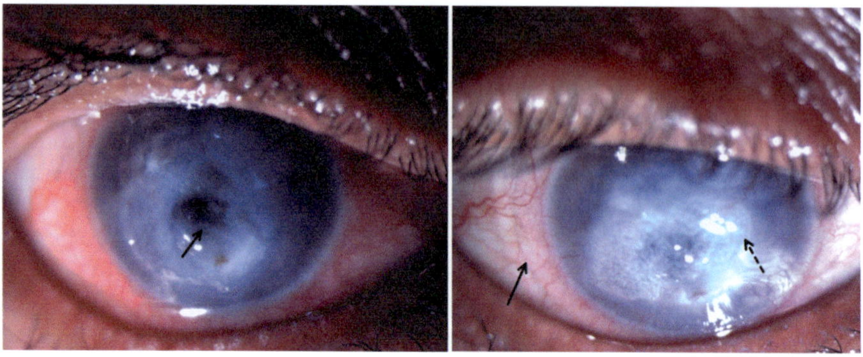

Fig. 8.4 Slit lamp picture with central perforation. Note the Cyanoacrylate glue in situ with bandage contact lens

Technique

Various successful techniques for gluing the cornea have been described. In general, the surgeon should first dry the wound and then use as little glue as possible to seal the wound and stop the leak. The wound must be dried well prior to application of the glue, as moisture in the wound greatly decreases the adhesion of the glue. Care must be taken to not drop any additional cyanoacrylate glue onto the conjunctiva or eyelids, as this can lead to significant irritation. Using a minimal amount of glue is important for multiple reasons: (1) glue that bulges anteriorly may cause more foreign body sensation and may be more prone to becoming dislodged; (2) glue does not adhere well to epithelium, so if too much glue is applied, great adhesion may not be obtained if the outer ring of glue is touching epithelium; (3) if too much glue is used and becomes dislodged, repeated applications may destabilize the wound, worsen the epithelial defect, or even increase the size of the perforation.

One technique for gluing involves the use of a sterile disposable drape. Gluing should be performed in sterile conditions, and a microscope is beneficial for visualization. A dermatological punch can be used to punch out a disc from a sterile disposable drape—usually a 2 mm punch is sufficient, but this can be adjusted based on the size of the perforation. This disc can then be placed on top of a cellulose eye spear or cotton tip applicator that has a small amount of sterile ophthalmic ointment on it. Once this has been prepared, attention can be turned to the eye. After topical anesthesia is obtained, a non-compressing lid speculum should be placed in the eye. Cellulose eye spears or jewelers forceps can be used to carefully debride 1–2 mm of epithelium around the perforation to improve adhesion. Vitreous should be cut if present at the wound. The wound should be dried completely using the cellulose eye spear or cotton tip applicator. Depending on the stability of the globe, any incarcerated tissue in the wound can be separated from the wound using air, viscoelastic devices, or simply mechanical separation. One small drop of adhesive can then be placed on the dry side of the previously made disc of sterile drape. The attached cotton tip applicator or cellulose eye spear can then be used to place the disc onto the cornea, with the glue facing the perforation. Polymerization can occur in seconds to minutes. The wound can be re-checked for a leak at this point; if still leaking, the glue can be revised or replaced at this time. Once the glue has solidified, a bandage contact lens can be placed over the eye. The patient should be checked at least 30 min after the procedure to check the positioning of the glue and deepening of the anterior chamber.

Outcomes

An early study of corneal gluing noted lower enucleation rates in non-traumatic corneal perforations compared to treatment with other modalities [28]. Despite the efficacy in stopping leaks, corneal glue is primarily a temporizing treatment [29]. Glue may be the definitive treatment in small, peripheral perforations, but most patients with central perforations will still require keratoplasty in the future. If glue fails to seal the wound, then repeat gluing or therapeutic keratoplasty may be the next step. One study demonstrated poor success (37% of eyes) of gluing in herpetic keratitis perforations, but gluing is still a valid first surgical management even for such eyes [8].

The two most common glues used in corneal perforations are cyanoacrylate glue and fibrin glue. Cyanoacrylate glue is nonbiodegradable, resulting in a longer presence on the cornea, and has some bacteriostatic properties, which may help its efficacy in perforations in bacterial keratitis. Due to its rough edges that do not degrade and smoothen over time, cyanoacrylate glue leads to increased foreign body sensation after it falls off. Additionally, cyanoacrylate glue has been reported to be pro-inflammatory, sometimes inducing necrosis and neovascularization of the cornea. Other complications that have been reported in association with cyanoacrylate glue include cataract, glaucoma, worsening of keratitis, and symblepharon, among others [30].

In contrast, fibrin glue (containing fibrinogen and thrombin) is both biodegradable and biocompatible, resulting in faster healing of the cornea. Minimal adverse reactions and inflammation have been seen with fibrin glue. Due to its biocompatibility, fibrin glue may also be injected intracamerally to help seal defects without apparent toxicity [31].

Potential downsides to fibrin glue include the shortened duration of the glue on the cornea (as it dissolves over time), the lack of bacteriostatic properties, and a significantly longer time for adhesive plug formation [32]. For defects up to 2 mm, the efficacy of fibrin glue appears similar to cyanoacrylate glue; for defects between 2 and 3 mm, cyanoacrylate glue appears superior. Fibrin glue has also been successfully used in conjunction with amniotic membrane transplantation, discussed later in this chapter.

8.8.2.2 Tenon's Patch Graft

Tenon's patch graft is an effective technique to manage corneal perforations between 3 and 6 mm in size using autologous Tenons tissue. A thin layer of Tenon's layer is harvested from the patient's own eye which is used as a scaffold to close the perforation (Fig. 8.5).

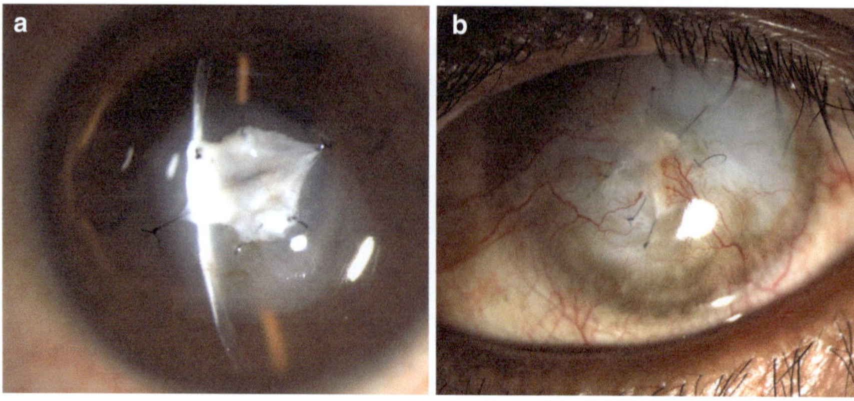

Fig. 8.5 Slit lamp picture (**a**) showing leucomatous corneal opacity with central perforation sized 2 * 3 mm with sutured Tenon's patch graft in situ. Subsequent postoperative picture (**b**) showing healed perforation with the formation of vascularised leucomatous corneal opacity. (Image courtesy Dr. Prafulla K Maharana; RP Centre for Ophthalmic Sciences AIIMS New Delhi)

Technique

Tenons capsule can be harvested about 2 mm posterior to the limbus. The superficial conjunctiva in the inferonasal or inferotemporal quadrant about 2 mm behind the limbus is incised to expose the underlying Tenon's capsule. The desired size of Tenon's capsule is excised and placed out on a flat plate. The graft should be slightly oversized than the corneal defect. Any debris over the corneal surface and surrounding the corneal perforation is cleared off followed by removing about 2 mm of epithelium around the perforation.

The Tenons graft is placed over the perforation and overlapping the edges of the corneal defect. If the edges of graft get rolled at the margin, they can be teased to open with the help of blunt cannula. The graft can be adhered to the application site with the help of fibrin glue or by 10'O suture. Cyanoacrylate glue is applied to the edge of the graft followed by putting a bandage contact lens over the surface.

8.8.2.3 Keratoplasty

Indication

Corneal transplantation is the definitive treatment for the majority of perforations, and therapeutic keratoplasty may be indicated in large perforations (>3 mm) that may not be amenable to gluing. The size and location of the perforation along with the underlying corneal pathology will dictate what method of keratoplasty may be best for the situation. Keratoplasty can be penetrating (full-thickness) or lamellar (partial thickness), small diameter (tectonic or patch graft) or large diameter, central or peripheral, and therapeutic (provide stabilization of globe or decrease infective burden) or optical (to improve vision). Graft survival and clarity is improved if surgery could be delayed for both traumatic and infectious perforations [33].

Technique

This chapter will not focus on in-depth techniques of keratoplasty in general, but rather some pearls to consider when planning for or performing keratoplasty on eyes with corneal perforations.

Lamellar keratoplasty is typically preferred over penetrating keratoplasty in cases of descemetocele or 2–3 mm size perforations. Partial thickness transplantation avoids the potential risk of endothelial rejection, which is often a harbinger of failure in keratoplasty. Penetrating keratoplasty may be essential for large (>2–3 mm) perforations, small perforations with surrounding tissue necrosis, or for significant infectious keratitis. Preservation of the patient's limbus is critically important. When a large portion of the cornea is affected by the pathology, the surgeon should ideally preserve at least a portion of the host limbus. This may require grafting off-center so that the area with more pathology can be covered to the limbus, while the unaffected side retains its limbus.

Tectonic keratoplasties, or patch grafts, can be temporizing or definitive treatments depending on the pathology (Figs. 8.6 and 8.7). In a small peripheral perforation, patch grafts are more likely to serve as a definitive treatment. Some peripheral corneal issues may require a crescentic graft rather than a circular graft. Tectonic keratoplasties can be lamellar or penetrating and have even been used to patch areas of scleral thinning. In central perforations, patch grafts are usually temporary until a later optical penetrating keratoplasty can be performed when the eye is stable and quiet. Because tectonic grafting is typically performed as a temporizing measure or for peripheral defects, surgeons have the choice to use grafts that are preserved differently. Traditional corneal grafts are preserved in media such as Optisol; however, glycerin-preserved, cryopreserved and gamma-irradiated corneal tissue can be used in tectonic grafting. These alternative methods of preservation allow the use of

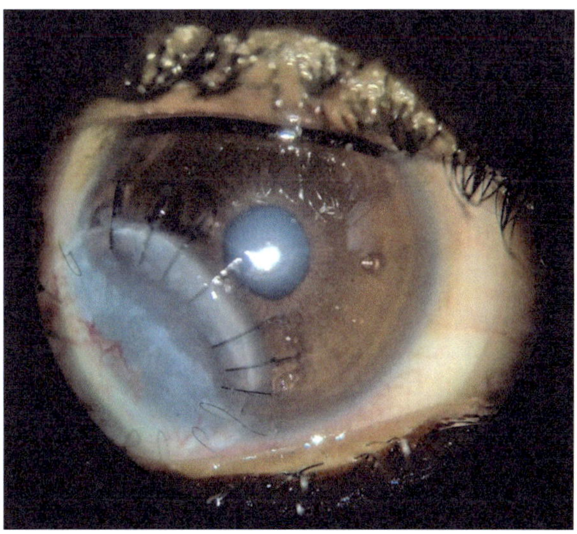

Fig. 8.6 Slit lamp picture showing peripheral patch graft done in corneal perforation secondary to peripheral ulcerative keratitis

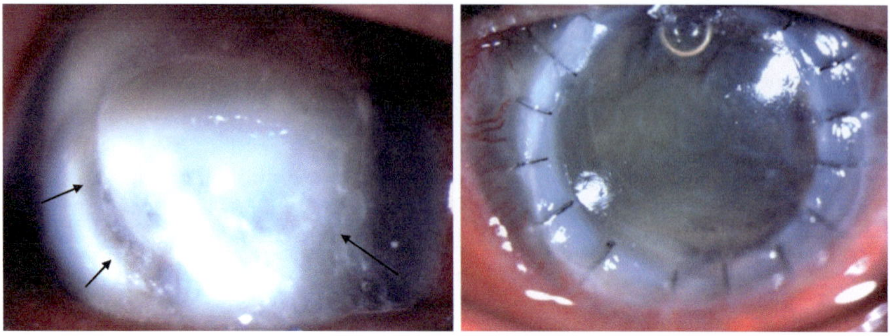

Fig. 8.7 Total penetrating keratoplasty done in sloughing corneal ulcer involving more than three quarters of the cornea

otherwise nonviable tissues (i.e., without fresh endothelium) and allows prolonged storage of the tissues for use in emergency surgery [34].

During surgery, the corneal button excision should remove all necrotic or diseased tissue, but in some cases this may not be possible. Care should be taken to debride any additional necrotic or melting corneal tissue outside of the trephinated area, as this will decrease the stability of sutures over time. Ideally, suture passes may need to incorporate sclera if the pathology is near the limbus and the peripheral cornea's integrity is diminished. If scleral bites are needed for stability, peritomy prior to passing those sutures should be performed so that appropriate suture tension can be achieved.

In eyes that have already perforated that are not holding pressure, it may be difficult to trephinate into the cornea. Viscoelastic can be injected into the anterior chamber to provide some intraocular pressure to trephinate and cut against; alternatively, fibrin glue has been injected intracamerally to provide stabilization during trephination [35].

Outcomes

Although emergent therapeutic keratoplasty can help stabilize the globe and potentially prevent enucleation or evisceration, the optical outcome and survival of these grafts is inferior to those when keratoplasty could be safely delayed. A second keratoplasty is often necessary after an emergent therapeutic keratoplasty to provide the desired optical outcome.

Some complications from keratoplasty include persistent epithelial defects, cataract, ulceration, epithelial keratopathy, and graft rejection. There is always a possibility of the need for repeat keratoplasty or other surgery, though this risk is increased in eyes that underwent urgent or emergent (rather than delayed) keratoplasty.

8.8.2.4 Amniotic Membranes

Indication

Amniotic membrane transplantation has proven to be an efficacious way to treat small corneal perforations since it was first used to treat epithelial defects in 1997 [36]. Amniotic membranes are rich in growth factors and cytokines that are thought to promote healing and they have been used to treat numerous ocular surface disorders (Fig. 8.8). Although often reserved for smaller defects, some amniotic membrane transplantation techniques have been successful in treating perforations up to 2–3 mm in diameter. Amniotic membranes come in fresh frozen and dry preserved variants.

Technique and Outcomes

Numerous surgical techniques have been described since the introduction of amniotic membranes as treatment for corneal perforations. As surgical techniques have been refined, amniotic membrane transplantation procedures have been reported to be very successful in perforations <3 mm. A 2016 study described a technique where 100% of corneal perforations (46 eyes) up to 3 mm in diameter were successfully treated [37]. The techniques suggested by the author vary depending on the size of the perforation. In larger perforations, a 2x4 mm rectangle is amniotic membrane is rolled up and plugged into the wound, and then another bilayered (folded onto itself) amniotic membrane is placed on top of the roll, with the epithelial side up. This bilayer membrane is sutured into place with interrupted 10-0 nylon sutures. A large amniotic membrane is sutured into position over the entire cornea using running 10-0 nylon sutures. Finally, 0.3 mL of 20% perfluoropropane (C_3F_8) is then injected intracamerally to reform the anterior chamber. For smaller perforations, the roll of the amniotic membrane is pushed into the defect and sutured using cross-stitch fixation. A similar technique using fibrin glue to help the amniotic membrane adhere was successful in repairing perforations up to 2 mm in diameter with overlying ulcers ranging from 2 to 5 mm in diameter [38].

8.8.2.5 Conjunctival Flaps

A multitude of conjunctival flaps have been used in eyes with corneal perforation or progressive corneal thinning, and their overall efficacy depends on the location of the perforation. Pedicle conjunctival flaps can be a useful technique for small, peripheral ulcers and perforations, as the overlying conjunctiva can provide serum growth

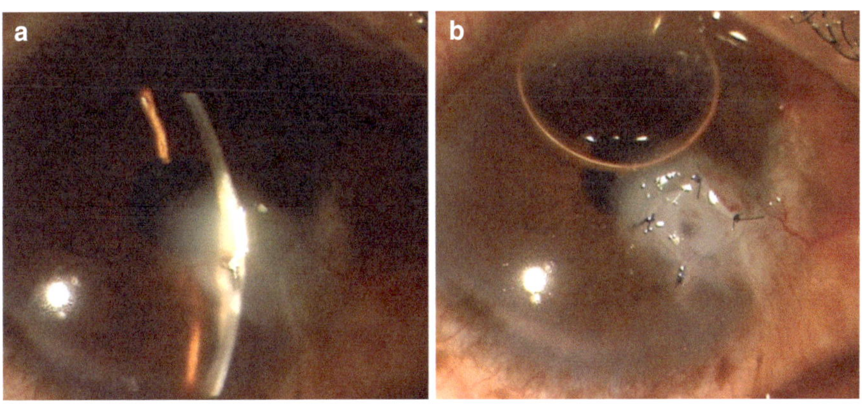

Fig. 8.8 Slit lamp picture (**a**) showing leucomatous corneal opacity with central perforation sized 2 × 1 mm, managed with appropriately sized multilayered amniotic membrane graft in situ (**b**). (Image courtesy Dr. Prafulla K Maharana; RP Centre for Ophthalmic Sciences AIIMS New Delhi)

factors to the cornea (via neovascularization) to facilitate healing. Covering the defect with the patient's own conjunctiva also provides a fair amount of analgesia for the patient. Despite positive results in healing persistent defects and neurotrophic ulcers, or sealing small perforations, neovascularization will increase the risk of potential graft rejection if required in the future [39]. Additionally, large conjunctival flaps that cover a central defect, such as a Gundersen flap, may result in a poor cosmetic result. For these reasons, conjunctival flaps for central perforations are less ideal than the aforementioned methods. Additionally, large conjunctival flaps that cover a central defect, such as a Gundersen flap, may result in a poor cosmetic result. Finally, in acutely worsening suppurative keratitis, perforations may continue to leak underneath the conjunctiva, increasing the risk for endophthalmitis and other complications. Other potential complications include flap dislocation and perforation.

Key Points

- Corneal perforations can be secondary to traumatic, infectious, and non-traumatic/non-infectious causes.
- Keratolysis, or corneal melting, usually involves proteolytic enzymes such as matrix metalloproteinases that lead to the breakdown of the corneal stroma.
- Neurotrophic keratopathy is an underdiagnosed cause of ocular surface disease that can lead to corneal perforation if not detected early.
- Non-surgical management of corneal perforations may include antimicrobials, anti-collagenases, anti-inflammatories, aqueous suppressants, and bandage contact lenses. Surgical management of corneal perforations may include gluing, keratoplasty, amniotic membrane, and conjunctival flaps.
- Cyanoacrylate glue is nonbiodegradable and has some bacteriostatic properties; however, it can cause foreign body sensation and is known to be pro-inflammatory. Fibrin glue is biodegradable and anti-inflammatory; limitations include a shorter duration of action, a longer time for plug formation, increased cost, and lack of bacteriostatic properties.
- A minimum amount of glue is required to seal a perforation; excessive glue can be irritating to the eye.
- Gluing is often a temporizing measure prior to keratoplasty, which is preferable to perform outside of the acute setting when the eye is less inflamed. Therapeutic keratoplasty is indicated in large perforations (>3 mm) that may not be amenable to gluing.
- Penetrating, lamellar, tectonic, and patch graft keratoplasties may all be used depending on the type, size, and location of perforation.

References

1. Hsu JK, Johnston WT, Read RW, McDonnell PJ, Pangalinan R, Rao N, Smith RE. Histopathology of corneal melting associated with diclofenac use after refractive surgery. J Cataract Refract Surg. 2003;29:250–6.

2. Chandler JW, Gillette TE. Immunologic defense mechanisms of the ocular surface. Ophthalmology. 1983;90:585–91.
3. Dawson CR. How does the external eye resist infection? Investig Ophthalmol. 1976;15:971.
4. Stuchell RN, Farris RL, Mandel ID. Basal and reflex human tear analysis. Ophthalmology. 1981;88:858.
5. Perkins RE, Kundsin RB, Pratt MV, Abrahamsen I, Leibowitz HM. Bacteriology of normal and infected conjunctiva. J Clin Microbiol. 1975;1:147–9.
6. Ormerod LD, Fong LP, Foster CS. Corneal infection in mucosal scarring disorders and Sjögren's syndrome. Am J Ophthalmol. 1988;105:512–8.
7. Kenyon KR. Decision-making in the therapy of external eye disease: noninfected corneal ulcers. Ophthalmology. 1982;89:44–51.
8. Moorthy S, Jhanji V, Constantinou M, Beltz J, Graue-Hernandez EO, Vajpayee RB. Clinical experience with N-butyl cyanoacrylate tissue adhesive in corneal perforations secondary to herpetic keratitis. Cornea. 2010;29:971–5.
9. Doymaz MZ, Foster CM, Destephano D, Rouse BT. MHC II-restricted, CD4+ cytotoxic T lymphocytes specific for herpes simplex virus-1: implications for the development of herpetic stromal keratitis in mice. Clin Immunol Immunopathol. 1991;61:398–409.
10. Hyndiuk RA. Experimental pseudomonas keratitis. Trans Am Ophthalmol Soc. 1981;79:541–624.
11. Hirst LW, Smiddy WE, Stark WJ. Corneal perforations: changing methods of treatment, 1960–1980. Ophthalmology. 1982;89:630–5.
12. Xie L, Zhai H, Shi W. Penetrating keratoplasty for corneal perforations in fungal keratitis. Cornea. 2007;26:158–62.
13. Lalitha P, Prajna NV, Kabra A, Mahadevan K, Srinivasan M. Risk factors for treatment outcome in fungal keratitis. Ophthalmology. 2006;113:526–30.
14. Prajna VN, Prajna L, Muthiah S. Fungal keratitis: the Aravind experience. Indian J Ophthalmol. 2017;65:912–9.
15. Cavanagh HD. Herpetic ocular disease: therapy of persistent epithelial defects. Int Ophthalmol Clin. 1975;15:67–88.
16. Foster CS, Duncan J. Penetrating keratoplasty for herpes simplex keratitis. Am J Ophthalmol. 1981;92:336–43.
17. Siracuse-Lee D, Saffra N. Peripheral ulcerative keratitis in sarcoidosis: a case report. Cornea. 2006;25:618–20.
18. Riley GP, Harrall RL, Watson PG, Cawston TE, Hazleman BL. Collagenase (MMP-1) and TIMP-1 in destructive corneal disease associated with rheumatoid arthritis. Eye (Lond). 1995;9:703–18.
19. Feroze KB, Patel BC. Neurotrophic keratitis. Treasure Island (FL): StatPearls Publishing; 2020.
20. Durrani AF, Atta S, Bhat AK, Mammen A, Dhaliwal D, Kowalski RP, Jhanji V. Methicillin-resistant staphylococcus aureus keratitis: initial treatment, risk factors, clinical features, and treatment outcomes. Am J Ophthalmol. 2020;214:119–26.
21. Smith VA, Cook SD. Doxycycline-a role in ocular surface repair. Br J Ophthalmol. 2004;88:619–25.
22. McElvanney AM. Doxycycline in the management of pseudomonas corneal melting: two case reports and a review of the literature. Eye Contact Lens. 2003;29:258–61.
23. Ramaesh T, Ramaesh K, Riley SC, West JD, Dhillon B. Effects of N-acetylcysteine on matrix metalloproteinase-9 secretion and cell migration of human corneal epithelial cells. Eye (Lond). 2012;26(8):1138–44.
24. Kessler E, Mondino BJ, Brown SI. The corneal response to pseudomonas aeruginosa: histopathological and enzymatic characterization. Invest Ophthalmol Vis Sci. 1977;16:116–25.
25. Wilhelmus KR, Gee L, Hauck WW, Kurinij N, Dawson CR, Jones DB, Barron BA, Kaufman HE, Sugar J, Hydiuk RA, et al. Herpetic eye disease study. A controlled trial of topical corticosteroids for herpes simplex stromal keratitis. Ophthalmology. 1994;101:1883–96.
26. Squirrell DM, Winfield J, Amos RS. Peripheral ulcerative keratitis 'corneal melt' and rheumatoid arthritis: a case series. Rheumatology (Oxford). 1999;38:1245–8.

27. Tatlipinar S, Akpek EK. Topical ciclosporin in the treatment of ocular surface disorders. Br J Ophthalmol. 2005;89:1363–7.
28. Hirst LW, Smiddy WE, De Juan E. Tissue adhesive therapy for corneal perforations. Aust J Ophthalmol. 1983;11:113–8.
29. Leahey AB, Gottsch JD, Stark WJ. Clinical experience with N-butyl cyanoacrylate (Nexacryl) tissue adhesive. Ophthalmology. 1993;100:173–80.
30. Jhanji V, Young AL, Mehta JS, Sharma N, Agarwal T, Vajpayee RB. Management of corneal perforation. Surv Ophthalmol. 2011;56:522–38.
31. Scalcione C, Ortiz-Vaquerizas D, Said D, Dua H. Fibrin glue as agent for sealing corneal and conjunctival wound leaks. Eye. 2018;32:463–6.
32. Sharma A, Kaur R, Kumar S, Gupta P, Pandav S, Patnaik B, Gupta A. Fibrin glue versus N-butyl-2-cyanoacrylate in corneal perforations. Ophthalmology. 2003;110:291–8.
33. Nobe JR, Moura BT, Robin JB, Smith RE. Results of penetrating keratoplasty for the treatment of corneal perforations. Arch Ophthalmol. 1990;108:939–41.
34. Lin H, Ong S, Chao A. Eye preservation tectonic graft using glycerol-preserved donor cornea. Eye. 2012;26:1446–50.
35. Por YM, Tan YL, Mehta JS, Tan DT. Intracameral fibrin tissue sealant as an adjunct in tectonic lamellar keratoplasty for large corneal perforations. Cornea. 2009;28:451–5.
36. Lee SH, Tseng SC. Amniotic membrane transplantation for persistent epithelial defects with ulceration. Am J Ophthalmol. 1997;123:303–12.
37. Fan J, Wang M, Zhong F. Improvement of amniotic membrane method for the treatment of corneal perforation. Biomed Res Int. 2016;2016:1693815.
38. Kim HK, Park HS. Fibrin glue-assisted augmented amniotic membrane transplantation for the treatment of large noninfectious corneal perforations. Cornea. 2009;28:170–6.
39. Deshmukh R, Stevenson LJ, Vajpayee R. Management of corneal perforations: an update. Indian J Ophthalmol. 2020;68:7–14.

Emergencies in Corneal Refractive Surgeries

9

Sridevi Nair, Manpreet Kaur, and Jeewan Singh Titiyal

9.1 Introduction

Cornea-based refractive surgeries are one of the most commonly performed surgical procedures for the correction of myopia, hypermetropia and astigmatism. The safety, efficacy and predictability of these surgeries are well-established with high levels of patient satisfaction. Rarely, corneal complications and emergencies may be observed in the intraoperative or postoperative period that require urgent intervention to prevent vision-threatening sequelae [1]. In this chapter we discuss the intraoperative and postoperative emergencies observed in association with various corneal refractive procedures along with their management and prevention.

9.2 Intraoperative Corneal Emergencies

Intraoperative corneal emergencies may be related to the application of suction during femtosecond-laser assisted refractive procedures, flap creation during laser-assisted in situ keratomileusis (LASIK), lenticule dissection during small-incision lenticule extraction (SMILE) or inadvertent corneal perforation during incisional surgeries or implant of intracorneal ring segments.

S. Nair · M. Kaur · J. S. Titiyal (✉)
Cornea, Cataract and Refractive Surgery Services, Dr R P Centre for Ophthalmic Sciences, All India Institute of Medical Sciences, New Delhi, India

B. Sharma, J. S. Titiyal (eds.), *Corneal Emergencies*,
https://doi.org/10.1007/978-981-16-5876-1_9

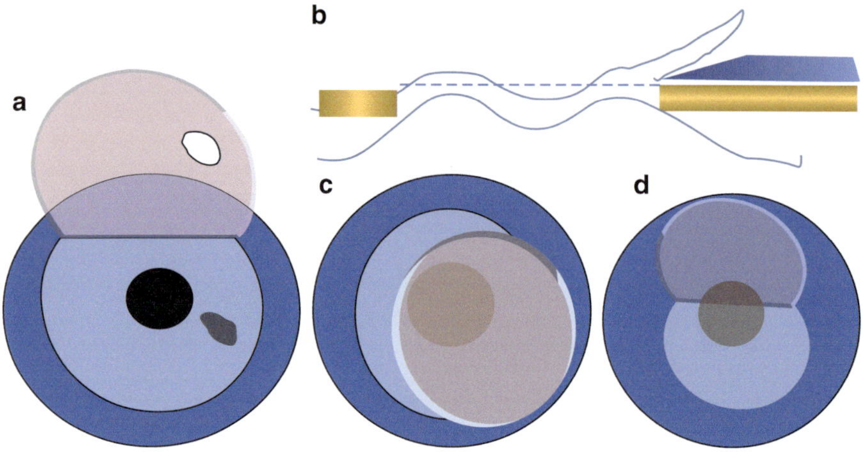

Fig. 9.1 Schematic diagram depicting the intraoperative flap complications commonly seen while using the microkeratome to create the LASIK flap. (**a**) Intraoperative flap buttonhole. (**b**) Buckling of the cornea under the microkeratome blade resulting in a flap buttonhole. (**c**) Intraoperative free Cap. (**d**) Intraoperative incomplete flap

9.2.1 Corneal Emergencies Related to Microkeratome-Flap Creation

Flap-related complications during LASIK are more commonly observed with the use of microkeratomes as compared with femtosecond laser. Free cap, incomplete flaps and buttonholes are corneal emergencies that may interfere with subsequent excimer laser ablation and adversely affect the anatomical integrity of the cornea and visual outcomes (Fig. 9.1) [1].

9.2.1.1 Incidence

An incomplete or partial flap formation is the most commonly seen intraoperative flap complication with an incidence ranging from 0.04% to 3.6% [2, 3]. The reported incidence of free caps during LASIK flap creation ranges from 0.08% to 4.9% [4]. Flap buttonholes are relatively uncommon and may be observed in 0.04–2.6% of cases [2, 3].

9.2.1.2 Risk Factors

Inadequate suction during the microkeratome pass may result in irregular flaps, buttonholes or free caps. Anatomical factors such as conjunctival chemosis, small palpebral fissure with inadequate exposure and deep-set eyes predispose to suction-related complications during microkeratome-assisted LASIK. In addition, patient factors such as excessively anxious, non-cooperative patients and surgeon factors related to lack of expertise, incorrect placement of the suction ring or inadvertent release of suction may lead to suction loss [5]. Machine and microkeratome malfunction including reduced motor power, blunt blades or jamming can predispose to flap-related complications. Extremes of keratometry predispose to flap irregularities, with free cap observed with flat corneas and buttonholes observed with excessively steep corneas. In addition, dry ocular surface, larger diameter flaps and use of same microkeratome for second eye surgery can result in flap irregularities and complications [6].

9.2.1.3 Diagnosis

The diagnosis of flap buttonholes, free cap and incomplete flaps is established clinically under the operating microscope. Flap buttonholes result from a superficial passage of the microkeratome blade which exits through the epithelium midway and appear as a doughnut-shaped flap. Incomplete flaps occur as a result of the microkeratome head not completing its full excursion. The flap appears smaller, with a hinge which is wider and situated closer to the centre than intended. A free cap may be observed lying on the corneal surface or jammed within the microkeratome blade head [1].

9.2.1.4 Treatment

Flap buttonholes, once detected, should not be lifted. The surgery is aborted, bandage contact lens (BCL) is placed to allow corneal healing and retreatment may be planned after at least 3 months to allow for refractive stabilization [5]. In case the flap edges are misaligned, the flap should be refloated and repositioned without disturbing the central area of uncut corneal tissue to ensure proper alignment of the flap buttonhole with the uncut corneal tissue.

Incomplete flap with hinge in periphery may not adversely affect the completion of the surgical procedure, and excimer laser ablation may be performed in the same sitting, either by shielding the hinge while performing the ablation, decreasing the size of the treatment zone or manually completing the lamellar dissection of the flap [6]. There is an increased risk of irregular corneal astigmatism in these cases. In case of an incomplete flap with a hinge lying within the central 5–6 mm of the cornea, the surgery should be aborted, flap carefully repositioned and retreatment planned after 3 months with a larger and thicker flap.

In patients with free caps, ablation may be performed if the area of the exposed stroma is larger than the intended optical zone (OZ). The cap is repositioned at the end of surgery, carefully aligned and a BCL is placed over the cornea. If the exposed stromal area is less than the OZ or the cap cannot be retrieved, the surgery is aborted, and retreatment planned after 3 months [7].

Customized ablation may often be required during retreatment owing to the significant incidence of irregular astigmatism in these cases.

9.2.1.5 Prevention

Proper patient counselling helps to ensure compliance during surgery and prevent patient-related complications. Ocular surface should be adequately hydrated to prevent dry spots. Flap creation may be avoided in cases with extremes of keratometry and a surface ablation may be preferred in those cases. Alternatively, femtosecond laser flaps may be created in difficult cases. Avoiding reuse of microkeratome blades, choosing an appropriately sized suction ring and regular servicing of the microkeratome to ensure proper functioning are essential to prevent machine-related complications.

9.2.2 Corneal Emergencies Related to Femtosecond-Laser Assisted Flap

Femtosecond laser is increasingly being employed to create corneal flaps during LASIK, owing to the enhanced predictability and safety. Flap irregularities, free caps and buttonholes conventionally observed with microkeratome-assisted flaps are not usually observed with femtosecond laser flaps; however, intraoperative complications such as suction loss and vertical gas breakthrough may be observed and require urgent management.

9.2.2.1 Suction Loss

Incidence

Intraoperative suction loss during femtosecond laser application may be observed in *0.2%–4.4%* of cases undergoing LASIK which leads to incomplete formation of the LASIK flap [8].

Risk Factors

Risk factors for intraoperative suction loss include an uncooperative, anxious patient with excessive head movement or forceful squeezing lids. In addition, anatomical factors including small palpebral apertures, deep-set eyes and flat keratometry (K-readings <42.00 D) predispose to suction loss. Excessive fluid in the conjunctival sac and improper placement of the suction ring can also interfere with adequate suction build-up and lead to complications [9].

Diagnosis

Intraoperative suction loss is observed as a halt of the femtosecond-laser raster progression with incomplete flap bed or side-cuts as a result of premature vacuum loss and separation of the applanation cone from the eye [8].

Treatment

The treatment strategy depends on the step at which suction loss occurred. When the suction loss occurs during the flap bed creation, it is advisable to reinitiate the treatment from the start with the same settings. In cases where it occurs during the side-cut creation only the side-cut programme need be reactivated after reducing the flap diameter by 0.5–1 mm [9]. The surgeon can redock and retreat in the same sitting using a new suction ring and the same cone.

Prevention

Preoperative patient counselling and adequate anesthesia ensure compliance during surgery and minimize complications related to patient movements. Preoperative testing and proper calibration of the machine is vital. Keeping the ocular surface optimally hydrated and maintaining adequate exposure of the eye is important.

9.2.2.2 Vertical Gas Breakthrough

Incidence

Femtosecond laser leads to the creation of cavitation bubbles at the site of laser application, which coalesce to form cleavage planes in the cornea. Vertical gas breakthrough occurs due to escape of cavitation gas bubbles from the intended laser dissection plane towards the subepithelial space and may be observed in 0.14% of cases undergoing LASIK (Fig. 9.2) [10].

Risk Factors

Thin flaps, stromal weakening or stromal scars at the level of the dissection plane, basement membrane dystrophy and focal defects in the Bowman's membrane predispose to the development of vertical gas breakthrough [10].

Diagnosis

Full-thickness vertical gas breakthrough constitutes a corneal emergency as the air bubble appears between the epithelium and applanation interface as a black spot, resulting in focal areas of uncut flap. A small buttonhole may be seen in the area of gas breakthrough.

Management

In cases with significant full-thickness vertical gas breakthrough involving the centre, it is advisable to abort the surgery and perform a repeat LASIK with a deeper cut or surface ablation after 3 months. When the area of vertical gas breakthrough is

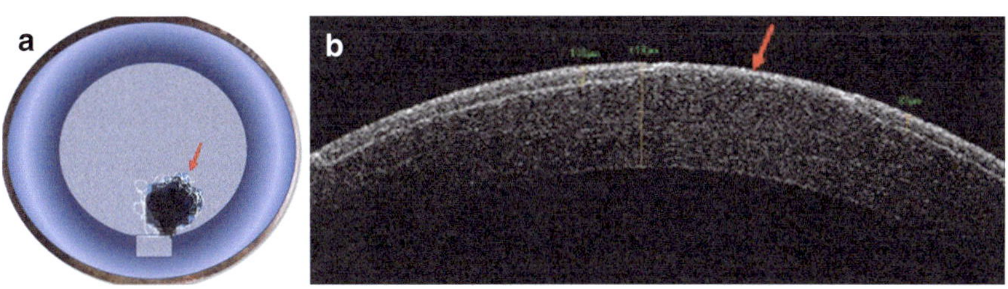

Fig. 9.2 (**a**) A schematic diagram depicting intraoperative vertical gas breakthrough (VGB) near the flap hinge (arrow). (**b**) Anterior Segment Optical Coherence Tomography showing a focal area of uncut flap corresponding to the location of the VGB (arrow)

small and peripheral, one may attempt to lift the flap by dissecting around it and proceed with the stromal ablation; however, there is a future risk of epithelial ingrowth [10].

Prevention

Preoperative assessment of corneal thickness with anterior segment optical coherence tomography (ASOCT) should be considered in cases such as corneal scars and basement membrane dystrophy to rule out corneal irregularities and focal thinning.

9.2.2.3 Flap Tears

Flap tears are more commonly observed with femtosecond-laser assisted LASIK as compared with microkeratome LASIK due to thinner femtosecond flaps with a higher incidence of adhesions and tissue bridges [11].

Incidence

The reported incidence of flap tear in FS-LASIK ranges from 0.4% to 0.5% of cases [11].

Risk Factors

Extremely thin flaps and persistent focal flap adhesions predispose to the development of an intraoperative flap tear. Inadvertent patient movement during flap lifting and improper surgical technique may also result in inadvertent flap tears. Laser systems using higher energy and lower frequency are more prone to develop persistent adhesions [8]. Excessive opaque bubble layer formation also causes difficulties during lamellar separation.

Diagnosis

A flap tear may be observed under the operating microscope while dissecting or lifting the flap and is often preceded by resistance due to its inadequate separation from the stromal bed. A complete tear at the hinge site results in a free cap.

Treatment

Surgery may be completed uneventfully in cases with small, peripheral tears by gently dissecting around the area involved. It is advisable to postpone the surgery in cases with large tears involving the pupillary area. The flap should be reposited carefully and a BCL placed over it. Customized surface ablation may be planned after 6–12 weeks [11].

Prevention

The flap should be adequately separated from the stromal bed before attempting to lift it. Caution should be exercised when dissecting thin flaps or flaps with extensive areas of adhesion.

9.2.3 Corneal Perforation During Excimer Laser Ablation

Intraoperative corneal perforation is an extremely rare corneal emergency that may be observed during excimer laser ablation in flap-based corneal ablative procedures. It characteristically presents with aqueous leakage during excimer laser application [12].

9.2.3.1 Risk Factors

Risk factors include thin residual stromal bed consequent to an excessively thick flap, excessive drying of the stromal bed and excimer laser machine malfunction causing repeated ablation at a single point [12].

9.2.3.2 Treatment

The procedure should be stopped immediately, and the flap should be reposited. Small perforations may be managed conservatively using a BCL and pressure patching. Sutures can be placed to better secure the flap and stop the aqueous leakage [12].

9.2.3.3 Prevention

Accurate preoperative pachymetry, preventing excessive drying of the stromal bed and proper preoperative excimer laser machine calibration help prevent intraoperative corneal perforation.

9.2.4 Lenticule Extraction Related Corneal Emergencies

Small-incision lenticule extraction involves the femtosecond-laser assisted creation of a refractive stromal lenticule which is then extracted via a small side-cut incision. The visual outcomes of SMILE are comparable to that of conventional corneal ablative procedures and there is no risk of flap-related complications. Intraoperative suction loss and lenticule mis-dissection are important corneal emergencies that may be observed during femtosecond laser application and subsequent dissection.

9.2.4.1 Suction Loss

Suction loss may occasionally be observed during femtosecond laser application and constitutes an emergency.

Incidence

The incidence of intraoperative suction loss ranges from 0.17% to 6.38% [13].

Risk Factors

Risk factors for intraoperative suction loss may be related to the patient cooperation, surgeon expertise, functioning of the machine and orbital anatomy. Patient-related factors include an anxious or uncooperative patient with excessive lid squeezing or head movements. Machine-related factors are longer suction time associated with SMILE and lower suction pressures. The patient interface 'acurvates' rather than applanates the cornea and is more prone to be disengaged with slight patient movements. Surgeon related factors are related to the learning curve, surgical expertise and improper docking technique. Anatomical factors include narrow palpebral apertures, deep sockets, excessively dry cornea, large cap diameter, large cylinder power and small corneal diameter.Loose conjunctival tissue and fluid ingress between the suction ports of the contact glass and the cornea may also lead to suction loss [14].

Diagnosis

A premature halt of the femto-laser application is seen when the patient interface is inadvertently disengaged from the patient's cornea during surgery.

Treatment

Management of the suction loss essentially depends on the stage at which it occurs. The 'Restart' treatment module in the Zeiss Visumax software is equipped to deal with such a scenario. In cases when suction loss occurs at <10% of the posterior lenticule cut, the surgery can be reinitiated from the start; however, in cases where more than 10% of posterior cut is completed it is advisable to abort the surgery. FS-LASIK may be attempted in the same sitting or retreatment may be planned after 6–12 weeks. If suction loss occurs during the lenticule side-cut, anterior cap-cut or the cap side-cut, the patient may be redocked and surgery continued from that particular step with minor modifications of the parameters. In cases where the procedure is re-started in the same sitting, the contact lens should be cleaned before re-docking. It is advisable to re-start the procedure as soon as possible before the reference bubble layer disappears [13].

Prevention

Preoperative calibration of the machine and choosing the correct contact lens as per the patient's corneal diameter should be ensured before starting the procedure. Proper patient counselling and positioning is imperative to ensure an uneventful surgery. The cornea should be optimally hydrated, and the speculum and drape should be applied in the correct fashion to ensure that the central field is free of any loose conjunctiva.

9.2.4.2 Lenticule Mis-Dissection and Cap-Lenticular Adhesion

Lenticule dissection and extraction is the most challenging step during SMILE and may be especially challenging for a novice surgeon.

Incidence

The reported incidence of difficult lenticule dissection varies from 1.8% to 9% and decreases with surgeon experience [15]. Lenticule mis-dissection with cap-lenticular adhesion requires timely diagnosis and urgent management to ensure optimal visual and anatomical outcomes.

Risk Factors

Risk factors for lenticule mis-dissection and cap-lenticule adhesion include surgeon related factors such as surgeon inexperience and incorrect surgical technique. Laser related factors such as low energy setting, dense opaque bubble layer and black spots can lead to increased microadhesions or insufficient lamellar separation. Thin lenticules usually seen in a lower refractive error patient are difficult to handle and have a higher risk of cap-lenticular adhesion, especially during the initial learning curve [16].

Diagnosis

Lenticule mis-dissection with a cap-lenticular adhesion may be challenging to diagnose. An ASOCT helps in the identification of the lamellar dissection planes and a hand-held OCT or intraoperative OCT is a useful adjunct to establish the diagnosis of a lenticule stuck to the overlying cap. In the absence of these diagnostic modalities, a clinical diagnosis may be established by nudging the underside of the cap in the periphery with a Sinskey hook, wherein observing a crescentic-shaped gap confirms the presence of a lenticule adherent to the overlying cap [16].

Treatment

The creation of a crescentic area of separation between the adherent lenticule and the cap confirms the presence of a cap-lenticular adhesion and provides a plane to enable further dissection and separation of the lenticule. A similar crescentic separation with the Sinskey hook may be created on the opposite side at 9'oclock and the lenticule may be extracted by gently peeling it off from the overlying cap with a microforceps. Alternatively, a lenticulorhexis may be performed to separate the lenticule from the cap [16].

In cases with unclear dissection planes or a false stromal passage, the procedure should be abandoned. Retreatment with FS-LASIK, cap-flap conversion using the CIRCLE software or surface ablation may be performed after refractive stability is achieved [16].

Prevention

Various signs have been described to help the surgeon prevent and identify lenticule mis-dissection such as the 'shimmer sign', 'white ring sign' and 'meniscus sign'. Surgical techniques such as sequential segmental dissection, Chung's swing technique and 'push-down' with a Y-shaped instrument have been described to enable safe lenticule extraction [16].

9.2.5 Corneal Perforation During Intracorneal Ring Segments Implantation

Corneal perforation during intracorneal ring segments (ICRS) implantation is rare complication that may be observed during the creation of channels (manual or femtosecond-laser assisted) or while forcefully inserting the rings.

9.2.5.1 Incidence

The incidence of endothelial perforation ranges from 0.1% to 0.6%, whereas an anterior corneal perforation may be observed during a forceful ring insertion in 1.8% of cases [17].

9.2.5.2 Risk Factors

Incorrect preoperative pachymetry measurements at the optical zone, excessively deep or superficial channel creation due to incorrect knife setting or FS laser depth and surgeon inexperience increase the risk of inadvertent perforation.

9.2.5.3 Diagnosis

The appearance of air bubbles in the anterior chamber is noted during endothelial perforation by the ring. Acute hydrops can occur as a consequence of intraoperative DM perforation during segment implantation [17].

9.2.5.4 Treatment

The surgery should be aborted as soon as sign of perforation is observed. A BCL may be placed. The perforation usually heals in about 4 weeks following which the procedure may be reattempted. In cases with endothelial perforation, the new channel should be made at least 30–90 μm anterior to the previous channel [17].

9.2.5.5 Prevention

Accurate preoperative pachymetry, proper setting of femtosecond-laser depth parameters and gentle manoeuvring while inserting the segments help prevent intraoperative corneal perforation duriing ICRS implantation.

9.2.6 Corneal Emergencies Related to Radial Keratotomy

Radial keratotomy (RK) is an incisional corneal refractive surgery that has fallen out of favour with the advent of corneal ablative procedures. The associated intraoperative emergencies are less relevant in the current scenario as the surgery is of historical importance. Intraoperative corneal perforations may be observed during RK that may necessitate discontinuation of the procedure with placement of sutures to seal the perforation. Accurate preoperative pachymetry and ensuring that the correct knife length is set while using a guarded blade are crucial in preventing this complication.

9.3 Postoperative Corneal Emergencies

Corneal emergencies may be observed in the immediate or late postoperative period after refractive surgeries. Infectious keratitis is a potentially sight-threatening complication that may be observed after any surgical procedure and may progress to phthisis bulbi if untreated. In addition, rupture or dehiscence of RK incisions, extrusion of ICRS implants, acute hydrops, diffuse lamellar keratitis and corneal melts may be observed.

9.3.1 Infectious Keratitis

Infectious keratitis is a serious complication which may be observed after any refractive surgery, including LASIK, photorefactive keratectomy (PRK), RK and ICRS implantation.

9.3.1.1 Incidence

Post-LASIK microbial keratitis is a rare but serious complication seen after LASIK surgery with a reported incidence of 0–1.5%.Post-PRK infectious keratitis is more common with the reported rate of infections 2–6 times higher than observed in post-LASIK cases [18]. Microbial keratitis may be observed after implant of ICRS in 0.1–4.8% of cases [19]. Post-SMILE and post-RK microbial keratitis are relatively rare with isolated case reports [20, 21].

9.3.1.2 Causative Organisms

Early onset postoperative infections are usually caused by Gram positive bacteria, with staphylococcus and streptococcus species being the most common. Atypical microorganisms, including atypical mycobacteria and fungi are frequently implicated in late-onset infections after LASIK. Pseudomonas species may be commonly isolated in delayed post-RK keratitis [18, 20, 21].

9.3.1.3 Risk Factors

Risk factors associated with microbial keratitis after corneal refractive procedures may be related to the preoperative ocular and systemic co-morbidities, intraoperative surgical technique and contamination, and postoperative wound healing. Preoperatively, history of past corneal surgeries, systemic co-morbidities such as uncontrolled diabetes mellitus and immunosuppressed state and ocular co-morbidities such as dry eyes, viral keratitis and blepharitis increase the risk of postoperative infectious keratitis. Intraoperatively, surface or interface contamination, epithelial defect and reuse of microkeratomes for flap creation predispose to infections. Horizontal implantation of ICRS rings with perpendicular wound creation is associated with slower healing after ICRS implant. In addition, superficial implantation of ICRS and inadvertent introduction of intrastromal foreign bodies are risk factors for the development of post-ICRS infections. Postoperative risk factors include delayed epithelial healing, prolonged topical steroid use, BCL use and incomplete eyelid closure. Epithelial pseudocysts or erosions at site of RK incisions are associated with increased risk of delayed infections [18–21].

9.3.1.4 Diagnosis

The onset of infection may be early (within 2 weeks) or delayed (2 weeks to 3 months). The diagnosis of infectious keratitis may be established in the presence of typical signs and symptoms. The patients present with diminution of vision, pain, redness and watering; examination reveals interface infiltrates that may progressively involve the stromal bed and overlying cap or flap. Epithelial defects are commonly observed in PRK but may not be observed at initial presentation in LASIK or SMILE [18, 20].

Post-ICRS infections usually present within the first 2 weeks with infiltrates appearing first at the incision site, then progressing around the ring and into the tunnel with a characteristic wound gap. Ring extrusion may be observed in severe cases [19].

Delayed infectious keratitis may be observed years after the initial surgery in post-RK cases with infiltrates along the RK incisions involving the inferior quadrant of cornea [21].

9.3.1.5 Treatment

Empirical broad-spectrum fortified antibiotics should be initiated at presentation, and the antimicrobial treatment may be tailored based on the culture and sensitivity reports. Frequent instillation of topical antibiotics on an hourly or two-hourly basis is advocated. Topical steroids should be discontinued. A high index of suspicion for atypical microorganisms should be kept, especially in cases with a delayed presentation. Post-LASIK keratitis refractory to medical therapy may require interface irrigation with antibiotics or flap amputation to remove the source of infection and improve penetration of antibiotics [18]. Post-ICRS infections may require explant of the ring segment followed by tunnel irrigation with antibiotics [19]. Therapeutic keratoplasty may be required in non-responsive cases with progressive stromal melt and perforation.

9.3.1.6 Prevention

Prevention of microbial keratitis after corneal refractive surgery entails adequate treatment of preoperative lid or adnexal infection prior to LASIK. Preoperative betadine cleaning of the patient's eye, maintaining surgical field sterility, proper sterilization of the operating instruments and the use of broad-spectrum antibiotics like fourth generation fluoroquinolones for pre- and post-operative prophylaxis help to reduce the incidence of postoperative infections [18].

9.3.2 Rupture or Dehiscence of Radial Keratotomy Incisions

Radial Keratotomy has been rendered obsolete with the advent of safer and more predictable refractive procedures; however, the postoperative complications may still be observed for the next few decades. As the cohort of RK patients that underwent their primary surgery in the 1980s–90s undergo phacoemulsification or other intraocular surgeries, the surgeons are increasingly likely to encounter the incision-related corneal emergencies. Any subsequent ocular surgery like penetrating keratoplasty, phacoemulsification, LASIK or even vitrectomy in a post-RK patient may result in intraoperative rupture or dehiscence of the RK incisions [22].

9.3.2.1 Risk Factors

Radial incisions created during RK are susceptible to dehiscence in the presence of inciting factors such as trauma or surgery, even after several years of surgery. Multiple incisions (24–32) with increased depth are more likely to dehisce. Creation of clear corneal or limbal incisions during phacoemulsification that transect the previous RK incisions increases the incidence of dehiscence of radial incisions. In addition, initiation of infusion after inserting the phacoemulsification probe in the anterior chamber can lead to the RK incisions 'giving way'. During penetrating keratoplasty the peripheral part of the RK incisions may partially or fully dehisce while performing host trephination or while cutting the host cornea with a corneal scissor. During LASIK, splaying of RK incision resulting in radial peripheral flap tears may be seen while creating the flap with microkeratome or manipulation during the lifting of the flap. Corneal laceration or even globe rupture along the RK incisions has been reported after blunt or penetrating trauma [23, 24].

9.3.2.2 Diagnosis

The diagnosis is established clinically on observing a gaping RK incision with aqueous leak observed under the microscope.

9.3.2.3 Management

Ruptured RK incisions should be sutured as in a corneal perforation to restore the integrity of the globe. The approximating sutures should not be too tight, otherwise the tension exerted by the sutures itself may lead to dehiscence of the adjacent RK incisions [23]. Anti-torque 10-0 or 11-0 nylon sutures are placed to straddle the radial incision during approximation of partially dehisced radial incision during penetrating keratoplasty [24]. Cases of post-traumatic corneal perforation or global rupture seen post-RK require immediate repair of corneal and the scleral tears. Splaying of RK incisions observed during LASIK requires the flap to be carefully reposited back with proper alignment of the RK and LASIK flap wound edge, and placement of a BCL.

9.3.2.4 Prevention

In phacoemulsification, a posterior limbal incision is recommended in cases with 4–12 RK incisions with sufficient space between two adjacent radial incisions. A scleral or sclero-corneal tunnel may be preferred in cases with 16 or more RK incisions to avoid transection of the radial incisions by phacoemulsification incision. Placement of a prophylactic suture across the RK incision adjacent to the main wound may be considered. Manoeuvring of the instruments in and out of the wound should be done gently. Post-operative intraocular pressure (IOP) should be managed appropriately to prevent incision rupture after surgery due to IOP spikes. Main wound should be sutured, and the patient should be reviewed for any delayed RK incision dehiscence even if the surgery was uneventful [23].

During penetrating keratoplasty, the use of preplaced transverse sutures across each radial incision, one 0.5 mm peripheral to the graft wound and the other 1.0 mm from the corneal limbus, or a preplaced purse-string suture to stabilize the peripheral RK incisions of the host cornea helps prevent its dehiscence. Placement of interrupted cardinal sutures or bites of a continuous suture between the RK incisions; meticulous closing of the radial keratotomy-graft wound junctions using a combination of apposition and overlying compression sutures, double-crossed interrupted and double-running anti-torque suturing techniques have also been described [24].

In post-RK patients undergoing LASIK, femtosecond laser may be used to create the flap instead of microkeratome. A thicker flap of around 130 microns is preferred with careful, gentle dissection while lifting the flap to prevent splaying of RK incisions.

9.3.3 Intracorneal Ring Segment Extrusion and Corneal Melt

Postoperative corneal emergencies associated with ICRS include ring extrusion and corneal melt overlying the ring segment. ICRS extrusion is a serious complication which may result from continual superficial migration of the implant or an overlying corneal stromal melt with full-thickness stromal defect. Deeper migration with endothelial perforation and acute hydrops may also be observed.

9.3.3.1 Incidence

Extrusion of ICRS segments may be observed in 0.5–30% of cases [25]. Corneal melt is relatively rare with an incidence of 0.1–0.7% [17].

9.3.3.2 Risk Factors

Local ocular factors such as thin corneas, dry eye disease, eye rubbing or atopy, advanced stage of keratoconus may predispose to extrusion of the ICRS implant and corneal melt. Risk factors associated with the surgical technique include an increased arc length, thick segments, manually created channels with shallow tunnel depth and superficial placement of ring, simultaneous cross-linking session and placing the segment too close to the incision site [17]. ICRS segment extrusion may also be observed in association with postoperative trauma [25].

9.3.3.3 Treatment

Immediate removal of the segment with topical antibiotic and steroid therapy is required in cases of corneal melt or segment extrusion [25]. In addition, systemic anti-collagenolytic agents are recommended in cases with corneal melt [17].

9.3.3.4 Prevention

Comprehensive preoperative assessment including accurate preoperative pachymetry with optimization of ocular co-morbidities such as dry eye disease and ocular atopy help prevent ICRS extrusion or corneal melt. Good surgical technique and surgical expertise is essential to ensure optimal depth of the channel. Femtosecond laser-assisted creation of intrastromal channels is associated with increased predictability and safety.

9.3.4 Acute Hydrops

Acute hydrops may rarely be observed in post-LASIK or post-RK cases, especially in association with localized ectasia.

9.3.4.1 Risk Factors

Acute hydrops may be observed in cases that develop post-LASIK or post-RK ectasia and may be associated with vigorous eye rubbing or trauma. Various factors predispose to the development of post-refractive surgery ectasia, such as preoperative keratoconus, family history of keratoconus, trauma, history of multiple corneal refractive procedures with inadequate residual bed thickness, young age and history of eye rubbing [26, 27].

9.3.4.2 Diagnosis

Acute hydrops after LASIK or RK presents with marked stromal oedema and the presence of stromal aqueous clefts [26, 27]. In LASIK, a separation of the flap from the stromal bed due to interface fluid accumulation may be observed. Stromal aqueous clefts are visible as translucent spaces in the corneal stroma communicating with the anterior chamber via a rupture in the Descemet's membrane. Aqueous leaking around the edge of the flap and shallowing of AC may be observed [26].

9.3.4.3 Management

Most cases of corneal hydrops resolve in 2–4 months on conservative management including topical steroids, antibiotics, cycloplegics and antiglaucoma medications The use of intracameral air or isoexpansile gases (SF6/C3F8) with or without intraoperative OCT guided anterior stromal punctures has been described in cases unresponsive to medical management or with extensive fluid clefts [27].

Post-LASIK ectasia with stromal perforation should be managed appropriately with pressure patching, BCL, cyanoacrylate tissue adhesives or patch grafting depending on the size and severity of perforation [26].

9.3.4.4 Prevention

Prevention of post-RK/LASIK ectasia and hydrops entails a comprehensive preoperative evaluation to rule out subclinical or clinical keratoconus. Management of allergic eye diseases is essential to prevent eye rubbing.

9.3.5 Acute Corneal Haze After Photorefractive Keratectomy

Acute corneal haze after phototherapeutic keratectomy (PRK) may be observed in 2–4% of cases with high magnitude of refractive errors [28].

9.3.5.1 Risk Factors

Risk factors for post-PRK corneal haze include high magnitude of refractive errors with subsequent greater ablation depths. More than 6D of myopia and 4D of hyperopia correction are associated with significant postoperative haze. In addition, intraoperative factors such as use of larger spot-sized laser and mechanical epithelial debridement and predispose to the development of acute corneal haze. Postoperative delayed epithelial healing, stromal surface irregularity, use of oral contraceptives, mechanical trauma and ultraviolet exposure are also associated with corneal haze. Corneal haze may also be observed in association with ocular and systemic factors such as atopy, autoimmune conditions and allergic conjunctivitis [28].

9.3.5.2 Diagnosis

Reticular opacities are observed at the corneal subepithelial level on slit lamp examination. The haze usually appears 1 week post-surgery, peaks at 3 months and then gradually resolves over the first year [28].

9.3.5.3 Treatment

The frequency and potency of topical steroids should be increased. In unresponsive cases, transepithelial PTK/PRK or manual keratectomy with mitomycin C (MMC) application (0.02%) may be required [28].

9.3.5.4 Prevention

Use of intraoperative MMC (0.02%) application during PRK in cases with high refractive errors helps minimize the incidence of postoperative haze. Avoidance of mechanical epithelial debridement and adequate use of post-operative steroids help to reduce the occurrence of post-PRK haze.

9.3.6 Flap Macrostriae and Flap Dislocation

Post-LASIK flap macrostriae may be observed in 0.2–4.39% of cases and result in significant visual disturbances [11]. The creation of a flap during LASIK permanently weakens the corneal integrity with a lifetime risk of flap slippage or dislocation.

9.3.6.1 Incidence

The reported incidence of flap dislocation ranges from 0.01% to 5.8% [11].

9.3.6.2 Risk Factors

Flap macrostriae and early dislocations may be observed in association with thin, desiccated flaps, misaligned flaps or free caps. Microkeratome-assisted flaps are more prone to develop postoperative striae and dislocations. Patient-related factors include high refractive error with deeper ablation causing a tenting effect, tear film insufficiency, postoperative eye rubbing, mechanical trauma and forceful squeezing. Late flap dislocations are usually incited by trauma or iatrogenic factors such as debriding the epithelium during vitrectomy [11].

9.3.6.3 Diagnosis

Flap macrostriae appear as wrinkling of the flap with full-thickness flap folds on slit lamp examination (Fig. 9.3). Dislocated flaps appear displaced from their intended site revealing the bare stromal bed in the periphery. The flap is often oedematous with folds. Early flap dislocations are more common and occur within a week of surgery while late dislocations are mostly incited by trauma and may be observed years after surgery [11].

9.3.6.4 Treatment

Flap dislocation and macrostriae require immediate intervention to prevent sight-threatening sequelae. Flap lifting, refloating and interface wash followed by its repositioning should be performed. Epithelial debridement may be needed if the patient presents after 24 h of onset with fixed folds. Gentle repeated stretching of the flap after repositioning in the direction perpendicular to the striae helps in optimal alignment of the flap. Suturing the flap may be required in some cases [11].

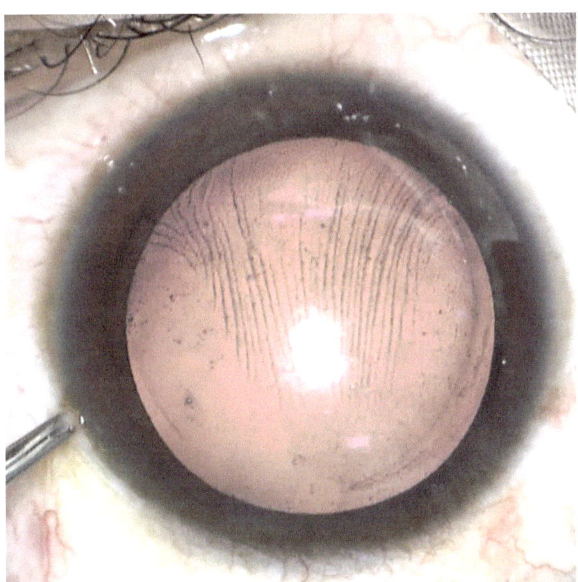

Fig. 9.3 Postoperative LASIK flap macrostriae seen as flap wrinkling with full thickness folds involving the visual axis on slit lamp examination

9.3.6.5 Prevention

Good surgical technique with maintenance of flap alignment and hydration while removing the interface fluid at the end of surgery promotes optimal flap adherence. Patients should be counselled properly to avoid forceful eye squeezing or rubbing in the immediate postoperative period. Patients who are prone to contact injury should be advised to wear protective eye wear and explained the possible lifetime risk of late flap dislocation.

9.3.7 Diffuse Lamellar Keratitis

Diffuse lamellar keratitis (DLK) is a sterile inflammatory response observed at flap-stromal interface in the absence of anterior chamber inflammation.

9.3.7.1 Incidence

The incidence varies from 0.1% to 7.7% with microkeratome-assisted LASIK to 0.08–19.4% with femtosecond-laser assisted LASIK [29].

9.3.7.2 Risk Factors

Patient-related risk factors for DLK include high degree of preoperative ametropia, peripheral immune infiltrates and atopy. Risk factors associated with surgical technique include the use of high energy femtosecond laser system, larger optical zones, perioperative flap epithelial defect and larger flap diameter. Introduction of contaminants in the interface can lead to DLK, including blood or meibomian gland secretions, bacterial endotoxins and exotoxins, chemical toxins produced during autoclaving, surgical marker pen, povidone-iodine, microkeratome oil and surgical glove contaminants. Postoperative infections including keratitis and conjunctivitis, collagen cross-linking, trauma, flap manipulations and enhancement procedures may incite DLK [30].

9.3.7.3 Diagnosis

DLK presents within 1 week of LASIK, typically within the initial 24 h with wave-like lines of white, granular inflammatory cell deposits in the interface (Fig. 9.4). There is minimal conjunctival inflammation and no anterior chamber reaction. It is an emergency as untreated severe DLK may progress to corneal melt and irreversible visual loss.

9.3.7.4 Treatment

Intensive topical corticosteroids are the mainstay of treatment. Oral steroids and flap lifting with interface irrigation may be required in severe cases. Stage 4 patients with corneal melt require adjunctive therapy with oral doxycycline, Vitamin C, topical sodium citrate drops and hyperosmotic drops to hasten resolution [30].

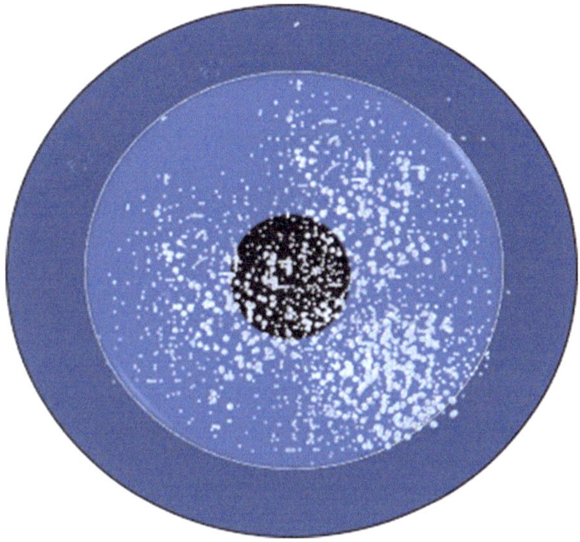

Fig. 9.4 Schematic representation of postoperative Diffuse Lamellar Keratitis after LASIK, with extensive whitish granular inflammatory cell deposits in the interface involving the visual axis

9.3.7.5 Prevention

Preventive measures include thorough interface wash before repositing the flap, careful cleaning of instruments and avoidance of contaminants. Lower energy, higher frequency femtosecond laser systems have a lower risk of DLK.

9.3.8 Central Toxic Keratopathy

Central toxic keratopathy (CTK) is a rare, acute, non-inflammatory condition observed rarely in post-LASIK patients [29]. No definite inciting factors have been linked to CTK; however, these cases are often preceded by diffuse lamellar keratitis (DLK) [31].

9.3.8.1 Incidence

The reported incidence of CTK varies from 0.01% to 0.7% of cases [29].

9.3.8.2 Diagnosis

Patients present 3–9 days after LASIK with loss of vision, associated with variable degrees of foreign body sensation, photophobia and pain. On examination, characteristic dense opacification in the central cornea is observed extending beyond the interface into the stroma, associated with striae, stromal tissue loss and a hyperopic shift [31].

9.3.8.3 Treatment

The central stromal opacity usually clears gradually, sometimes over a period of several months. Oral doxycycline, Vitamin C, topical sodium citrate drops and hyperosmotics may help prevent flap melt and hasten resolution [31]. CTK is unresponsive to steroid therapy and surgery is thought to have a limited role.

9.3.9 Pressure-Induced Intralamellar Stromal Keratitis

Pressure-induced Intralamellar Stromal Keratitis (PISK)is an extremely rare complication which after LASIK. It presents with DLK-like interface haze but is caused by steroid-induced ocular hypertension after LASIK [32].

9.3.9.1 Diagnosis

Patients present 2 weeks after surgery with loss of vision and corneal stromal haze subsequent to corneal oedema resulting from a raised IOP. Fluid accumulation may be observed on ASOCT in the potential space between the flap and the stromal bed [32].

9.3.9.2 Treatment

Treatment consists of discontinuation or tapering of steroids and antiglaucoma medications to control the IOP.

9.4 Conclusion

Modern-day refractive surgeries are associated with a high degree of safety, efficacy, predictability and patient satisfaction. Over the decades the techniques of corneal refractive surgery have undergone a remarkable change. Advances in laser technology have allowed newer lasers with higher frequencies to be employed in corneal refractive surgery, associated with a better precision and lower complication rate. The seemingly perfect refractive outcomes go hand in hand with high patient expectations, and a thorough preoperative counselling is essential to educate the patients about potential risks and their sequelae. Corneal emergencies may rarely be observed both intraoperatively and postoperatively after refractive surgeries and require prompt diagnosis with urgent management to restore the visual acuity and anatomical integrity.

Key Points

- Emergencies associated with corneal refractive surgeries may be seen in the intraoperative or the postoperative stage.
- In patients undergoing LASIK, flap-related complications comprise the major intraoperative complications.
- The incidence of intraoperative flap-related emergencies in LASIK has significantly reduced with advent of Femtosecond Laser for flap creation.
- Suction loss and lenticule mis-dissection are the important intraoperative complications seen during SMILE surgery.

- Postoperative flap striae or dislocation are complications unique to LASIK and require urgent intervention if affecting the patient's vision or involving the visual axis.
- Post-LASIK diffuse lamellar keratitis and microbial keratitis need to be differentiated from each other based on time of presentation and clinical features, as both warrant urgent, albeit different management strategies.
- Prompt diagnosis and appropriate treatment are the keys to managing emergencies in patients undergoing corneal refractive surgeries and can help prevent significant vision loss and long-term sequelae in these patients.

Financial Disclosures and Conflicts of Interest None.

References

1. Schallhorn SC, Amesbury EC, Tanzer DJ. Avoidance, recognition, and management of LASIK complications. Am J Ophthalmol. 2006;141(4):733–9.
2. Carrillo C, Chayet AS, Dougherty PJ, Montes M, Magallanes R, Najman J, et al. Incidence of complications during flap creation in LASIK using the NIDEK MK-2000 microkeratome in 26,600 cases. J Refract Surg. 2005;21(5 Suppl):S655–7.
3. Romero-Diaz-de-Leon L, Serna-Ojeda JC, Navas A, Graue-Hernández EO, Ramirez-Miranda A. Intraoperative flap complications in LASIK surgery performed by ophthalmology residents. J Ophthalmic Vis Res. 2016;11(3):263–7.
4. Nakano K, Nakano E, Oliveira M, Portellinha W, Alvarenga L. Intraoperative microkeratome complications in 47,094 laser in situ keratomileusis surgeries. J Refract Surg. 2004;20(5 Suppl):S723–6.
5. Al-Mezaine HS, Al-Amro SA, Al-Obeidan S. Incidence, management, and visual outcomes of buttonholed laser in situ keratomileusis flaps. J Cataract Refract Surg. 2009;35(5):839–45.
6. Rao SK, Padmanabhan P, Sitalakshmi G, Rajagopal R, Lam DS. Timing of retreatment after a partial flap during laser in situ keratomileusis. J Cataract Refract Surg. 1999;25(11):1424–5.
7. Melki SA, Azar DT. LASIK complications: etiology, management, and prevention. Surv Ophthalmol. 2001;46(2):95–116.
8. dos Santos AM, Torricelli AAM, Marino GK, Garcia R, Netto MV, Bechara SJ, et al. Femtosecond laser-assisted LASIK flap complications. J Refract Surg. 2016;32(1):52–9.
9. Davison JA, Johnson SC. Intraoperative complications of LASIK flaps using the IntraLase femtosecond laser in 3009 cases. J Refract Surg. 2010;26(11):851–7.
10. Seider MI, Ide T, Kymionis GD, Culbertson WW, O'Brien TP, Yoo SH. Epithelial breakthrough during IntraLase flap creation for laser in situ keratomileusis. J Cataract Refract Surg. 2008;34(5):859–63.
11. Shah DN, Melki S. Complications of femtosecond-assisted laser in-situ keratomileusis flaps. Semin Ophthalmol. 2014;29(5–6):363–75.
12. Liu Q, Gong XM, Chen JQ, Yang B, Ge J, To CH. Laser in situ keratomileusis induced corneal perforation and recurrent corneal epithelial ingrowth. J Cataract Refract Surg. 2005;31(4):857–9.
13. Reinstein DZ, Archer TJ, Vida RS, Carp GI. Suction stability management in small incision lenticule extraction: incidence and outcomes of suction loss in 4000 consecutive procedures. Acta Ophthalmol. 2020;98(1):e72–80.

14. Osman IM, Awad R, Shi W, AbouShousha M. Suction loss during femtosecond laser-assisted small-incision lenticule extraction: incidence and analysis of risk factors. J Cataract Refract Surg. 2016;42(2):246–50.
15. Titiyal JS, Kaur M, Rathi A, Falera R, Chaniyara M, Sharma N. Learning curve of small incision lenticule extraction: challenges and complications. Cornea. 2017;36(11):1377–82.
16. Titiyal JS, Kaur M, Shaikh F, Sahay P. Double crescentic edge separation for the management of cap-lenticular adhesion in small incision lenticule extraction. Indian J Ophthalmol. 2020;68(5):897–9.
17. Mounir A, Radwan G, Farouk MM, Mostafa EM. Femtosecond-assisted intracorneal ring segment complications in keratoconus: from novelty to expertise. Clin Ophthalmol Auckl NZ. 2018;12:957–64.
18. Schallhorn JM, Schallhorn SC, Hettinger K, Hannan S. Infectious keratitis after laser vision correction: incidence and risk factors. J Cataract Refract Surg. 2017;43(4):473–9.
19. Tabatabaei SA, Soleimani M, Mirghorbani M, Tafti ZF, Rahimi F. Microbial keratitis following intracorneal ring implantation. Clin Exp Optom. 2019;102(1):35–42.
20. Sachdev GS, Diwan S, Sachdev MS. Unilateral fungal keratitis after small-incision lenticule extraction. JCRS Online Case Rep. 2019;7(1):11–3.
21. Levy J, Hirsh A, Klemperer I, Lifshitz T. Late-onset pseudomonas keratitis after radial keratotomy and subsequent laser in situ keratomileusis: case report and literature review. Can J Ophthalmol. 2005;40(2):211–3.
22. Jammal HM, Dolat WM. Ruptured globe 20 years after radial and transverse keratotomy. Int Ophthalmol. 2012;32(1):51–3.
23. Behl S, Kothari K. Rupture of a radial keratotomy incision after 11 years during clear corneal phacoemulsification. J Cataract Refract Surg. 2001;27(7):1132–4.
24. McNeill JI, Wilkins DL. A purse-string suture for penetrating keratoplasty following radial keratotomy. Refract Corneal Surg. 1991;7(5):392–4.
25. Mounir A, Farouk MM, Abdellah MM, Mohamed ME. Extrusion of femtosecond laser-implanted intrastromal corneal ring segments in keratoconic eyes: prevalence, risk factors, and clinical outcomes. J Ophthalmol. 2020;2020:8704219.
26. Chen C-L, Tai M-C, Chen J-T, Chen C-H, Chang C-J, Lu D-W. Acute corneal hydrops with perforation after LASIK-associated keratectasia. Clin Exp Ophthalmol. 2007;35(1):62–5.
27. Sharma N, Sachdev R, Jindal A, Titiyal JS. Acute hydrops in keratectasia after radial keratotomy. Eye Contact Lens. 2010;36(3):185–7.
28. Efthymios K, Genovefa M, John A, Michael M. Very late onset corneal haze in a photorefractive keratectomy patient associated with presumed viral keratoconjuctivitis. Indian J Ophthalmol. 2020;68(6):1186.
29. Choe CH, Guss C, Musch DC, Niziol LM, Shtein RM. Incidence of diffuse lamellar keratitis after LASIK with 15 KHz, 30 KHz, and 60 KHz femtosecond laser flap creation. J Cataract Refract Surg. 2010;36(11):1912–8.
30. Randleman JB, Shah RD. LASIK interface complications: etiology, management, & outcomes. J Refract Surg. 2012;28(8):575–86.
31. Moshirfar M, Hazin R, Khalifa YM. Central toxic keratopathy. Curr Opin Ophthalmol. 2010;21(4):274–9.
32. Rosa N, De Bernardo M, Lanza M. Pressure-induced stromal keratitis. J Refract Surg. 2013;29(2):81–2.

Acute Chemical Injuries of the Cornea

10

Monika Balyan, Arun Kumar Jain, and Chintan Malhotra

10.1 Introduction

Ocular chemical injuries can be categorized under true ophthalmic emergencies and require urgent intervention. The clinical presentation varies widely, with sight-threatening complications highly likely at the distal end of the spectrum. The incidence of chemical injuries as stated by the two major epidemiological studies from the United States and the United Kingdom are 51.10 new cases/million per year and 56 new cases/million/year, respectively [1, 2]. Most of the data from the developed countries suggest that about two-thirds of the injuries occur at the workplace, with the majority of victims being males in the age of 20–40 years. Apart from the workplace, most other incidents happen at home or as a result of criminal assault. Alkali injuries are more common than acid injuries as the alkali is more commonly found as a constituent of household and industrial products. About 70–80% of the chemical injuries are attributed to alkaline chemicals; this figure is worrisome as alkalis are known to cause severe injuries as compared to acids [3–5]. No definite epidemiological data can be reproduced for a majority of the developing countries due to the lack of a central database, and the data from the developed countries cannot be rightly extrapolated for developing countries as the legislations for work safety, population awareness, and availability of protective equipment vary considerably.

10.2 Causative Agents of Ocular Chemical Injury

Nearly 25,000 chemical substances with the potential to cause chemical injuries to the eyes have been identified [6]. The majority of these injuries are caused by acids or alkalis, as these substances are commonly used in factories, construction sites,

M. Balyan · A. K. Jain (✉) · C. Malhotra
Cornea, Cataract and Refractive Services, Advanced Eye Center, PGIMER, Chandigarh, India

B. Sharma, J. S. Titiyal (eds.), *Corneal Emergencies*,
https://doi.org/10.1007/978-981-16-5876-1_10

and are accessible even for household use. Some of the acids and alkalis commonly responsible for causing ocular burns are enlisted in Table 10.1. Ocular chemical injuries caused by acid-alkali will be discussed in detail in this chapter, besides these, some other common agents attributed to ocular chemical burns are briefly described here.

10.2.1 Classification of Common Agents Responsible for Causing Ocular Chemical Injuries

- Corrosives:
  (a) *Acids or oxidizing agents*
  Strong acids, e.g., Hydrochloric acid, Nitric acid, Sulfuric acid.
  Weak acids, e.g., Acetic acid, Carbonic acid
  (b) *Alkali or reducing agents*
  e.g. Ammonia, lye, Potassium hydroxide, Calcium hydroxide
- Vesicants
- e.g. Sulfur mustard, Mustard/lewisite, Nitrogen mustard
- Plant-based irritants
- e.g. *Calotropis Procera, Euphorbia lathyris*
- Lacrimatory or riot control agents
- e.g. Bromobenzyl cyanide, Chloroacetophenone, Chloropicrin, Dibenzoxazepine.

10.2.1.1 Vesicants

Vesicants are oily liquids that get aerosolized when released from an explosion or at high temperatures. E.g. sulfur, nitrogen mustard. These are lipophilic substances and therefore get concentrated in the lipid layer of the tear film and cause prolonged ocular surface exposure [7]. Ocular effects can be seen in the form of lid edema, conjunctivitis, punctate epitheliopathy, or sloughing up of epithelium [8]. Most of the cases (90%) recover without any sequelae. Severe injury (10%) destroys conjunctival and limbal blood supply resulting in limbal ischemia and limbal stem cell deficiency (LSCD) [9]. After exposure to the vesicants, the affected individual should be shifted under open air, away from the exposure site. The rest of the treatment course is similar to any corrosive injury and will be discussed in detail, later in this chapter.

10.2.1.2 Lacrimatory Agents

These are aerosol dispersed agents that cause ocular irritation and are mainly deployed for crowd control during riots. These agents activate transient receptor potential (TRP); TRPA1 &TRPV1 ion channel present in the nociceptors of the peripheral sensory nerves which are also stimulated by intense heat, therefore causing a feeling of intense burning. These agents also cause neurogenic inflammation by the release of substance P [10, 11].

Table 10.1 Acids and Alkali commonly responsible for causing ocular chemical injuries, with their uses and characteristic properties

Acids			
Strength	Compound	Uses	Properties
Strong acids	Sulfuric acid (H_2SO_4)	Car batteries, making other acids, fertilizers, explosives, dyes, petroleum refining	Open globe injury in cases of blast injuries. Chemical injury compounded with thermal injury
	Nitric acid (HNO_3)	Fertilizers, rocket propellant, explosives	Yellow discoloration of exposed tissue
	Hydrochloric acid (HCL)	Household cleaning, plastic manufacturing	Hydrogen chloride gas fumes cause ocular irritation and profuse lacrimation
Weak acids	Chromic acid (H_2CrO_4)	Chrome plating industry	Brown discoloration of the exposed tissue. Produces chronic conjunctival inflammation
	Acetic acid (CH_3COOH)	Vinegar	Concentration >10% can be harmful to the eye. The essence of vinegar (80% acetic acid) and glacial acetic acid (90%) causes severe damage to the eye
	Sulfurous acid (H_2SO_3)	Meat mincing, preservative, bleach, refrigerant	Highly soluble in lipid and water
	Hydrofluoric acid (HF)	Semiconductor production, rust remover, glass etching	Causes severe ocular injury by dissolving cell membranes

Alkali			
Rate of penetration	Compound	Uses	Comments
Fastest (<3 min)	Ammonia (NH_3)	Fertilizers, cleaning agents, refrigerants	Forms fumes with water, high solubility, and rapid penetration
3–5 min	Sodium hydroxide/lye [NaOH]	Drain cleaners, paper, and textile industries, hair straightening	Easy availability at home, therefore frequently used for assault
>5 min	Potassium hydroxide (KOH)	Caustic potash	Dissolution in water is an exothermic reaction
Slightly less rapid then KOH	Magnesium hydroxide [$Mg(OH)_2$]	Sparklers	Can cause combined chemical and thermal injury
Slowest/variable depends upon precipitation	Calcium hydroxide/Lime [$Ca(OH)_2$]	Cement, mortar, whitewashing	The most common agent causing alkali injury. Reacts with epithelial cell membranes to form calcium soaps

- Tear gas—Common agents used in tear gas are Chloroacetophenone, Dibenzoxazepine, chlorobezylidenemalononitrile.
- *Chemical Mace* is a mixture of tear gas (original formula consisted of 1% chloroacetophenone) with a chemical solvent. These agents can cause lacrimation, epithelial edema, stromal clouding, and epithelial sloughing [12].
- Oleoresin Capsicum, commonly known as pepper spray is commonly used for self-defense. The active agents are lipophilic substances grouped as capsaicinoids, mainly capsaicin and dihydrocapsaicin, which bind to the vanilloid type 1 receptor; TRPV1 [11, 13, 14].
- Exposure may lead to an inability to open eyes, stinging, pain, and lacrimation. If the victim is wearing contact lenses, they should be removed immediately. Capsaicin is insoluble in water; therefore, the symptoms are not relieved by irrigation with water. However, the role of immediate irrigation cannot be excluded. There is no specific antidote; therefore, treatment aims at decontamination followed by symptoms specific supportive measures.

10.2.1.3 Plant-Based Toxins

- *Calotropis procera* (Sodom apple): The latex of the plant contains alkaloids like *calotropin, calcilin, catotoxin* which cause caustic injury to the eye [15]. Patients usually present with painless diminution of vision since the latex has anesthetic properties. Other findings are the presence of punctate epitheliopathy, corneal edema, presence of Descemet's folds (Fig. 10.1). Unlike most of the other chemicals, Calotropis causes more damage to the endothelial cells as compared to the epithelium [16].
- Euphorbia species: The sap of the Euphorbia plant is toxic to the skin and the eyes and causes alkaline chemical injury [17]. Ocular toxicity due to accidental exposure to the sap may manifest in the form of mild conjunctivitis to severe keratouveitis [18–20].

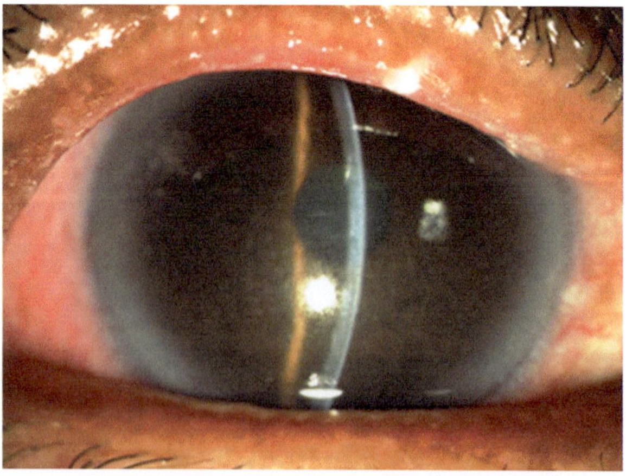

Fig. 10.1 A 34-year-old female with accidental exposure to *Calotropis* sap. The anterior segment showed the presence of corneal edema with multiple Descemet's folds. Endothelial involvement is notably more than epithelial affection

10.2.1.4 Other Common Agents Responsible for Ocular Chemical Injuries

During the festive week of Holi, ocular chemical injuries due to synthetic colors are very commonly encountered in India. Oxidized metals or industrial dyes are sometimes added to these to impart a specific color. E.g. copper sulfate—green color, mercury sulfide—red color, aluminum bromide—yellow color. The watercolors which are used mostly contain an alkaline base with the potential to cause chemical injuries [21].

Cosmetics like hair colorants contain ammonia as an alkylating agent and hydrogen peroxide as an oxidizing agent, likely to cause ocular burns on exposure [22]. Commonly used products like the depilatorycrèmes contain calcium thioglycolate along with calcium hydroxide and can possibly cause severe caustic injury (Fig. 10.2) [23].

At the tertiary care centers, ophthalmic consultations are commonly sought for motor vehicle accidents (MVA) with associated ocular injuries. Injuries resulting due to sudden deployment of the airbags may lead to severe ocular burns due to the sudden release of chemicals like sodium hydroxide during the deployment [24]. If left ignored, these injuries may result in sight-threatening complications.

10.3 Pathophysiology of a Corrosive Injury

The severity of the injury caused by a chemical agent and final visual outcomes depend on the area of exposure, nature, concentration, and quantity of the substance as well as on efficacy and timing of the emergency treatment. Chemical substances cause tissue destruction through the dissociated ions which accumulate in the tear film, destroy the adnexa, and penetrate the cornea to reach the aqueous humor. Pain, lacrimation, and blepharospasm occur as a result of direct injury to the free nerve

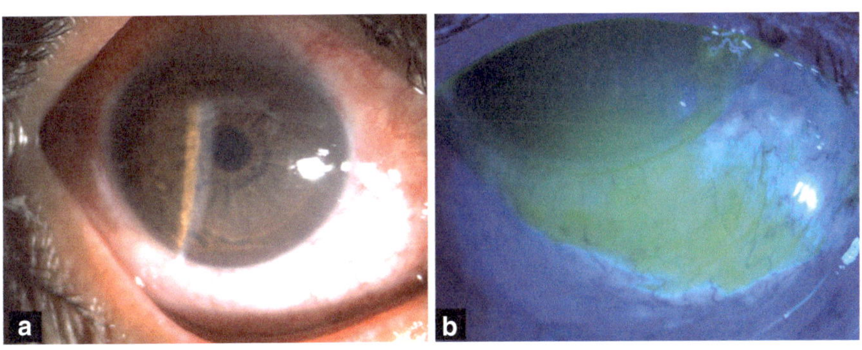

Fig. 10.2 (**a**) A 25-year-old male with a history of accidental smearing of depilatory crème in the eye. The picture shows an epithelial defect involving almost three-fourths of the cornea along with multiple Descemet's folds. The presence of limbal ischemia can be noted from 3 to 9 clock hours. (**b**) The corneal and conjunctival epithelial defect stained with fluorescene dye and visualized under the cobalt blue filter

endings located in the conjunctiva, lid, and the cornea. The strength of an oxidizing and reducing agent depends on its ability to readily give hydrogen and hydroxyl ions in the solution; therefore, a stronger acid or alkali causes more tissue destruction than the weaker ones [25]. An exception to this is the Hydrofluoric acid, which is a weak inorganic acid, but is a strong solvent, therefore dissolves cellular membranes and rapidly penetrates the eye. It also chelates calcium and magnesium ions, thereby halting cellular metabolic activities [26].

The difference in the severity of the acid and alkali injuries lies in their different tissue interactions. Acid results in the precipitation of proteins within the cornea and conjunctiva which acts as a partial barrier for deeper penetration of the offending agent [27] (Figure 10.3a). On the other hand, in cases of alkali injuries, hydroxyl ions rapidly penetrate the eye, causing saponification of cellular membranes with massive cell death, partial hydrolysis of corneal glycosaminoglycans and collagen, and rapid corneal clouding (Figure 10.3c). An increase in aqueous humor pH because of rapid penetration of alkali agent into anterior chamber results in lysis of cells lining the anterior chamber along with the compromisation of the blood–aqueous barrier, and release of necrotic debris into the anterior chamber [28]. Among the alkali, ammonia has the fastest penetration rate (<3 min) and is known to cause severe ocular burns [29]. Alkali burns due to lime [$Ca(OH)_2$] are much more common but less severe due to its property to precipitate over the surface, but it may act as a chemical reservoir and cause prolonged exposure if not removed from the fornices or the other potential spaces (Fig. 10.4). Chuna packets (edible calcium hydroxide paste), a popular additive to chewing tobacco in India can cause severe ocular alkali burns in children as a result of bursting of chuna packets while playing with them.

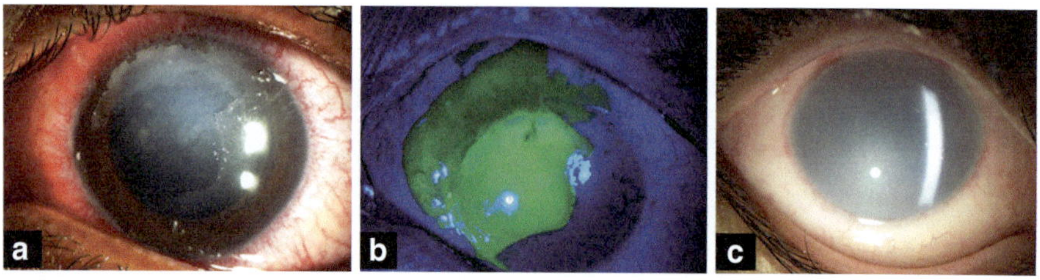

Fig. 10.3 (**a**) An eye post-acid injury showing the presence of an epithelial defect along with the formation of a whitish plaque due to the coagulation of surface proteins. In the setting of chemosis and perilimbal hemorrhage, assessing the degree of limbal ischemia can be difficult and may show significant inter-observer variations. On the other hand, a limbal epithelial defect can be clearly demarcated using fluorescence staining under a cobalt blue filter in the same case (**b**). (**c**) shows an eye post alkali injury, with severe limbal ischemia extending 360° with the presence of sclerosed limbal vessels, implying poor prognosis. Note the presence of diffuse stromal haze with no view of the anterior chamber structures

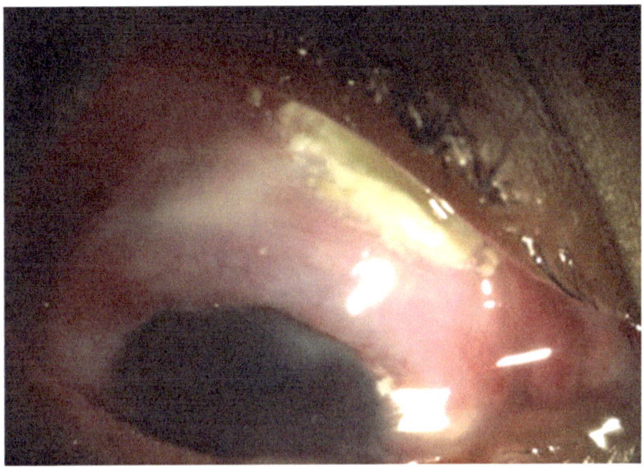

Fig. 10.4 A16-year-girl with a history of accidental fall of lime ($Ca(OH)_2$) into the eye. Lime particles sequestered here if not removed immediately may act as a prolonged source of chemical exposure, resulting in intractable damage to the eye

10.3.1 Rise in Intraocular Pressure (IOP)

The rise in IOP post intraocular chemical injury is a biphasic response. Shrinkage of the collagenous envelope of the eye due to the injury causes an immediate rise in intraocular pressure. The secondary rise in IOP occurs due to prostaglandin release in the aqueous humor, which stays for a longer duration. The necrotic debris clogs the trabecular meshwork and hinders the aqueous outflow. Sometimes even direct injury may occur to the trabecular meshwork. Later on, the organization of the debris occurs in the outflow channels, and cicatricial changes set in, leading to permanent destruction of the trabecular meshwork and synechial closure of the angles [30]. Glaucomatous optic neuropathy is often a cause of grave visual outcomes in the patients who later undergo keratoplasties or keratoprosthesis.

10.3.2 Inflammatory Process

Chemical injuries to the eye result in the release of pro-inflammatory mediators and infiltration of the involved tissue with the polymorphonuclear (PMN)cells. There are two waves of inflammation associated with a chemical injury and the first wave is considered crucial in initiating the second wave. The first wave occurs in the initial 24 h. Change in pH beyond the buffering capacity causes lysis of the corneal cells, disruption of the blood–aqueous barrier, and release of necrotic debris into the aqueous humor, leading to a severe fibrinous inflammatory reaction in the entire anterior segment of the eye. The second wave begins at around 2–3 weeks and coincides with the phase of tissue breakdown and repair. The change in the balance between the two may either result in healing or necrosis of the ocular structures [31].

10.3.3 Fall in the Aqueous Ascorbate Levels

An active transport mechanism, located in the ciliary epithelium, is responsible for concentrating ascorbic acid in the aqueous humor, almost 15–20 times to that of the plasma. The deficiency of ascorbic acid in the aqueous following an alkali burn may occur from direct injury to the ciliary epithelium or through damage to the small blood vessels perfusing the ciliary body [32]. Ascorbic acid is an essential co-factor for collagen synthesis, and its deficiency can cause impaired wound healing and a higher risk of corneal perforation.

10.4 Clinical History

- Nature of the chemical agent (patients sometimes may bring an image of the offending agent, or carry the chemical holder itself).
- Nature of the injury. History of high-velocity injuries, e.g. battery blast, explosions, firecracker injuries should raise suspicion of open globe injury or intraocular foreign body.
- Whether any protective glasses or shields were on at the time of injury.
- If emergency irrigation was performed and for how long.

10.5 Immediate Treatment and Transfer

10.5.1 Treatment at the Injury Site

In the event of a chemical injury, the bystanders or the first responders should take measures to ensure that additional exposure to the offending agent should be immediately cut off. Patient should be shifted to a clean, non-contaminated site, the soiled clothes should be taken off and the emergency irrigation should be started without any further delay. Clean tap water is easily available in such situations, and a copious amount should be used for the irrigation. Delay in lavage for obtaining the irrigants of choice or for transferring the patient to a higher facility is not warranted. The irrigation should continue while the patient is being transferred to the higher center, which can be made possible with the use of an irritating contact lens, e.g. Morgan therapeutic lens (Fig. 10.5).

10.5.2 Treatment in Ophthalmic Emergency

The emergency treatment should *precede* the examination to classify or grade the chemical injury. To optimize patient comfort while irrigation, a drop of proparacaine 0.5% can be instilled. If the injury is unilateral, then the other eye should be patched and the head of the patient should be tilted slightly toward the involved eye to prevent the fluid from accidentally flowing into the normal eye. In cases

Fig. 10.5 A Morgan contact lens (MorTan Inc.) is a "hands-free" emergency irrigation device that enables continuous irrigation of the ocular surface. The attached tube has a luer lock which couples to an intravenous delivery system. *Image used with permission

with bilateral injury, a nasal cannula, laid over the bridge of the nose, with its prongs directed toward both the inner canthus can be used to provide simultaneous irrigation to both the eyes, avoiding any further delay in the emergency treatment. The eye can be held open using gauze or a lid speculum can be applied to facilitate irrigation. Careful attention must be directed to the regions where the presence of extreme chemosis may likely hide some particulate matter. Double eversion of the lid should be performed and fornices should be properly swiped to dislodge the sequestered particles. Lime particles get precipitated and may require removal using forceps and sometimes cotton-tipped applicators soaked in Ethylenediaminetetraacetic acid (EDTA) may help. Care should be taken while manipulating the eyes with the history of blast injuries, e.g. a battery blast or other explosive injuries, as ocular integrity may be compromised in such situations.

10.5.2.1 Choice of Fluid and Duration of Irrigation

The American National Standards Institute recommends irrigation starting with a maximum delay of 10 s after eye burns and to be carried out for no <15 min with a sufficient quantity (500–1000) mL of the isotonic physiological saline, or the available solution [33]. The ideal duration of external lavage may vary according to the severity of the injury and should be continued until the tear pH measured from lower fornix reaches almost close to the normal physiological pH of 7.4. The various fluids used for irrigation differ as per their tonicity and buffering capacity. An alkali should never be used to neutralize an acid and vice versa.

- *Amphoteric substances*: An amphoteric substance has the property to neutralize acid as well as an alkali, e.g. Diphoterine (Prevor laboratories, France). The non-availability of these buffers is the main reason, why they are not readily used.
- *Non-buffering substances*: e.g. tap water, 0.9% normal saline. Tap water is usually hypotonic (may slightly vary with the geographic region) and normal saline is isotonic. There is a controversy regarding the optimum tonicity of irrigating fluid to be used. Studies done on rabbit models suggest that a hypotonic substance causes stromal swelling, therefore dilutes and flushes out the chemical [34], while some study suggests that it may cause deeper penetration of the chemical substance along with cell lysis [35]. Normal saline is isotonic, there-

fore it does not cause stromal swelling and it does not have any buffering ability, hence it is considered inferior to some of the other fluids.

- *Agent specific buffers*: Unlike the amphoteric substances which work for both acids and alkali, these substances work against either acids or alkali. Ringers lactate has lactate as a buffer for acid burns. Balanced saline solution (BSS) is another buffering solution. It contains both acetate and citrate. Citrate gives it the ability to bind to non-specific metallic ions. BSS has the protective property of a weak buffer and prevents the swelling of the cornea under healthy conditions, and at the same time protects the endothelium [36–38].

10.5.2.2 Aqueous Humor Replacement

The utility of external lavage alone is arguable when the chemical has reached into the aqueous humor. Removal of the aqueous humor having a non-physiological pH, with or without replacing it with saline has been suggested in the literature. Studies done in animal models with alkali injury recorded a drop in pH by1.5 units after paracentesis alone and subsequently replacing it by phosphate buffer solution further reduced it by 1.5 units [28]. Although it is not a routinely performed procedure while managing these cases but can be considered in cases with moderately severe to severe grades of chemical injuries, especially for the cases presenting within 2 h of injury.

10.6 Clinical Examination and Classification of Chemical Injuries

Once a thorough external lavage has been performed, a detailed ocular examination should be carried out, starting from the blinking, examination of lids for lid defects, lagophthalmos, presence of any eschar preventing the complete closure of the lids. Globe should be properly examined for its integrity in cases of blast injuries. Visual acuity and intraocular pressure have to be recorded. Presence of limbal ischemia, corneal and conjunctival epithelial defect, degree of stromal edema should be recorded. If visible, the details of the anterior chamber like the presence of cellular reaction or fibrin, iris changes, opacification of the lens should be put down in the patient's record.

While assessing limbal ischemia it is important to note that the presence of thrombosed vessels around the limbus should not be confused with the patient perilimbal vessels. Thrombosed vessels are deep red to brown with the presence of broken, stationary blood columns in between.

The staging of the injury can precisely be performed 24–48 h after the injury, as the actual degree of limbal ischemia becomes evident after the chemosis settles down and the level of stromal hydration induced by the external lavage also subsides by then. Well-documented diagrams representing the extent of the injury, describing the clock hours, and measurements of the corneal and conjunctival defects should be drawn in the patient's record. If possible, anterior segment

Table 10.2 Roper–Hall classification of severity of ocular surface chemical burns [39] (Reprinted with permission: Roper-Hall MJ. Thermal and chemical burns. Trans Ophthalmol Soc U K. 1965;85:631–53. PMID: 5227208)

Grade	Prognosis	Cornea	Limbus
I	Good	Corneal epithelial damage	No limbal ischemia
II	Good	Cornea haze, iris details visible	<1/3 limbal ischemia
III	Guarded	Total epithelial loss, stromal haze, iris details obscured	1/3–1/2 limbal ischemia
IV	Poor	Poor cornea opaque, iris and pupil obscured	>1/2 limbal ischemia

Table 10.3 Dua et al. classification of ocular surface chemical burns (Reprinted with permission: Dua HS, King AJ, Joseph A. A new classification of ocular surface burns. Br J Ophthalmol. 2001; 85(11):1379–83)

Grade	Prognosis	Clinical findings	Conjunctival involvement[a]	Analog scale
I	Very good	0 clock hours of limbal involvement	0%	0%
II	Good	≤3 clock hours of limbal involvement	≤30%	0.1–3/1–29.9%
III	Good	>3–6 clock hours of limbal involvement	>30–50%	3.1–6/31–50%
IV	Good to guarded	>6–9 clock hours of limbal involvement	>50–75%	6.1–9/51–75%
V	Guarded to poor	>9–<12 clock hours of limbal involvement	>75–< 100%	9.1–11.9/75.1–99.9%
VI	Very poor	Total limbus (12 clock hours) involved	Total conjunctiva (100%)	12/100%

[a]For calculating the conjunctival involvement area, only involvement of bulbar conjunctiva [excluding palpebral conjunctiva], up to and including the conjunctival fornices is considered. The analog scale is calculated by recording the limbal involvement in clock hours/percentage of conjunctival involvement

photographs should be taken. That would act as a guide toward recovery and plays an important role in cases with medicolegal implications.

Classification systems serve as an aid to grade the injury, help in tailoring the treatment methodology, and foreseeing the visual prognosis. The commonly used classification systems are the Roper–Hall classification which is a modification of a classification system developed by Ballen et al. [39, 40] and Dua's classification system. Roper–Hall system considers the extent of corneal involvement and the limbal ischemia in terms of clock hours as the markers to grade the severity of the chemical injury (Table 10.2), and it does not take the conjunctival involvement as a criterion for the grading. On the other hand, Dua's classification system does not take into account the corneal involvement, instead, it is based on the percentage of conjunctiva involved along with the extent of limbal epithelial defect in clock hours (Table 10.3). As the presence of limbal ischemia has long been recognized as an indirect marker of limbal stem cell damage [41], Roper–Hall system considers the presence of perilimbal ischemia as the marker of stem cell damage, while Dua's system considers the presence of limbal epithelial defect to mark the same [42]. They suggest that sometimes even in the presence of limbal vascularity there might be an underlying stem cell damage.

Therefore, fluorescein staining is required to grade the limbal involvement as per Dua's system. It reduces the inter-observer bias which can be commonly encountered while assessing the perilimbal ischemia, especially during early hours, in the presence of severe conjunctival chemosis. An analog scale is thus calculated which acts as a guide to monitor improvement or worsening during treatment. It is an important guide toward the treatment response as the analog scale will show a change even when the grade of the injury remains the same.

Another shortcoming of the Roper–Hall system is that all the injuries with more than 50% of limbal ischemia are labeled as grade IV severity. Therefore, a patient with limbal ischemia involving 7 clock hours is labeled to be of equal severity as a patient with 12 clock hours involvement, however, this implication might not stand correct for most of the cases. Also important to note here is that none of these classification systems takes into account the depth of the injury.

10.7 Phases of Chemical Injury

Mc Culley divided the course of chemical injury into four phases [42] as described in Table 10.4. The treatment in different stages might overlap or differ according to the ongoing pathophysiological changes in the eye.

Table 10.4 Phases of chemical injury

Phase	Time in days	Findings
Immediate	0	Immediate effects of injury in the form of raised IOP, corneal or conjunctival epithelial defect with or without limbal ischemia, and intraocular findings like lens opacification
Acute	0–7	Signs of inflammation start to appear. In mild injuries, the epithelium starts to heal. IOP may rise due to inflammation, rapid change occurs in corneal transparency
Early reparative	7–21	This is the transition phase. Epithelial healing gets completed in the milder form of injuries. Acute inflammation transits into chronic inflammation, stromal repair process and scarring starts making its way
Late reparative	>21	Cases with mild injuries heal completely, and inflammation subsides. In eyes with severe injuries, sequelae of LSCD start appearing in the form of pseudo pterygium, corneal neovascularization. Conjunctival cicatrization and lid abnormality start to develop. The persistent epithelial defect either heals with scarring or leads to secondary infection or corneal melt. Raised IOP often missed, can lead to glaucomatous damage

10.8 Treatment

10.8.1 Acute and Early Reparative Treatment

Once the emergency treatment has been provided, the acute and early reparative treatment aims at reducing the inflammation, halting the stromal breakdown, consequently promoting re-epithelialization and providing patient comfort.

10.8.1.1 Broad-Spectrum Topical Antibiotics

Topical broad-spectrum antibiotics are given to prevent superadded infectious keratitis in the presence of an epithelial defect. Preservative-free topical fluoroquinolones instilled 4–6 times a day provide good antimicrobial coverage and can be continued till the time the defect heals.

10.8.1.2 Artificial Lubricants and Cycloplegics

Severe chemical injuries lead to the destruction of conjunctival goblet cells and damage to Meibomian glands, resulting in poor mucin and lipid components in the tear film. Preservative-free artificial tear substitutes and gel increase patient comfort, prevent drying and further epithelial breakdown, thereby promotes re-epithelialization. Cycloplegic agents should be added to the initial treatment regimen for mydriasis and to provide relief from the painful ciliary body spasm.

10.8.1.3 Oral and Topical Sodium Ascorbate (10%)

Ascorbate is a reducing agent required by fibroblasts to hydroxylate proline during collagen synthesis. As mentioned earlier, a significant reduction in ascorbate level develops in the aqueous humor post chemical injury, which can in turn inhibit collagen synthesis by fibroblasts leading to corneal thinning and perforation. Therefore, ascorbate supplementation significantly reduces the risk of corneal perforation [43]. Topical ascorbate has better anterior segment penetration than the oral form [44]. Maintaining compliance with topical ascorbate eye drops can be challenging due to ocular pain and burning on the instillation of drops, therefore oral ascorbate should always be given along, and patient education and reinforcement would help them to comply with the treatment. Instilling topical sodium ascorbate 10% solution 1–2 hourly along with 500–1000 mg of oral ascorbic acid four times a day may maintain aqueous ascorbic acid at levels high enough to reduce the risk of corneal ulceration.

10.8.1.4 Corticosteroids

Post chemical injury, severe inflammation is the key factor around which most of the complications revolve. Steroids reduce the inflammatory cell infiltration and Polymorphonuclear lysosomal enzyme release into the stroma. They are also helpful in the treatment of associated iridocyclitis. In an animal study, the use of steroids after 6 days has been reported to increase the risk of stromal melting [45], however studies published later supported that no increased risk of corneoscleral melting was seen when the steroids were concurrently used with ascorbic acid [46]. Potent topical steroids in the form of 1% prednisolone acetate or 0.1% dexamethasone should be started from the first day of the injury and instilled every 1–2 hourly and the frequency can be reduced as per the inflammatory reaction.

10.8.1.5 Oral Tetracyclines and Topical Citrate

Inflammatory cell release proteinases, collagenase, and stromelysin causing collagen breakdown leading to corneal or scleral melts [47]. Tetracyclines and citrate have shown a definite role in suppressing the release of proteolytic enzymes and in scavenging free oxygen radicals released in animal models of chemical injuries. Topical citrate is a calcium chelator, it depletes the intracellular calcium from neutrophils thereby inhibiting chemotaxis, phagocytosis, and release of proteolytic enzymes [48]. Tetracyclines have anti-inflammatory and anti-collagenolytic activity besides their antimicrobial properties. Doxycycline inhibits MMP 9 activity and downregulates the release of pro-inflammatory cytokine IL-1b and tumor necrosis factor [49].

10.8.1.6 Ocular Hypotensive Agents

Depending upon the IOP antiglaucoma medications either in the form of oral carbonic anhydrase inhibitors or topical agents can be prescribed. Aqueous suppressants are considered as preferred agents as the outflow channels are mostly clogged or sometimes even damaged due to direct injury.

10.8.1.7 Blood Derived Topical Agents

Autologous peripheral blood serum (PBS), platelet-rich plasma (PRP), and umbilical cord serum (UCS) have been reported to hasten epithelial healing in chemical injuries. These are rich in various growth factors like epidermal growth factor (EGF), transforming growth factor-beta (TGF-β), surface immunoglobulin A, and fibronectin [50]. Issues with blood-derived topical therapy are difficulties in obtaining and preparing the treatment, lack of a standardized preparation protocol, potential risk of contamination and infection, shorter shelf life, and higher cost.

10.8.2 Surgical Treatment in the Acute Phase

10.8.2.1 Amniotic Membrane Transplantation (AMT)

Human amniotic membrane transplantation (AMT) may help in accelerating re-epithelialization of corneal and conjunctival surfaces, reducing ocular surface inflammation and pain. It may help to alleviate some potential sequelae like a non-healing defect and symblepharon formation and also help partially restore the limbal stem cell function [51]. The amniotic membrane (AM) serves as a basement membrane for epithelial cell migration and provides various growth factors like epidermal growth factor, transforming growth factor, and hepatocyte growth factor [52]. AM reduces scarring by the release of anti-inflammatory cytokines and inducing apoptosis of inflammatory cells [53]. Suturing in an acutely inflamed eye is a difficult task and requires expertise. Advancement has been made toward sutureless

AMT, e.g. devices like Prokera (Scope Ophthalmics Ltd) which contains an amniotic membrane clipped between transparent flexible rings is helpful in such cases. Placement of AM sutured over a symblepharon ring is another non-traumatic alternative when the other sutureless AM devices are not available. In cases with large areas of conjunctival defects and forniceal involvement, placement of a symblepharon ring with suturing of the AM to the lid margins can be performed. It has been seen that re-epithelialization is significantly faster in medium severity injuries (Dua's stage II-III) with AMT [54, 55]. However, no additional benefit was observed in cases with severe chemical injuries. When applied in the acute stage, a severe inflammatory state of the eye may lead to the rapid dissolution of AMT, necessitating several repeat procedures.

The prophylactic approach should be followed for the prevention of symblepharon formation in all cases involving conjunctival burns. Transudation of intravascular fluid in an inflamed eye often results in the formation of fibrin bridges. The raw surfaces get adhered to each other and later scarring and contractures develop, leading to the formation of symblepharon or ankyloblepharon. Periodic removal of these adhesions in the initial phases using a glass rod greased in antibiotic ointment or applying a symblepharon ring or covering the raw surfaces with an AMT helps in preventing these sequelae [56]. However, these approaches might not be effective in cases with severe burns.

10.8.2.2 Tenonplasty

Severe chemical burns can lead to extensive destruction of the limbal vascular supply, leading to sterile necrosis and corneoscleral melt [57]. AMT may fail to re-epithelialize the conjunctival defects in cases where there is ischemia due to the destruction of episcleral vasculature [58, 59]. In cases with scleral ischemia, tenonplasty is considered to be a useful way to provide a vascular pedicle for the migration of conjunctival epithelial cells, in the early period [60, 61]. After complete excision of the dead, necrosed tissue, careful separation of the viable tenons tissue is done while preserving the vascular supply of the capsule which is located posteriorly [62]. Advancement of these vascularized tenons from the orbital region is performed up to the limbus, thereby covering the avascular area by healthy vascularized tissue. The procedure can be combined with AMT to provide an additional advantage of its anti-inflammatory and healing properties (Fig. 10.6). Anterior segment angiography can be utilized to demarcate the area with limbal ischemia and perform a selective tenonplasty [63]. Important to note here is that Tenon's advancement may be difficult in patients with acute injury due to the presence of inflamed, friable conjunctival, and Tenon's tissue.

10.8.2.3 Glued-On Contact Lens

Animal studies have shown that covering the corneal surface with methyl methacrylate lens with cyanoacrylate glue application in the initial period of chemical injury prevented PMN infiltration of the stroma and stromal ulceration. Glued-on lenses applied to already ulcerating corneas arrested further ulceration by prohibiting additional PMN infiltration. The epithelium should not be allowed to grow on

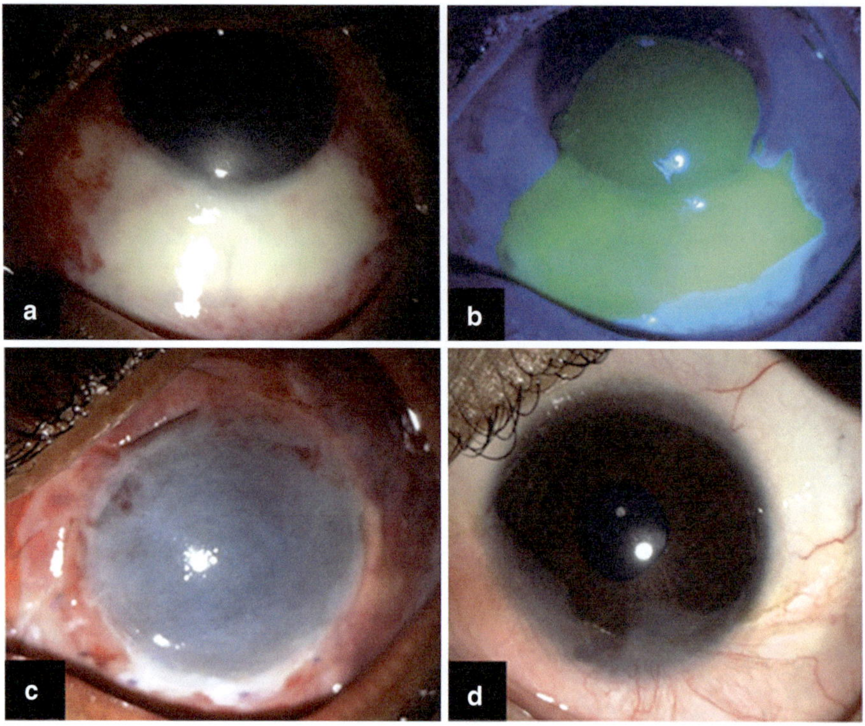

Fig. 10.6 A patient presenting after 48 h of exposure to acetic acid, after receiving primary treatment elsewhere. By this time chemosis has grossly subsided, making perilimbal ischemia clearly demarcated, which corresponds to the area of conjunctival defect taking fluorescence stain (**a**, **b**). Sectoral tenonplasty and AMT were performed for this eye (**c**, **d**) postoperative picture shows vascularization of the necrosed area with localized growth of conjunctival tissue, sparing the visual axis

the affected area; therefore, a complete 360° seal is required between the periphery of the lens and the corneal surface. The efficacy of this procedure is based on the possibility that epithelium stimulates the infiltration of the stroma by PMNs which then participate in stromal matrix degradation [64].

10.8.3 Treatment in the Intermediate Stage

The treatment in the intermediate stage is directed toward promoting re-epithelialization, reducing inflammation, and managing the complications arising after the acute stage, e.g. non-healing defect, descemetocoele formation, corneal perforation, microbial keratitis, corneal-scleral melt, etc. [65].

Even in the mild form of injury, recurrent epithelial erosions may develop when there is damage to the basal lamina or anterior stroma. In some cases, even when the limbal stem cells are intact, adhesion problems can occur due to faulty epithelial–stromal interaction due to the accelerated degradation of fibrinogen by plasminogen activator [66]. The further epithelial movement does not occur in the absence of adhesion of the leading edge of the epithelium and thereafter it peels off.

Several strategies may help in treating a non-healing epithelial defect, apart from the conservative treatment. Performing a tarsorrhaphy helps in minimizing the mechanical rubbing of the eyelids with the friable healing epithelium. Application of a well-fitted bandage contact lens would serve the same function; however, an increased risk of microbial keratitis limits its use. AMT serves its purpose well in acute as well as intermediate stages in promoting epithelial healing. For smaller corneal perforation up to 3 mm, closure with cyanoacrylate glue is the least invasive and effective way of re-establishing the integrity of the eye. Larger perforations and corneal melts require keratoplasty. The issue of non-healing defects does not spare even the implanted grafts; therefore, performing an intraoperative or early postoperative tarsorrhaphy is advisable.

10.8.4 Chronic Sequelae and Treatment

A summary of the chronic sequelae of ocular chemical injuries has been provided in Table 10.5; Fig. 10.7. Treatment of chronic sequelae and an attempt for visual rehabilitation should start with optimizing the ocular surface first. Lid-globe congruity, presence of a near-normal tear film, and a quiet eye without intractable glaucoma are the obligatory requirements before visual restorative procedures are undertaken. Lid abnormalities like lagophthalmos, ectropion, entropion, and dystrichiasis should be corrected first before going ahead with keratoplasty or stem cell transplant. Symblepharon lysis and expansion of cul-de-sac should be performed. Punctual plugs can be used to address the aqueous tear deficiency.

Table 10.5 Chronic sequelae of ocular chemical injuries

Ocular structures	Associated complications
Eyelids and related structures	Meibomian gland destruction Lagophthalmos, lid defects Trichiasis Ectropion, entropion
Conjunctiva	Goblet cell loss, dry eyes Symblepharon, ankyloblepharon Subconjunctival scarring
Cornea and limbus	Limbal stem cell deficiency Conjunctivalization of cornea Corneal neovascularization, corneal scarring Corneal melt, microbial keratitis Recurrent erosions, non-healing epithelial defect
Intraocular structures	Chronic inflammation Damage to the trabecular meshwork, ocular hypertension Anterior synechiae Damage to iris tissue Cataract formation Ciliary body damage, hypotony/phthisis bulbi Glaucomatous optic neuropathy

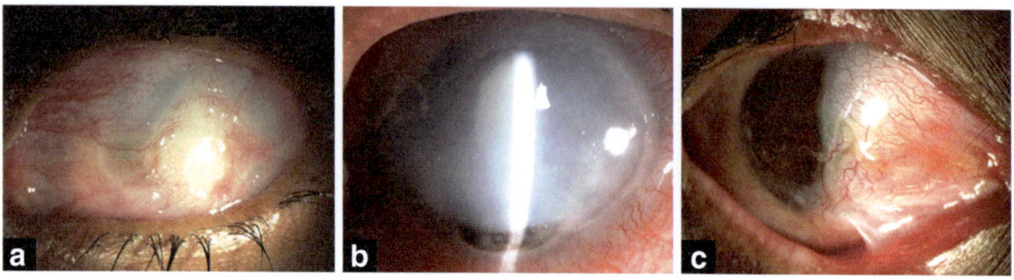

Fig. 10.7 Various chronic sequelae after ocular chemical injury in the form of; (**a**) Total conjunctivalization of the cornea due to extensive limbal stem cell damage. (**b**) A sterile melt of the cornea due to stromal lysis with iris prolapsing inferiorly near the limbus. A flat anterior chamber with the presence of a cataractous lens can be noted. (**c**) kerato-blepharon identified nasally along with conjunctivalization of the cornea seen from 6 to 9 clock hours

10.8.4.1 Limbal Stem Cell Transplant

Limbal stem cell deficiency (LSCD) is one of the devastating complications of severe ocular chemical injuries, resulting due to irreversible damage to the stem cells population residing deep in a protected microenvironment within the limbal epithelium. Various manifestations of LSCD are recurrent corneal erosions or non-healing epithelial defects, corneal neovascularization, and conjunctivalization of the cornea. Limbal stem cell transplant (LSCT) should only be done once the inflammation remains subsided for at least 3 months; this provides time for recovery of existing stem cells damaged by chemical injury [67]. In general, LSCTs are either autologous or allogeneic, Table 10.6 provides a summary of various techniques for LSCT.

10.8.4.2 Keratoplasty

In chemical injuries, keratoplasty may be required in early stages for tectonic or therapeutic purposes and for visual rehabilitation in the late phase. In an inflamed, vascularized eye, the risk of graft rejection is higher for the cases undergoing penetrating keratoplasty, therefore anterior lamellar keratoplasty is preferred over full-thickness corneal grafting wherever possible, to reduce the risk of endothelial rejection. In cases with LSCD, performing a staged procedure with LSCT performed 6 weeks before the corneal transplantation is seen to be associated with an 80% survival rate after 12 months. This is in distinct contrast to the 25% success rate for non-staged procedures [68].

10.8.5 Treatment of the End-Stage Disease

10.8.5.1 Keratoprosthesis

In cases with the end-stage disease which are not suitable for keratoplasty or have had multiple failed grafts, keratoprosthesis is the final treatment that can be offered to these patients. However, the patient should be thoroughly explained about the need for prolonged prophylactic antibiotic therapy, the need for regular replacement of the bandage contact lens, long-term complications, and the need for a lifelong

Table 10.6 Various techniques for treating limbal stem cell deficiency

Extent of LSCD	Laterality	Procedure	Donor source	Need for systemic immunosuppression
Partial LSCD		Pannus excision with AMT		No systemic immunosuppression required
Total LSCD	Unilateral LSCD	Conjunctival–limbal autograft (CLAU)	Limbal stem cells harvested from the patient's other eye	
		Cultivated limbal epithelial transplantation (CLET).		
		Simple limbal epithelial transplantation (SLET)		
		Cultivated oral mucosal epithelial transplantation (COMET)	Graft derived from autologous oral mucosal cells	
	Bilateral LSCD	Living related conjunctival–limbal allograft (lr-CLAL),	Limbal stem cells Harvested from an immediate family member	Requires systemic immunosuppression
		Keratolimbal allograft (KLAL)	Stem cells harvested from cadaver eyes	
		Allogenic cultivated limbal epithelial transplantation (allo-CLET)	Stem cells from a donor with ex vivo expansion	

follow-up. As mentioned earlier, previously missed, untreated glaucoma remains a leading cause of poor visual outcome after a successful keratoprosthesis. The post-operative management sometimes can be exhaustive and may demand a great deal of dedication and patience from the surgeon as well as the patient's part.

10.8.5.2 Enucleation or Evisceration

This might be required for a worn out, painful blind eye in which all other treatment options have been failed.

10.8.6 Experimental Treatment Modalities

More recently proposed treatment agents for promoting corneal wound healing like TNF-α antibodies (Infliximab), growth factors (e.g. fibronectin, EGF, retinoic acid), subconjunctival progesterone, thiol dipeptides have shown promising results in animal studies. However, clinical trials will be needed before any of these approaches can be considered for human use [64, 69, 70].

The devastating nature of ocular chemical injuries may result in severe personal, social, and economic loss to the victim. Many of these injuries are preventable, emphasizing the importance of public health measures, education, and safekeeping in the prevention of such incidents. Widespread media campaigns may prove helpful in educating the public about early irrigation and emergency treatment.

Key Points

- Time to initial irrigation has the greatest impact on the visual prognosis and ensures the best possible outcome for this potentially blinding condition.
- In an eye post chemical injury, the degradative and the reparative process are ongoing simultaneously. A shift in the balance between the two decides the ultimate outcome.
- Therefore, the treatment aims at reducing the degradative process and accelerating the reparative process.
- The visual rehabilitation in the form of keratoplasty should be undertaken only when the inflammation has subsided and ocular surface reconstruction should be performed before the keratoplasty.
- Prevention of such injuries by promoting safety protocols should be the primary aim. As the prognosis in severe cases is mostly unfavorable and demands exhaustive efforts from patients as well as the surgeon's end.

References

1. White ML, Chodosh J, Jang J, Dohlman C. Incidence of Stevens-Johnson syndrome and chemical burns to the eye. Cornea. 2015;34(12):1527–33.
2. Ghosh S, Salvador-Culla B, Kotagiri A, Pushpoth S, Tey A, Johnson ZK, et al. Acute chemical eye injury and limbal stem cell deficiency–a prospective study in the United Kingdom. Cornea. 2019;38(2):198–202.
3. Kuckelkorn R, Kottek A, Schrage N, Reim M. Poor prognosis of severe chemical and thermal eye burns: the need for adequate emergency care and primary prevention. Int Arch Occup Environ Health. 1995;67(4):281–4.
4. Hong J, Qiu T, Wei A, Sun X, Xu J. Clinical characteristics, and visual outcome of severe ocular chemical injuries in Shanghai. Ophthalmology. 2010;117(12):2268–72.
5. Macdonald EC, Cauchi PA, Azuara-Blanco A, Foot B. Surveillance of severe chemical corneal injuries in the UK. Br J Ophthalmol. 2009;93(9):1177–80.
6. National Health Portal (NHP). Chemical injuries to the eyes (internet). India; 2016. www.nhp.gov.in/disease/eye-ear/chemical-injuries-to-the-eyes.
7. Solberg Y, Alcalay M, Belkin M. Ocular injury by mustard gas. Surv Ophthalmol. 1997;41(6):461–6.
8. Maumenee AE, Scholtz RO. The histopathology of ocular lesions produced by sulfur and nitrogen mustards. Bull Johns Hopkins Hosp. 1948;82(2):121–47.
9. Safarinejad MR, Moosavi SA, Montazeri B. Ocular injuries caused by mustard gas: diagnosis, treatment, and medical defense. Mil Med. 2001;166(1):67–70.
10. Bessac BF, Sivula M, von Hehn CA, Caceres AI, Escalera J, Jordt SE. Transient receptor potential ankyrin 1 antagonists block the noxious effects of toxic industrial isocyanates and tear gases. FASEB J. 2009;23(4):1102–14.

11. Brône B, Peeters PJ, Marrannes R, et al. Tear gasses CN, CR, and CS are potent activators of the human TRPA1 receptor. Toxicol Appl Pharmacol. 2008;231(2):150–6.
12. Gross DA. The forgotten history of mace, designed by a 29-year-old and reinvented as a police weapon. Smithsonian Magazine; 4 November 2014.
13. Reilly CA, Crouch DJ, Yost GS. Quantitative analysis of capsaicinoids in fresh peppers, oleoresin capsicum, and pepper spray products. J Forensic Sci. 2001;46(3):502–9.
14. Hayman M, Kam PCA. Capsaicin: a review of its pharmacology and clinical applications. Curr Anaesth Crit Care. 2008;64(4):939–71.
15. Kuriachen PM, Dave Y. Structural, developmental, and histochemical studies in the collectors of *Calotropis procera* (Asclepiadaceae). J Phytol Res. 1989;2(4):7–14.
16. Basak Samar K, Arup B, Ayan M, Prashant S. Ocular toxicity by latex of *Calotropis procera* (Sodom apple). Indian J Ophthalmol. 2009;57(3):232–4.
17. Ioannidis AS, Papageorgiou KI, Andreou PS. Exposure to *Euphorbia lathyris* latex resulting in alkaline chemical injury: a case report. J Med Case Rep. 2009;3:115.
18. Grant WM, Schuman JS. Toxicology of the eye. 4th ed. Springfield, IL: Charles C Thomas; 1993. p. 680–2.
19. Scott IU, Karp CL. Euphorbia sap keratopathy: four cases and a possible pathogenic mechanism. Br J Ophthalmol. 1996;80(9):823–6.
20. Eke T. Acute kerato-uveitis associated with topical self-administration of the sap of the petty spurge (*Euphorbia peplus*). Eye. 1994;8(6):694–6.
21. https://www.holifestival.org/chemical-colors
22. https://www.poison.org/articles/2016-sep/hair-dye
23. Park R, Hansen T, Bell D. Self-inflicted chemical burns caused by depilatory cream use: the price of beauty. Indian J Burns. 2019;27(1):44–8.
24. Barnes SS, Wong W Jr, Affeldt JC. A case of severe airbag-related ocular alkali injury. Hawaii J Med Public Health. 2012;71(8):229–31.
25. Krachmer J, Mannis M, Holland E. Chapter 98 - acid injuries of the eye. In: Cornea fundamentals and medical aspects of cornea and external disease. 2nd ed. Elsevier.
26. McCulley JP. Ocular hydrofluoric acid burns: animal model, mechanism of injury, and therapy. Trans Am Ophthalmol Soc. 1990;88:649–84.
27. Friedenwald JS, Hughes WF Jr, Herrmann H. Acid burns of the eye. Arch Ophthalmol. 1946;35:98–108.
28. Paterson CA, Pfister RR, Levinson RA. Aqueous humor pH changes after experimental alkali burns. Am J Ophthalmol. 1975;79(3):414–9.
29. Grant WM, Thomas CC. Toxicology of the eye. Cutan Ocul Toxicol. 1987;6(3):155–6.
30. Paterson CA, Pfister RR. Intraocular pressure changes after alkali burns. Arch Ophthalmol. 1974;91(3):211–8.
31. Wagoner MD. Chemical injuries of the eye: current concepts in pathophysiology and therapy. Surv Ophthalmol. 1997;41(4):275–313.
32. Pfister RR, Paterson CA. Ascorbic acid in the bums treatment of alkali of the eye. Ophthalmology. 1980;87(10):1050–7.
33. Schrage N. Rinsing therapy of eye burns. In: Schrager, et al., editors. Chemical ocular burns: new understanding and treatments. Heidelberg: Springer; 2011. p. 77–92.
34. Kompa S, Schareck B, Tympner J, et al. Comparison of emergency eye-wash products in burned porcine eyes. Graefes Arch Clin Exp Ophthalmol. 2002;240(4):308–13.
35. Kuckelkorn R, Schrage N, Keller G, Redbrake C. Emergency treatment of chemical and thermal eye burns. Acta Ophthalmol Scand. 2002;80(1):4–10.
36. Kompa S, Redbrake C, Hilgers C, Wüstemeyer H, Schrage N, Remky A. Effect of different irrigating solutions on aqueous humor pH changes, intraocular pressure and histological findings after induced alkali burns. Acta Ophthalmol Scand. 2005;83(4):467–70.
37. Rihawi S, Frentz M, Reim M, Schrage NF. Rinsing with isotonic saline solution for eye burns should be avoided. Burns. 2008;34(7):1027–32.
38. Herr RD, White GL Jr, Bernhisel K, Mamalis N, Swanson E. Clinical comparison of ocular irrigation fluids following chemical injury. Am J Emerg Med. 1991;9(3):228–31.

39. Roper-Hall MJ. Thermal and chemical burns. Trans Ophthalmol Soc UK. 1965;85:631–53.
40. Ballen PH. Treatment of chemical burns of the eye. Eye Ear Nose Throat Mon. 1964;43:57–61.
41. Dua HS, King AJ, Joseph A. A new classification of ocular surface burns. Br J Ophthalmol. 2001;85(11):1379–83.
42. McCulley JP. Chemical injuries. In: Smolin G, Thoft RA, editors. The cornea: scientific foundation and clinical practice. Boston, MA: Little Brown; 1987. p. 527–42.
43. Levinson RA, Paterson CA, Pfister RR. Ascorbic acid prevents corneal ulceration and perforation following experimental alkali burns. Investig Ophthalmol. 1976;15(12):986–93.
44. Pfister RR, Paterson CA. Ascorbic acid in the treatment of alkaliburns of the eye. Ophthalmology. 1980;87(10):1050–7.
45. Donshik PC, Berman MB, Dohlman CH, Gage J, Rose J. Effect of topical corticosteroids on ulceration in alkali-burned corneas. Arch Ophthalmol. 1978;96(11):2117–20.
46. Davis AR, Ali QH, Aclimandos WA, Hunter PA. Topical steroid use in the treatment of ocular alkali burns. Br J Ophthalmol. 1997;81(9):732–4.
47. Reim M, Bahrke C, Kuckelkorn R, Kuwert T. Investigation of enzyme activities in severe burns of the anterior eye segment. Graefes Arch Clin Exp Ophthalmol. 1993;231(5):308–12.
48. Hughes WF Jr. Alkali burns of the eye; clinical and pathologic course. Arch Ophthalmol. 1946;36:189–214.
49. Ralph RA. Tetracyclines and the treatment of corneal stromal ulceration: a review. Cornea. 2000;19(3):274–7.
50. Yoon KC, Heo H, Im SK, You IC, Kim YH, Park YG. Comparison of autologous serum and umbilical cord serum eye drops for dry eye syndrome. Am J Ophthalmol. 2007;144(1):86–92.
51. Meller D, Pires RT, Mack RJ, et al. Amniotic membrane transplantation for acute chemical or thermal burns. Ophthalmology. 2000;107(5):980–9.
52. Koizumi N, Inatomi T, Sotozono C, Fullwood NJ, Quantock AJ, Kinoshita S. Growth factor mRNA and protein in preserved human amniotic membrane. Curr Eye Res. 2000;20(3):173–7.
53. Shimmura S, Shimazaki J, Ohashi Y, Tsubota K. Antiinflammatory effects of amniotic membrane transplantation in ocular surface disorders. Cornea. 2001;20(4):408–13.
54. Tamhane A, Vajpayee RB, Biswas NR, et al. Evaluation of amniotic membrane transplantation as an adjunct to medical therapy as compared with medical therapy alone in acute ocular burns. Ophthalmology. 2005;112(11):1963–9.
55. Tandon R, Gupta N, Kalaivani M, Sharma N, Titiyal JS, Vajpayee RB. Amniotic membrane transplantation as an adjunct to medical therapy in acute ocular burns. Br J Ophthalmol. 2011;95(2):199–204.
56. Merle H, Gérard M, Schrage N. Brûluresoculaires [Ocular burns]. J Fr Ophtalmol. 2008;31(7):723–34.
57. Gicquel J-J. Management of Ocular Surface Chemical Burns. Br J Ophthalmol. 2011;95(2):159–61.
58. Joseph A, Dua HS, King AJ. Failure of amniotic membrane transplantation in the treatment of acute ocular burns. Br J Ophthalmol. 2001;85(9):1065–9.
59. Lopez-Garcia JS, Rivas Jara L, Garcia-Lozano I, et al. Histopathologic limbus evolution after alkaline burns. Cornea. 2007;26(9):1043–8.
60. Kuckelkorn R, Redbrake C, Reim M. Tenonplasty: a new surgical approach for the treatment of severe eye burns. Ophthalmic Surg Lasers. 1997;28(2):105–10.
61. Iyer G, Srinivasan B, Agarwal S, et al. Visual rehabilitation with keratoprosthesis after tenonplasty as the primary globe-saving procedure for severe ocular chemical injuries. Graefes Arch Clin Exp Ophthalmol. 2012;250(12):1787–93.
62. Reim M, Overkamping B, Kuckelkorn R. 2 years experience with tenon-plasty. Ophthalmologe. 1992;89(6):524–30.
63. Tabatabaei SA, Soleimani M, Mirshahi R, Zandian M, Ghasemi H, Hashemian MN, et al. Selective localized tenonplasty for corneal burns based on the findings of ocular surface fluorescein angiography. Cornea. 2017;36(8):1014–7.

64. Kenyon KR, Berman M, Rose J, Gage J. Prevention of stromal ulceration in the alkali-burned rabbit cornea by glued-on contact lens. Evidence for the role of polymorphonuclear leukocytes in collagen degradation. Invest Ophthalmol Vis Sci. 1979;18(6):570–87.
65. Dua HS, Forrester JV. The corneoscleral limbus in human corneal epithelial wound healing. Am J Ophthalmol. 1990;110(6):646–56.
66. Berman M, Leary R, Gage G. Evidence for a role of the plasminogen activator- plasmin system in corneal ulceration. Invest Ophthalmol Vis Sci. 1980;19(10):1204–21.
67. Bizrah M, Yusuf A, Ahmad S. An update on chemical eye burns. Eye. 2019;33(9):1362–77.
68. Baradaran-Rafii A, Eslani M, Haq Z, Shirzadeh E, Huvard MJ, Djalilian AR. Current and upcoming therapies for ocular surface chemical injuries. Ocul Surf. 2017;15(1):48–64.
69. Zhou C, Robert MC, Kapoulea V, Lei F, Stagner AM, Jakobiec FA, et al. Sustained subconjunctival delivery of infliximab protects the cornea and retina following alkali burn to the eye. Invest Ophthalmol Vis Sci. 2017;58(1):96–105.
70. Cejkova J, Olmiere C, Cejka C, Trosan P, Holan V. The healing of alkali-injured cornea is stimulated by a novel matrix regenerating agent (RGTA, CACICOL20): a biopolymer mimicking heparan sulfates reducing proteolytic, oxidative and nitrosative damage. Histol Histopathol. 2014;29(4):457–78.

11 Emergencies Associated with Corneal Transplantation

Rinky Agarwal, Surya Dev Tayal, and Namrata Sharma

Keratoplasty is the most common and most successful of all organ and tissue transplants [1, 2]. In this procedure, the diseased host cornea is removed and replaced by a corneal graft obtained from a human cadaveric donor. It can involve either full-thickness (penetrating keratoplasty, PKP) or partial-thickness (lamellar keratoplasty, LK) replacement of the host cornea. In anterior lamellar keratoplasty (ALK), only the anterior opacified stromal layer is replaced with an analogous donor tissue. While in endothelial keratoplasty (EK), pathogenic host endothelial cell layer is swapped with a donor Descemet membrane (DM)-endothelial complex with or without the inclusion of stromal layers.

The success of any keratoplasty procedure depends on numerous factors such as the etiology, age of presentation, type of surgery, surgical expertise, and patient compliance. An overview of complications associated with different keratoplasty techniques, presenting as emergencies is described in Table 11.1 [3, 4].

11.1 Intraoperative Emergencies

Intraoperative complications can be either host related or graft related.

R. Agarwal (✉) · S. D. Tayal
Saraswathi Institute of Medical Sciences, Hapur, Uttar Pradesh, India

N. Sharma
Dr Rajendra Prasad Centre for Ophthalmic Sciences, AIIMS, New Delhi, India

B. Sharma, J. S. Titiyal (eds.), *Corneal Emergencies*,
https://doi.org/10.1007/978-981-16-5876-1_11

Table 11.1 Complications associated with keratoplasty

Complications
A. Intraoperative
I. *Host related*
Posterior capsule rent Suprachoroidal hemorrhage
II. *Donor related*
Reversal Loss Buttonholing Eccentric trephination
B. Postoperative
I. *Common to all keratoplasties*
Anterior segment inflammation Wound leak Glaucoma Suture-related complications Persistent-epithelial defect Posterior segment complications Graft infection Graft rejection Graft failure
II. *Specific to Lamellar keratoplasties*
Interface-related problems Graft detachment

11.1.1 Host Related

11.1.1.1 Posterior Capsule Tear With or Without Vitreous Loss

During combined procedures involving corneal transplantation with cataract extraction, posterior capsule (PC) can be inadvertently damaged, with or without subsequent vitreous loss. This may be more common in open-globe surgeries and in individuals with the frail capsule or positive vitreous pressure. Surgical inexperience and poor corneal visibility during LK can also lead to this complication.

Presentation and Diagnosis

Accidental PC tear during open-globe surgery usually occurs while delivering the lens or while aspirating the cortical matter. In lamellar surgeries, the tear may occur during phacoemulsification or during sub-incisional cortical matter aspiration.

The margins of the tear can be identified in retro-illumination mode of the microscope and vitreous strands in the anterior chamber (AC) can be assessed by staining with triamcinolone acetonide, peaking of previously round pupil or by use of dry swab stick at wounds. It is important to maintain a high index of suspicion for this complication as it may be easily missed in eyes with overlying corneal haze.

Management

Small capsular tears without vitreous loss can be managed with the placement of an IOL either in the bag or in the ciliary sulcus. However, larger tears with vitreous loss warrant adequate anterior vitrectomy and intraocular lens (IOL) can be placed in the sulcus after assessing the status of the remaining posterior capsule. In the absence of adequate ciliary support, scleral fixation of IOL can also be attempted in the same sitting by an experienced surgeon. The choice of IOL is usually a three-piece lens for better stability. Infrequently, during lamellar surgeries, a single-piece IOL can also be placed in the bag in case of small tears. Very rarely, the patient may have to be left aphakic in the primary sitting and IOL implantation undertaken in the second sitting.

If the crystalline lens dislocates posteriorly, the wounds should be sutured without any delay and immediate help sought from the vitreoretinal specialist. If pars plana vitrectomy is not possible during primary sitting due to poor visibility, the corneal transplantation is undertaken as planned, and lens removal should be postponed to a later date based on corneal clarity. In the interim period, topical and systemic steroids should be administered to control the inflammation.

Use of intravenous mannitol preoperatively and general anesthesia intraoperatively may be preferred in high-risk patients.

11.1.1.2 Suprachoroidal. Hemorrhage

Suprachoroidal hemorrhage (SCH) is an extremely rare yet, the most feared, intraoperative complication of keratoplasty. Various risk factors are detailed in Table 11.2.

Presentation and Diagnosis

Intraoperatively, change in red-reflex. should raise suspicion of SCH. While appreciation of brown choroidal mounds succeeded by extrusion of intraocular contents suggests SCH in open-globe surgeries. The sudden rise of intraocular pressure (IOP) along with excruciating pain, nausea, and vomiting followed by shallowing of AC and iris prolapse indicates SCH in closed globe procedures.

Management

The emergency management includes prompt closure of the surgical incision with sutures (nylon/Vicryl/silk) along with digital compression of the globe to tamponade the expanding hemorrhage and intravenous mannitol administration for reducing IOP. Immediate SCH drainage by means of posterior sclerotomies carries the risk of rebleed from dislodgement of the clot. It is, therefore, preferable to delay the

Table 11.2 Risk factors for Suprachoroidal. hemorrhage (SCH)

Systemic risk factors	Ocular risk factors
Anti-coagulant drugs	Sudden decompression of eyeball
Anti-platelet medications	History of glaucoma
Advanced age	Axial myopia
Uncontrolled hypertension	Aphakia/Pseudophakia
Atherosclerosis	Prolonged or complicated surgery
Cardiovascular disease	Vitreous loss during surgery
Diabetes mellitus	History of SCH in the fellow eye
Valsalva-type maneuvre	Retrobulbar anesthesia

surgical drainage till liquefaction of the blood (around 5–14 days later) ensues. This can be assessed on serial B-scan ultrasonography. In the interim, ocular hypotensive agents (topical, oral, intravenous), topical steroids, topical cycloplegics, and oral analgesics can be administered.

Prevention

SCH can be prevented by adequate preoperative screening and management of the aforementioned risk factors. Adequate preoperative regulation of glaucoma and systemic hypertension, the institution of intravenous mannitol immediately before the surgery and conducting surgery under general anesthesia should be preferred in high-risk patients.

11.1.1.3 Descemet Membrane Perforation

Intraoperative perforation of DM is rare but serious complication specific to deep ALK. An accidental DM tear may occur while cleaving the pathogenic host stroma from the clear residual stroma.

Incidence and Risk Factors

It is reported to occur in 18.7% cases, around 15% of these are microperforations (<1 mm) [5]. Most of these occur during deep dissection (31.7%), stromal air injection (26.7%), and graft suturing (20.8%). It is more commonly seen with novice surgeons and thinner corneas.

Presentation

A high index of suspicion must be maintained for diagnosing intraoperative DM perforations. While large perforations can result in the frank leak of aqueous through the defect followed by abrupt shallowing of AC, small perforations, especially if peripheral, may be missed intraoperatively if not identified by fluorescein staining.

Management

Management of DM perforation depends on the size and location of the perforation and also on the stage of the surgery at which the perforation occurs. If perforation occurs initially during trephination, it is possible to tightly suture the site of perforation (full-thickness sutures including recipient DM and donor stroma) and continue lamellar dissection. If a perforation happens during stromal dissection, a careful layer-by-layer dissection can be attempted to prevent conversion to PKP. Care should be taken to dissect in the microperforation region only at the end to avoid any extension of the DM tears. DM perforations occurring while suturing are usually microperforations and can be managed by resuturing at a fresh site along with intracameral air tamponade.

Small and peripheral perforations can be managed conservatively with intracameral air tamponade, patching of a defect with residual stroma, fibrin glue, or heavy viscoelastic substance (VES) and by suturing of the defect. Intracameral air can also be injected to temporarily seal the perforation. Postoperatively, the pupil is fully dilated, and the patient is asked to lie supine for 2–3 days during the majority of the day.

A large or central perforation may mandate conversion to PKP. Rarely centripetal layered dissection may also be undertaken for such perforations to prevent conversion to PKP.

Outcome and Prevention

Postoperative outcomes are usually good with minimal effect on visual acuity or graft survival. Still, a high index of suspicion should be maintained for shallow AC, or double or triple AC formation in the postoperative phase.

In eyes at risk of DM perforations such as healed hydrops and corneal thickness <250 μm, general anesthesia and stromal dissection may be preferred over local anesthesia and big bubble formation. Accurate preoperative assessment of depth of stromal opacification by means of anterior segment optical coherence tomography (ASOCT), ultrasound biomicroscopy and intraoperative assessment by real-time intraoperative OCT can prevent DM perforation [1].

11.1.2 Donor Related

The corneal donor tissue can get misplaced or damaged during the process. of donor preparation (usually undertaken prior to host preparation). The incidence of these complications tends to decrease with the surgeon's experience and caution.

During PKP, a misplaced donor is commonly found adhering to the margins of the trephine. Reversed donor orientation while punching can be corrected by noting its curvature. These donors should be used cautiously as endothelial viability may be compromised in the entire process.

LK procedures are additionally prone to donor buttonholing (tear in donor), eccentric trephination (identified by noting irregularly thick graft margins or eccentric trephination marks on the residual donor rim), reversal (ALK grafts have convex upwards curvature and EK grafts usually fold inwards towards the stromal side, the reversal of these grafts can be identified by noting these findings) and loss, all of which can lead to irreversible graft trauma. It is best to defer any host manipulation in such cases until fresh tissue is available. Donor buttonholing is usually recognized by the presence of a tear that leaks fluid.

11.2 Postoperative Emergencies

Early postoperative complications usually occur within 1 month after surgery, while delayed complications are reported later. Careful clinical examination, high index of suspicion, regular use of anterior segment optical coherence tomography, and ardent patient compliance can aid in prevention as well as early diagnosis and timely management of these complications.

11.2.1 Complications Common to all Keratoplasties

11.2.1.1 Anterior Segment Inflammation

Anterior segment inflammation is a common finding after any intraocular surgery. Normally, mild to moderate AC reaction can also be commonly seen in the early postoperative phase of a keratoplasty, particularly PKP.

Risk Factors

Intense inflammation may sometimes be witnessed when concomitant procedures such as cataract extraction, IOL implantation, iris-related maneuvers, and anterior vitrectomy are undertaken. This risk may be less with LK procedures as these are relatively closed-chamber procedures that involve less trauma to the iris tissue.

Types

Depending on the indication and type of surgical procedure, anterior segment inflammation can present in varying grades of severity comprising of fibrin formation, toxic anterior shock syndrome (TASS), and Urrets-Zavalia syndrome (UZS).

TASS is an intense anterior segment inflammatory reaction secondary to the inadvertent introduction of potentially toxic non-infectious agents in anterior chamber. Incorrectly constituted intracameral preparations with inappropriate chemical composition, concentration, pH, or osmolality. Antibiotics, anesthetic agents, denatured VES, have been implicated in causing TASS. Organic contaminant residues in reusable cannulas, detergents, or non-ionized water employed for cleaning instruments, oxidized metal deposits are other causes. Rarely, the reaction can also occur to intracameral drug injection, capsule staining dyes and due to inadvertent seeping of antibiotic-steroid ointment instilled at the end of the surgery. The hallmark features include moderate to severe anterior uveitis, diffuse corneal edema, and raised IOP in the immediate postoperative phase. It. can be differentiated from postoperative acute endophthalmitis by its early onset (TASS usually manifests on the first postoperative day) and absence of posterior segment involvement.

UZS is a rare complication of corneal transplantation associated with mydriatic use in the immediate postoperative period. In deep ALK and EK, pupillary block due to large intracameral air bubbles can also lead to UZS. The presumed cause is iris tissue ischemia secondary to elevated IOP or inflammation. In the acute phase, UZS is associated with a fixed dilated pupil with or without adherence to the anterior lens capsule. Later on, formation of peripheral anterior synechiae (PAS), iris atrophy, anterior subcapsular cataract and secondary glaucoma can occur in UZS.

Management

The primary treatment of excess inflammatory response such as fibrin formation and TASS involves the urgent institution of intensive steroid therapy (topical ± oral/intravenous). High-potency steroids such as prednisolone or dexamethasone are preferred for topical application. They are begun on an hourly basis and then slowly tapered based on the clinical response. Additional methods of management such as cycloplegic agents, anti-glaucoma drugs, tissue plasminogen activator (smallest effective dose), hyphema drainage, synechiolysis, and iridectomy/iridoplasty can be supplemented whenever necessary. The most important step in preventing TASS is to formulate TASS prevention protocols and regularly train surgical staff about adequate cleaning and sterilization of ophthalmic surgical instruments. Switching to single-use disposable instruments is also an effective way to prevent contamination of ophthalmic instruments during cleaning and sterilization.

UZS involves immediate withdrawal of cycloplegic agents and the institution of topical steroids to control the inflammation. The dilated pupil in UZS does not respond to pilocarpine, sympatholytic agents or to alpha-adrenergic blockers and hence the treatment is directed towards the symptomatic control of glare and photophobia. Cosmetic contact lenses can be employed for this purpose, and these also help in the concealment of anisocoria. Synechiolysis and surgical pupilloplasty can also be attempted to release PAS and mechanically pull the peripheral iris centrally. Certain steps such as thorough wash of VES and avoidance of massive intracameral air injection in phakic patients at the end of the surgery, cautious use of cycloplegic agents, adequate control of IOP and inflammation in the immediate postoperative phase may aid in preventing the occurrence of UZS. Sometimes iridectomy may be indicated in eyes with increased vitreous pressure, shallow AC, or the presence of voluminous air or gas in the AC.

11.2.1.2 Wound Leak

Wound leaks in the early postoperative period can occur from surgical incisions, suture tracts, or graft-host junction. A low IOP with or without a shallow AC should raise suspicion of a wound leak [6]. This is best diagnosed by positive Seidel test on fluorescein staining.

Wound leaks in the late postoperative phase can occur after trauma-associated wound dehiscence. More severe cases can witness gross hypotony, iris prolapse, loss of lens/IOL, choroidal detachment (CD) and loss of eyeball. These are less common with LKs due to the superior globe strength offered by residual partial-thickness host tissue.

Any wound leak deems urgent attention due to the risk of endophthalmitis and graft failure. In eyes with well-formed AC, conservative management such as pressure bandage and soft contact lens can be undertaken. These temporary measures can also be employed initially for eyes with shallow AC. However, if these methods fail, the definitive treatment involves securing the wound with sutures (intermittent 10-0 nylon sutures) or tissue adhesives (fibrin glue or cyanoacrylate glue). The prolapsed iris tissue should be excised if it is >24-h old or associated with signs of necrosis. Rarely, regrafting is required to salvage the globe's integrity.

Wound leaks, if untreated, can lead to endophthalmitis, endothelial cell loss, graft failure, suboptimal visual gain, fistula formation, and epithelial ingrowth due to astigmatism. These can be prevented by ensuring good wound construction at the beginning of the surgery and their adequate closure at the end of the surgery. Newer techniques of wound construction, such as femtosecond laser, can also decrease the incidence of wound leaks.

11.2.1.3 Glaucoma

Glaucoma is a sight-threatening complication and can lead to irreversible visual loss from optic nerve head damage [7]. Early postoperative rise of IOP can occur due to retained VES in the AC, intense anterior uveitis, hyphema, pupillary block, endophthalmitis, and worsening of pre-existing glaucoma. While delayed-onset glaucoma can be added due to vitreous in AC, progressive PAS formation, steroid use, epithelial ingrowth, and graft rejection.

Presentation

Acute onset rise of IOP due to pupillary block, PAS, and intense inflammation may be associated with sudden onset sleep-disturbing pain, nausea, vomiting, ocular congestion and loss of vision. While patients with chronic glaucoma are usually asymptomatic and present with constricted visual field or loss of central vision only in late phases. It is therefore important to measure IOP and evaluate optic nerve head status at every follow-up. Given the inaccuracy of Goldmann applanation tonometry in eyes with corneal edema and surface irregularities, Mackay-Marg electronic tonometer or dynamic contour tonometer is recommended to measure IOP in post-keratoplasty patients. Automated perimetry should also be undertaken whenever possible.

Management

The use of topical medications to control IOP remains the first-line treatment of post-keratoplasty glaucoma. Topical and systemic anti-glaucoma medications such as beta-adrenergic blockers (Timolol maleate 0.5% or Betaxolol 0.5% two times/day), alpha-2 adrenergic agonists (Brimonidine tartarate 0.2% two times/day), oral carbonic anhydrase inhibitors 250 mg three times/day), and osmotic agents (intravenous Mannitol 20% 1–2 g/kg, oral Glycerol 50% 1–1.5 g/kg) should be administered for control of IOP. The choice of therapy relies on the experience and discretion of the treating ophthalmologist.

However, the adverse effects of the above medications and their effect on graft survival must be considered before instituting the therapy. Beta-adrenergic blockers can lead to superficial punctate keratopathy, exacerbation of dry eyes and corneal anesthesia that can be detrimental to the graft. Alpha-2-adrenergic agonists are associated with allergic reactions, superficial punctate keratopathy and dry eyes. It is preferable to not use miotics as they aggravate inflammation and can stimulate graft rejection besides increasing the risk of retinal detachment in aphakics. Caution should also be exercised while administering prostaglandin analogs as they may result in uveitis, CME and reactivation of herpes simplex keratitis. Long-term use of topical carbonic anhydrase can lead to graft decompensation due to damage to donor endothelial cells, while their systemic use can cause tinnitus, gastrointestinal disturbances, paraesthesia, anorexia, nephrolithiasis and blood dyscrasias. Besides, all topical agents should be used judiciously as these can cause preservative (Benzalkonium chloride 0.01%) induced secondary epitheliopathy. Steroid-induced glaucoma involves either tapering of the ongoing steroids or shift to a lower potency steroid along with administration of anti-glaucoma agents.

Surgical modalities such as laser trabeculoplasty, peripheral iridectomy, filtering surgery supplemented with metabolites such as mitomycin C, tube shunts and cyclocryotherapy can be undertaken at the earliest for refractory cases to prevent donor failure and permanent blindness. The underlying cause, if any, should also be dealt with simultaneously. For example, PAS formation can be managed by syncehiolysis.

The risk of graft rejection is increased after filtering or tube surgery as the drainage site may provide a conduit for retrograde passage of inflammatory cells into the AC. Besides, postoperative complications such as shallow AC, iridocorneal touch, tube-endothelial touch may accelerate the process of graft failure.

Pupillary block glaucoma in the early postoperative phase is diagnosed by the presence of a shallow peripheral AC, deep central AC, 360° posterior synechiae, iris bombe, and PAS. A large air bubble left at the end of the surgery is an important cause of this condition. For air-induced pupillary block, intravenous injection of mannitol and pupillary dilatation allow air bubbles to move anteriorly and relieve the block. If not responding to conservative management, air bubbles can be brought anteriorly by tapping the iris with a Sinskey hook [8]. The routine use of mydriatic drops at the end of the surgery, titration of an air bubble that can clear the edge of the dilated pupil and inferior peripheral iridectomy can decrease the chances of postoperative pupillary block.

11.2.1.4 Suture Related Complications

Suture-related complications such as loose/broken/tight sutures, exposed suture knots, and suture abscess can cause wound leak, graft infection, graft rejection or astigmatism and need removal or replacement of affected sutures depending on wound healing (Figs. 11.1 and 11.2). If infected, the suture should be sent for microbiological evaluation after removal.

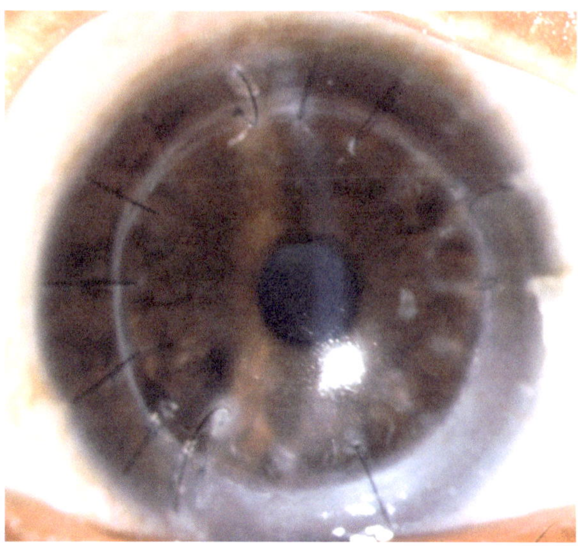

Fig. 11.1 Loose sutures post deep ALK

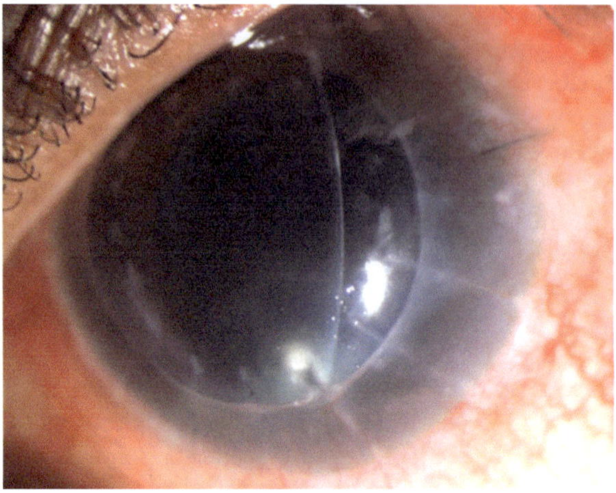

Fig. 11.2 Suture-related infection post deep ALK

Suture-related immune infiltrates are quite common in the early postoperative period and are differentiated from suture-related infections by their occurrence along with the host site of multiple suture tracts with an absence of an overlying epithelial defect.

While infections mandate immediate administration of antibiotics in a treatment similar to graft infection (described later), benign infiltrates usually resolve with an increased corticosteroid regimen similar to graft rejection (described later).

11.2.1.5 Persistent Epithelial Defect

The intact epithelium is essential for undisturbed wound healing and subsequent graft survival. Persistent-epithelial defects (PEDs) occur due to delayed/absent epithelial healing for more than 14 days and are relatively less common with EK procedures due to intact epithelial integrity [9, 10].

Risk Factors

Risk factors include prior ocular surface diseases, reactivation of herpetic keratitis, graft infection/rejection, and preservatives used in topical medications. Age >60 years, graft diameter >9 mm, and presence of comorbid systemic diseases, such as Rheumatic diseases, Diabetes mellitus, and cancer therapy are additional risk factors. To prevent PEDs, the best attempts should be made to preserve the donor epithelium during surgery.

Management

PEDs are usually refractory to standard therapy such as topical lubricants, prophylactic antibiotics, and steroids, and oral Tetracyclines. The current standard management includes a stepwise strategy of conservative management followed by an escalation of medical or surgical therapies if non-responsive.

Sodium hyaluronate-based preservative-free lubricant therapy (hourly artificial tears and ointments), pressure patching, and bandage contact lens should be attempted first. They not only lubricate the cornea but also minimize the risk of mechanical erosion from constant lid movement.

The next step involves the application of a punctal plug (permanent silicone or temporary collagen plugs), that will increase retention of tear-film and associated growth factors required for corneal epithelial healing.

Surgical interventions such as debridement and tarsorrhaphy (temporary suture tarsorrhaphy, or injection of Botulinum toxin A into Levator palpebrae superioris) are tried next. The former aids in the migration of new epithelial cells by removing inert and necrotic tissue from the margins of the PED, while the latter decreases the exposure of cornea by the closure of palpebral fissure. Temporary fibrin glue application with patching therapy can also be tried for re-epithelization.

Amniotic membrane grafting has proven to be extremely useful for PEDs. Amniotic membrane has anti-inflammatory properties, provides a mechanical scaffold for re-epithelialization, and contains many growth factors, proteinase inhibitors and proteins that facilitate corneal wound healing. Autologous serum drops (Patient's serum is diluted by 20% or 50% and used every 3 h daily) consisting of many growth factors, and whole blood-derived products, such as umbilical cord blood serum and platelet-rich fibrin tears, can also be used for treating PEDs. Recently, n*ovel treatments such as* topical fibronectin, Thymosin beta 4 (Tβ4) and Nexagonare are also being tried for refractory PEDs.

Outcome

If not treated timely, PEDs can progress to graft melt, perforation, neovascularization, infection, and failure. On resolution, anterior stromal scarring, and thinning can result in corneal astigmatism, thereby compromising visual gain.

11.2.1.6 Posterior Segment-Related Complications

Posterior segment complications are of infrequent occurrence as compared to anterior segment complications. However, they are a significant threat to graft outcome and are associated with a substantial risk of compromised visual potential. Endophthalmitis, Choroidal detachment (CD), retinal detachment (RD) and cystoid macular edema (CME) are posterior segment-related complications post-keratoplasty.

Endophthalmitis

Endophthalmitis is a rare but serious sight-threatening complication that can occur both in the early and late postoperative period [11, 12]. Around 27% of cases occur within the first 1 week of surgery, while 27% and 46% cases between 1 and 4 weeks and beyond 1 month, respectively. The incidence of endophthalmitis is greater post-EK than with PKP (0.23% after PKP vs. 0.34% after EK). The likelihood of graft survival is only 27% [11–14].

Causative Organism

Microorganisms commonly associated with postoperative endophthalmitis include Gram positive bacteria (82%, coagulase-negative *Staphylococcus* species), Gram negative bacteria (9%, *Streptococcus* species), fungal species (9%, *Candida albicans*), and miscellaneous organisms. Fungal endophthalmitis usually presents months after the surgery, whereas bacterial endophthalmitis presents early.

Risk Factors

Endophthalmitis is seen to be associated with both donors as well as host-related factors. The potential risk factors include PED, wound leak, graft infection, contaminated sutures, trauma, and secondary intraocular surgeries. The cause of donor's death, unsterile tissue retrieval practices, and indication for corneal transplantation also play a role in the occurrence of this complication.

Presentation and Diagnosis

A patient with acute endophthalmitis characteristically presents with sudden onset painful loss of vision, along with redness, watering, and photophobia. Lid edema, conjunctival congestion, corneal edema, uveitis and secondarily raised IOP are other clinical features. While patients with chronic endophthalmitis usually present with mild congestion and gradual onset diminution of vision. The diagnosis is aided by visualization of vitreous exudates on fundoscopy or on B-Scan ultrasonography.

Management

Urgent vitreous tap followed by administration of broad-spectrum intravitreal antibiotics (Vancomycin 1 mg in 0.1 mL, Ceftazidime 2.25 mg in 0.1 mL, and Amikacin 0.4 mg/0.1 mL) in combination should be undertaken to salvage visual and structural integrity. Antifungal agents (Amphotericin B 5 μg in 0.1 mL, Voriconazole 50 μg in 0.1 mL) should be administered in suspected cases. Vitreous samples obtained at the beginning of the surgery should be sent for microbiological examination inclusive of antibiotic susceptibility such that the treatment may be changed accordingly. Steroids in any route are absolutely contraindicated in fungal cases. For bacterial endophthalmitis, systemic steroids can be instituted along with antibiotic treatment.

Pars plana vitrectomy (PPV)can also be undertaken depending on the severity of the disease and clinical response. Eyes presenting with extremely poor vision (light perception) and eyes not responding to initial treatment are best handled by early PPV. A graft exchange may be required in eyes with poor corneal visibility or anterior extension of posterior infection.

Prevention

Prevention of endophthalmitis involves intraoperative painting of ocular surface with 5% Povidone-iodine solution and preoperative management of risk factors such as blepharitis, meibomitis, canaliculitis, keratitis sicca, etc., and use of prophylactic antibiotics (Moxifloxacin 0.5% four times per day form 3 days before surgery). The role of intracameral antibiotics at the end of the surgery for the prevention of endophthalmitis is also regarded as an important measure.

Choroidal Detachment

Choroidal detachment can present as a rare complication due to conditions that result in low IOP. Wound leak and unquantified dosage of aqueous suppressants are important causes of the same.CD can infrequently present in the early postoperative phase. It can be either serous CD or hemorrhagic CD.

Serous CD is suspected by the presence of hypotony (IOP <6 mmHg) in the absence of wound leak or shallow AC. They are usually self-limiting and can be managed medically with intensive topical steroid therapy and cycloplegic agents (atropine three times per day or homatropine four times per day). Oral steroids can be administered to battle anterior and posterior uveitis, if any. If choroidal detachment persists longer than 1 week, drainage of the suprachoroidal fluid should be considered. However, an immediate drainage is indicated when the lens touches the corneal endothelium. While, hemorrhagic CD overlies a raised IOP and shallow AC and requires drainage if it persists for >3 days, has angle closure, pupillary block, or other related complications. CDs can be appreciated on ophthalmoscopy as domed shape elevations restricted by vortex veins. B-scan ultrasonography confirms their diagnosis and aids in differentiating serous from hemorrhagic CDs (hyperreflective internal nodules reflect blood clots).

Retinal Detachment

Retinal detachment is an infrequent complication after corneal transplantation. RD after keratoplasty can be associated with high myopia, prior history of retinal detachment or ocular surgery, or intraoperative posterior dislocation of lens/IOL Additionally, patients who have had a complicated surgical procedures with vitreous handling are also at an increased risk of postoperative RD. High index of suspicion is required for RD which mandates urgent surgical intervention for preventing further loss of vision.

Cystoid Macular Edema

CME is more common in eyes with excess inflammation due to intraoperative manipulations or secondary interventions. Diagnosis of CME requires high index of suspicion as it may be missed in patients with suboptimal visual gain. These can be detected easily on macular OCT and fundus fluorescein angiography. Treatment includes topical nonsteroidal anti-inflammatory therapy (Ketorolac tromethamine 0.5%, Indomethacin 1%, and Diclofenac 1%,) or Corticosteroid therapy. Intravitreal injection of corticosteroids such as Triamcinolone acetonide and vascular endothelial growth factor inhibitors such as Bevacizumab, Ranibizumab, etc. Corticosteroid-based intravitreal implant (Dexamethasone, Triamcinolone acetonide and Fluocinolone acetonide biodegradable) and focal retinal laser can also be undertaken in resistant cases.

11.2.1.7 Graft Infection

Graft infection following corneal transplant surgery is a devastating corneal emergency with a potential for graft failure and poor visual outcome in the

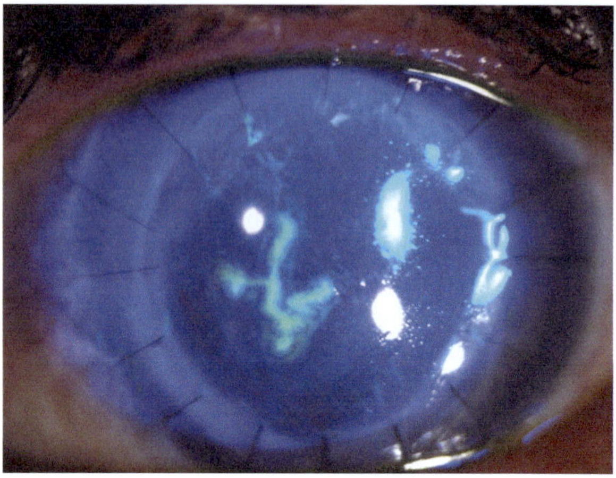

Fig. 11.3 Graft infection post PKP; Herpetic keratitis in this case

majority of patients. The infection usually occurs during the first six postoperative months. Early infection may arise because of recurrence of the host disease, infected donor tissues, or intraoperative contamination. While the late infection is usually caused by pathogens that are acquired from the environment. The incidence of graft infection after keratoplasty varies from 1.76% to 7.4%. Common causative organisms include bacteria (*Staphylococcus, Pseudomonas, Streptococcus),* fungi (*Candida, Aspergillus, Fusarium*) and herpes virus (primary or reactivation) (Fig. 11.3).

Risk Factors

Graft infection in the early postoperative period can occur due to transoperative contamination of the surgical field or donor graft or incomplete excision of infected tissue [13]. Other risk factors include PEDs, contact lens usage, suture-related complications, steroid use, ocular surface disease, older age, and diabetes mellitus and other immunosuppressive disorders.

Management

Post-keratoplasty microbial keratitis is challenging to manage, and donor rim cultures are rarely helpful. The treatment includes sending infected graft tissue for appropriate microbiological examination and starting broad-spectrum fortified antibiotics (Cefazolin 5%, Tobramycin 1.3%), which can later be modified based on drug sensitivity results and clinical response. Antifungal therapy (Natamycin 5%, Voriconazole 1%, Amphotericin B 0.15%) should be started for patients with suspected mycotic keratitis. The topical therapy is started on an hourly basis which is tapered according to patient response. Appropriate oral antibiotics should also be administered without any delay. Topical steroids should be temporarily stopped and resumed once the infection subsides. In case of an imminent rejection, systemic steroids should be administered. Re-graft should be considered for extensive infections.

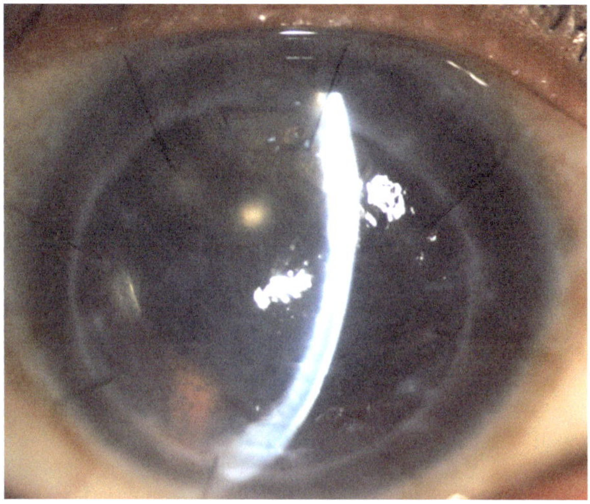

Fig. 11.4 Graft rejection post PKP; Note differential graft edema and keratitic precipitates

Outcome
Graft infection can lead to graft opacification, graft rejection, graft failure, endophthalmitis, glaucoma, and phthisis bulbi if not managed timely.

11.2.1.8 Graft Rejection
Allograft rejection ensues when the donor antigens initiate a cascade of immune modulatory changes in the host. Host antigen-presenting cells carry allo-antigens from the grafted tissue to the draining lymph nodes of the recipient via lymphatic vessels. Despite being an immune-privileged tissue, the cornea is prone to immune-mediated rejection like any other tissue transplant (Fig. 11.4) [8, 14–17]. Histologically, corneal graft rejection involves infiltration of donor tissue by CD4+ T-cells, macrophages, neutrophils, and natural killer cells (NK cells) and the invasion of blood and lymphatic vessels.

Incidence
The incidence of a graft rejection episode varies from 4% to 20% after low-risk PKP and 5.3–14% after Deep ALK (stromal rejection only). The incidence of rejection is low with LKs due to the less amount of antigenic load transferred. Five-year rejection episode rates are 7.9% after Descemet's stripping EK and 2.3% after DMEK [8, 14–17]. The incidence decreases with proper case selection, with a lesser amount of antigenic load transferred (PKP > Deep ALK> Descemet stripping EK > DMEK) and use of prophylactic steroids and immune suppressants (Cyclosporine and Azathioprine). The peak time for immunologic rejection occurs between 12 and 18 months after surgery.

Risk Factors
Risk factors include prior failed grafts, corneal neovascularization, active uveitis, glaucoma, PAS, large grafts, eccentric grafts, and young age (highly active immune

system). Additional risk factors for EK include cessation of topical corticosteroids and African-American descent.

Types

Depending on the duration, it is classified as hyperacute, acute, or chronic rejection. The hyperacute rejection is extremely rare and occurs within the first few days of transplantation. While acute and chronic rejection can occur weeks, months, or years later. While the majority of acute rejections post PKP are symptomatic, approximately 2/3rd and 1/3rd patients with rejected deep ALK and EK grafts, respectively, are diagnosed incidentally. Different types of corneal graft rejections are discussed in Table 11.3.

Management

Corticosteroids remain the mainstay of management, and hourly administration of topical steroids (Prednisolone acetate 1%, Dexamethasone 0.1%, Difluprednate 0.05%) should be undertaken immediately. These are then tapered gradually to a maintenance dose of one drop per day according to the extent of the resolution of the rejection episode. Single-dose pulse therapy with 100 mg Dexamethasone or 500 mg of Methylprednisolone in 150 mL of 5% dextrose solution as a slow intravenous infusion over 1–2 h can also be administered. Some eyes may be additionally treated with intracameral or sub-Tenon's injections. Oral steroids are not typically used to treat acute corneal graft rejection episodes. Infrequently, Bevacizumab injection, inhibitors of insulin receptor substrate-1, corneal collagen

Table 11.3 Types of immune-mediated corneal graft rejection

Type	Symptoms	Signs	Management
Epithelial rejection	Asymptomatic	– Elevated epithelial rejection line that stains with fluorescein or rose Bengal present – Supepithelial infiltrates – Absent with endothelial keratoplasty	Conservative
Stromal rejection	Decrease in vision	– Accompanied with endothelial rejection – Circumciliary congestion, stromal haze and edema in a previously clear graft – Absent with endothelial Keratoplasty	– Urgent pulse intravenous steroid + Intensive topical steroid therapy – Cycloplegics, osmotic agents, antiglaucoma medications
Endothelial rejection	Pain, redness, photophobia, decrease in vision	– Endothelial rejection line (Khodadoust line) – Keratic precipitates – Anterior uveitis – Circumciliary congestion – Differential stromal edema	Same as stromal rejection

crosslinking, photodynamic therapy, and fine-needle diathermy may be used to target neovascular endothelial cells and blood vessels.

Outcome

Although most patients with acute graft rejection respond successfully to medication management, around 25% may eventually require graft replacement.

11.2.1.9 Graft Failure

Donor failure signifies loss of donor function due to any cause [8, 18]. In primary graft failure (PGF), the donor fails to clear at any time after surgery (till 2 weeks post PKP, 3 months post-EK). It usually results from unhealthy donor tissue, prolonged donor tissue preservation time, or transoperative trauma (related to surgeon's experience and surgical complexity such as the presence of anterior chamber IOL, large iridectomies, and filtering tubes). In EK procedures, iatrogenic PGF can occur due to endothelial damage during tissue preparation and manipulation (insertion, centration and attachment).

Secondary graft failure can occur anytime beyond the duration of PGF, and any post-surgical complication can lead to donor failure. The incidence depends on the type of surgery, etiology, surgical expertise, recognition, and management of complications, and patient compliance for follow-up.

Management

A re-graft (LK, PKP or kerato-prosthesis) can be undertaken after graft failure based on the endothelial function, stromal clarity, and number of previous failures and their cause. It is advisable to wait for at least 6 months to 1 year before a repeat grafting is performed.

11.2.2 Complications Specific to Lamellar Keratoplasties

Lamellar keratoplasties have garnered much attention over the last decades owing to inherent advantages such as preservation of globe integrity and elimination of endothelial graft rejection and less stringent donor quality criteria. However, interface-related complications and donor detachments are unique to LK and pose a constant risk of corneal emergencies in the postoperative period.

11.2.2.1 Interface-Related Problems

Interface is created after LKs due to horizontal graft-host apposition (compared to vertical graft-host apposition in PKP) [19]. Figure 11.5 is illustrative of various interface-related problems.

Interface Fluid

Interface fluid accumulation may present as double or triple AC formation after ALK. These can be seen after intraoperative macro or micro perforations of DM and can be managed conservatively (shallow diffuse fluid collections, localized fluid

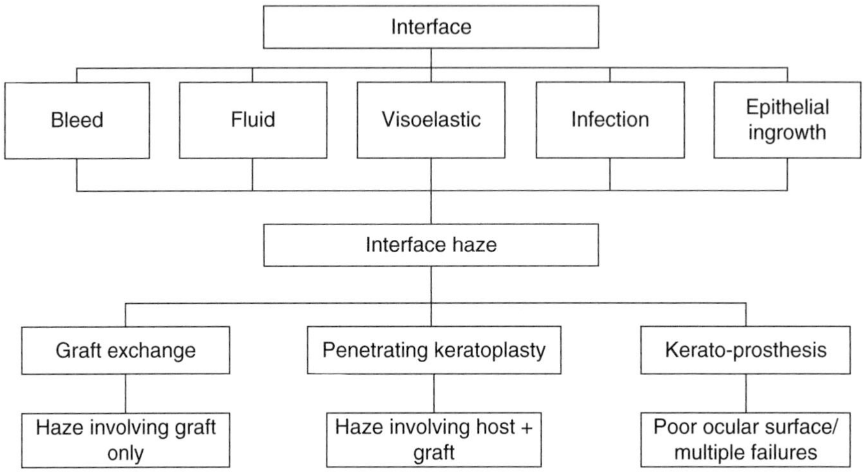

Fig. 11.5 Interface-related complications and management

pockets) or with intracameral air injection (large fluid collection, fluid persisting for weeks), based on the height and duration of the fluid. This is unlike retained VES that rarely resolves spontaneously and requires drainage.

Interface Bleed

Interface bleed may arise from trauma to the iris or corneal blood vessels. It usually resolves spontaneously, but sometimes may lead to interface haze or graft detachment. Topical steroids can be increased in frequency to hasten the absorption of blood constituents.

Interface Infection

The interface is a possible dead area where microorganisms can multiply without being detected by the host's immune system [20, 21]. Infection in interface might come from either the host or the graft. Because of the deep-seated nature of the infiltrates, the sequestration of the pathogens and scanty penetration of the currently available antimicrobial drugs usually results in a delayed diagnosis. Fungal keratitis is more common than bacterial or viral keratitis, and it typically manifests as white interface infiltrates that are not accompanied by considerable inflammation. Initially, conservative therapies such as topical antimicrobials and antibacterial interface irrigation may be used. However, most of the time condition is progressive, and the disease is difficult to control. Usually, it might necessitate partial graft excision, graft removal, graft exchange, or even penetrating keratoplasty. Highly virulent organisms can cause infection to spread quickly, necessitating evisceration in some cases.

Epithelial Ingrowth

Migration of epithelial cells with the graft or through ill-apposed incisions can lead to epithelial ingrowth in the interface that may extend deeper into the AC, particularly, if vitreous is attached to the wound. It is diagnosed clinically by its classic appearance of the nest of cells and by histopathological analysis. Treatment may range from observation of small epithelial nests not involving the visual axis to graft replacement for severe cases. Scraping of epithelial cells with mitomycin C application and laser-induced resolution has also been tried in literature. Minimizing the use of venting incisions and appropriate closure of all surgical incisions may help in preventing this complication.

11.2.2.2 Graft Detachment

The most common complication following EK is graft dislocation [8]. The reported incidence varies with different studies and can range from 1.5% to 35%. Risk factors include prior glaucoma surgery, surgical inexperience, postoperative hypotony, eye rubbing, interface fluid or retained VES, and DM folds. Usually, the graft detachment is detected within the first postoperative week, but occasionally, it may be detected after several weeks.

Many strategies such as scraping off the peripheral donor bed, air tamponade, supine positioning postoperatively, venting incisions, and suturing of side port incisions have been described to reduce the rate of graft detachment. Peripheral detachments ≤1/3rd graft surface area and not affecting the visual acuity may be managed conservatively. Intracameral air injection (re-bubbling) followed by strict supine positioning remains the mainstay of management. Long-acting gases such as sulfur hexafluoride (SF_6) and perfluoropropane (C_3F_8) may be required for prolonged tamponade in eyes with large, persistent, and inferiorly placed graft detachments. The presence of residual interface fluid may require venting incisions. In extremely rare cases with posterior dislocation of graft (eyes with aphakia, scleral/iris-sutured IOL with PC tear), prompt pars plana vitrectomy with lenticule removal is performed to prevent subsequent visual deterioration. Majority of graft detachments respond re-bubbling. In few cases where multiple re-bubbling attempts fail, a repeat EK or PKP may be required due to PGF.

11.3 Conclusion

It is not uncommon to experience corneal emergencies associated with corneal transplantation both in intraoperative and postoperative periods. Corneal emergencies encountered during corneal transplantation range from less serious entities like wound leak, postoperative inflammation and epithelial defect to more serious ones like graft infection, failure, and posterior segment complications. High index of suspicion and appropriate management remains the most important consideration while managing such cases to salvage visual and structural integrity.

Key Points

- The emergencies associated with keratoplasty can be intraoperative or postoperative.

- Intraoperative complications can be host related such as posterior capsular tear and suprachoroidal hemorrhage or donor related such as graft loss, damage, reversal, and buttonholing.
- Intense anterior segment inflammation, wound leak, glaucoma, suture-related complications, persistent-epithelial defect, posterior segment complications and graft infection/rejection/failure can be witnessed in the postoperative phase of any type of keratoplasty.
- Deep ALK procedures are particularly prone to intraoperative DM perforations and postoperative interface-related problems.
- EK procedures are prone to intra and postoperative graft detachment and dislocation.
- A familiarity with possible complications and knowledge of proper management techniques is important to promote long-term graft survival.

References

1. Sharma N, Agarwal R, Jhanji V, Bhaskar S, Kamalakkannan P, Nischal KK. Lamellar keratoplasty in children. Surv Ophthalmol. 2020;65(6):675–90.
2. Espandar L, Carlson AN. Lamellar keratoplasty: a literature review. J Ophthalmol. 2013;2013:894319.
3. Henein C, Nanavaty MA. Systematic review comparing penetrating keratoplasty and deep anterior lamellar keratoplasty for management of keratoconus. Cont Lens Anterior Eye. 2017;40(1):3–14.
4. Stechschulte SU, Azar DT. Complications after penetrating keratoplasty. Int Ophthalmol Clin. 2000;40(1):27–43.
5. Huang OS, Htoon HM, Chan AM, Tan D, Mehta JS. Incidence and outcomes of intraoperative descemet membrane perforations during deep anterior lamellar keratoplasty. Am J Ophthalmol. 2019;199:9–18.
6. Ma JF, Rapuano CJ, Hammersmith KM, Nagra PK, Dai Y, Azari AA. Outcomes of wound dehiscence post-penetrating keratoplasty. Cornea. 2016;35(6):778–83.
7. Dada T, Aggarwal A, Minudath KB, Vanathi M, et al. Post-penetrating keratoplasty glaucoma. Indian J Ophthalmol. 2008;56:269–77.
8. Basak SK, Basak S. Complications and management in Descemet's stripping endothelial keratoplasty: analysis of consecutive 430cases. Indian J Ophthalmol. 2014;62:209–18.
9. Fu Y, Liu J, Tseng SC. Ocular surface deficits contributing to persistent epithelial defect after penetrating keratoplasty. Cornea. 2012;31(7):723–9.
10. Vaidyanathan U, Hopping GC, Liu HY, et al. Persistent corneal epithelial defects: a review article. Med Hypothesis Discov Innov Ophthalmol. 2019;8(3):163–76.
11. Chen JY, Jones MN, Srinivasan S, Neal TJ, Armitage WJ, Kaye SB, NHSBT Ocular Tissue Advisory Group and Contributing Ophthalmologists (OTAG Audit Study 18). Endophthalmitis after penetrating keratoplasty. Ophthalmology. 2015;122(1):25–30.
12. Tran KD, Yannuzzi NA, Si N, et al. Clinical features, antimicrobial susceptibilities, and treatment outcomes of patients with culture positive endophthalmitis after penetrating keratoplasty. Am J Ophthalmol Case Rep. 2018;9:62–7.
13. Vajpayee RB, Sharma N, Sinha R, Agarwal T, Singhvi A. Infectious keratitis following keratoplasty. Surv Ophthalmol. 2007;52(1):1–12.

14. Pereira NC, Araújo M, Pinto NT, Moreira PB, Rocha GA, Moura GS, Sousa LB. Complications in endothelial keratoplasty performed by cornea fellows. Arq Bras Oftalmol. 2013;76(5):301–4. Portuguese
15. Liu H, Chen Y, Wang P, Li B, Wang W, Su Y, Sheng M. Efficacy and safety of deep anterior lamellar keratoplasty vs. penetrating keratoplasty for keratoconus: a meta-analysis. PLoS One. 2015;10(1):e0113332.
16. Sinha R, Agarwal R, Titiyal JS. Extraocular use of sodium hyaluronate 1% for preventing air/gas escape during descemetopexy. Indian J Ophthalmol. 2020;68(4):667–8.
17. Hos D, Matthaei M, Bock F, Maruyama K, Notara M, Clahsen T, Hou Y, Le VNH, Salabarria AC, Horstmann J, Bachmann BO, Cursiefen C. Immune reactions after modern lamellar (DALK, DSAEK, DMEK) versus conventional penetrating corneal transplantation. Prog Retin Eye Res. 2019;73:100768.
18. Barraquer RI, Pareja-Aricò L, Gómez-Benlloch A, Michael R. Risk factors for graft failure after penetrating keratoplasty. Medicine (Baltimore). 2019;98(17):e15274.
19. Fontana L, Moramarco A, Mandarà E, Russello G, Iovieno A. Interface infectious keratitis after anterior and posterior lamellar keratoplasty. Clinical features and treatment strategies. A review. Br J Ophthalmol. 2019;103(3):307–14.
20. Sharma N, Kaur M, Titiyal JS, Aldave A. Infectious keratitis following lamellar keratoplasty. Surv Ophthalmol. 2021;66(4):623–43.
21. Bhalerao SA, Mohamed A, Vaddavalli PK, Murthy SI, Reddy JC. Outcomes of rebubbling for graft detachment after Descemet's stripping endothelial keratoplasty or Descemet's stripping automated endothelial keratoplasty. Indian J Ophthalmol. 2020;68(1):48–53.

Acute Graft Rejection

12

Rajesh Fogla and Deepak Soni

12.1 Introduction

Corneal transplantation is among the most frequently performed and successful solid organ transplant procedures due to the relative immune privilege of the cornea. In 2019, approximately 85,600 corneal transplantation were performed in the USA [1]. Although traditional full-thickness penetrating keratoplasty is commonly performed, the past decade has witnessed an increasing trend towards lamellar corneal surgery, which provides better rates of graft survival, rejection reversibility, and visual outcomes [2]. The cornea is immunologically privileged being avascular and free of lymphatics, which prevents access of the immune system to the cornea. In addition, there is low expression of major histocompatibility antigen (MHC I & II) in the cornea, besides anterior chamber associated immune deviation (ACAID) [3]. This explains the high success rates of full-thickness penetrating keratoplasty with one-year survival rate of about 90% and 15-year survival rate of 55% in avascular, non-inflamed recipient cornea [4]. Immune-mediated corneal graft rejection still remains the most common cause for graft failure in the late post-operative period. Although the risk of rejection is lower with newer lamellar keratoplasty procedures, epithelial, subepithelial, and stromal immune reactions can occur following deep anterior lamellar keratoplasty (DALK), and endothelial immune reactions with Descemet stripping automated endothelial keratoplasty (DSAEK) or Descemet membrane endothelial keratoplasty (DMEK).

This article discusses in detail the incidence, risk factors, pathogenesis, clinical presentations, treatment, and recent advances in the management of corneal graft rejections.

R. Fogla (✉)
Eye Department, Apollo Hospitals, Hyderabad, India

D. Soni
All India Institute of Medical Sciences, Bhopal, India

B. Sharma, J. S. Titiyal (eds.), *Corneal Emergencies*,
https://doi.org/10.1007/978-981-16-5876-1_12

12.2 Incidence

Depending on the research design, risk factors for rejection, and the type of transplantation procedure done, the rate of graft rejection ranges from 2.3 to 68 per cent in the literature [5]. At a 5-year follow-up, the Cornea Donor Study (CDS) found that 23% of individuals experienced one rejection episode and 37% of these eyes had graft failure [6]. Graft rejection occurs in 33% of cases, according to the Australian Corneal Graft Registry [7]. In the presence of stromal neovascularisation, higher rejection rates up to 32% as has been reported as opposed to 14 per cent in avascular or mildly vascular corneas [8]. After the first, second, and third regrafts, patients may have rejection rates of 40, 68, and 80%, respectively [9].

Low-risk grafts have a near 90% 2-year survival rate, with survival rates of 90 and 82% after 5 and 10 years post-transplant [10]. Endothelial keratoplasty treatments such as DSAEK or DMEK have a low endothelial rejection rate of 10% to 4% and are frequently responsive to topical corticosteroids due to the absence of donor epithelium and stroma, as well as the lack of direct contact of donor endothelium with limbal vasculature [11, 12]. In eyes having Descemet stripping endothelial keratoplasty (DSEK), the risk of rejection was shown to be increased with African-American ethnicity (five times relative risk) and pre-existing glaucoma (two times relative risk) [13]. Because the healthy host endothelium is preserved with anterior lamellar keratoplasty, such as DALK, there is no risk of immune-mediated endothelial rejection. Immune reactions in the subepithelial and stromal layers can still occur, with reported rates ranging from 1 to 24% [14]. With DALK, the 3-year cumulative rate of stromal rejection episode was found to be 10% [15].

12.3 Risk Factors for Corneal Graft Rejection

12.3.1 Donor Characteristics

Donor cornea characteristics do not significantly affect rejection rates. Collaborative Corneal Transplantation Study (CCTS) did not find benefit of Human Leukocyte Antigen (HLA) matching, and proposed ABO matching in high-risk corneal transplantation to reduce risk of allogenic rejection [9]. Other studies have shown prolonged graft survival in type 1 HLA matched corneal transplant cases and recommend HLA matching for high-risk corneal grafts [4]. CCTS also did not find any impact on graft outcomes related to donor preservation methods and gender mismatch between donor and recipient.

12.3.2 Host Characteristics

12.3.2.1 Host Bed Vascularisation

Corneal neovascularization is one of the most important causes of corneal allograft rejection. In the presence of stromal neovascularisation, rejection rates rise from

14% in avascular or mildly vascular corneas to 32% in vascularised corneas [8]. Deep stromal blood vessels in two or more quadrants of the recipient cornea are considered high risk. The presence of stromal vascularization in all four quadrants doubles the risk of rejection, enhances the severity of the immune response, and shortens the time it takes for the graft to be rejected [9]. High-risk grafts account for about 10% of all grafts.

12.3.2.2 Failed Grafts

The risk of graft rejection increases with regraft, CCTS recognised this risk to be 1.2 for each successive graft [9]. Patients may have rejection rates of 40%, 68%, and 80% after first, second, and third regrafts [9]. This is usually related to pre sensitisation from previous graft, besides vascular host bed and increased inflammatory response to repeat surgery.

12.3.2.3 Pre-Existing Disease

Herpetic keratitis, uveitis, atopic dermatitis, and other inflammatory conditions increase the risk of immune reactions. Primary allograft rejection rates have been reported to be 29% in the first year and 46% at 2 years in eyes with a history of herpetic keratitis [16].

Pre-operative glaucoma, prior glaucoma surgery or other complex anterior segment surgery, iris synechiae, vitreous adhesions all increase the risk of rejection in the transplanted graft [7, 9]. Ocular surface disease, dry eye, limbal stem cell deficiency and neurotrophic keratopathy has been shown to increase the risk of graft rejection. Vernal keratoconjunctivitis increases the risk of stromal rejection following DALK [17].

12.3.3 Technical Factors

Large and eccentric grafts are associated with an increased risk of rejection owing to their close proximity to the limbus. Loose or broken sutures can predispose to vascularisation and localised inflammation and increased risk of rejection.

12.3.4 Other Factors

Younger age is associated with an increased risk of rejection due to a combination of a robust immune response and delayed reporting or recognition of rejection episodes [9]. Blood transfusions may also increase the risk of rejection episodes. There is also an increased risk of rejection during and after pregnancy [18]. Gender incompatibility has recently emerged as an important risk factor for graft rejection and failure. Cornea from a female donor can be used for male or female recipients without any increased risk, however, cornea from a male donor should not be used in female recipients as it is associated with increased risk of graft rejection [19].

When any of these risk factors are present, the patient should be considered at high risk for graft rejection, and any episode of inflammation should be suspected of being graft rejection and treated appropriately unless proven otherwise.

12.3.5 Low Risk Penetrating Keratoplasty

Penetrating keratoplasty performed in conditions with low-risk of graft rejection is mainly due to relatively preserved corneal immune and (lymph)angiogenic privileges seen in non-inflammatory and non-vascular diseases like keratoconus and Fuchs' endothelial dystrophy. Endothelial rejection is the most common type of rejection observed in such conditions, with most of the rejection episodes occurring between 11 and 18 months after PK [20]. Long-term low-dose topical steroids have been observed as a protective factor for reduced risk of rejection in such a scenario [21].

12.4 Pathogenesis

The immunological response of the host is directed towards antigens in the donor cornea, resulting in corneal graft rejection. This immune response can be directed at one or more layers of the cornea (epithelial, stromal, and endothelial) or can be directed against all the layers. Although epithelial and stromal rejection may typically be reversed, endothelium rejection causes irreversible loss of optical clarity and can lead to permanent graft failure [6]. Rejection begins with the host's sensitisation to donor antigens (induction phase), in which antigen-presenting cells (APC, dendritic cells) directly or indirectly sensitise T cells and stimulate proliferation in draining lymph nodes. Immune effectors are delivered to the graft via blood capillaries during the efferent phase. It is a T cell-dependent effector mechanism (CD4+ & CD8+ T cells) that causes graft rejection by releasing inflammatory cytokines such as interleukin (IL-2, IL-4, IL-10), and interferon gamma (IFN—Y) [5].

12.5 Clinical Presentation

Corneal graft rejection can have varied clinical presentations depending on the involvement of layers of the cornea [4, 5, 8]. Early recognition of clinical features is critical in the effective management of graft rejection.

12.5.1 Symptoms

The patient usually presents with symptoms of blurred vision, pain, redness, watering, and photophobia. However, a majority of patients may remain asymptomatic in the early phase of graft rejection, especially with lamellar keratoplasty procedures such as DALK, DSAEK, or DMEK.

12.5.2 Signs

Clinical features can vary depending on the type of corneal transplantation and the severity of the rejection episode. Circumciliary congestion along with anterior uveitis and raised intraocular pressure can be associated with graft rejection and be present before clinical appearance of cellular infiltrates in the cornea.

12.5.2.1 Epithelial Rejection

Epithelial rejection is usually asymptomatic / mildly symptomatic and seen in the early post-operative period up to 3 months. It is characterised by an elevated undulating line of greyish epithelium, staining with Fluorescein or Rose Bengal dye. This represents a region of the destruction of donor epithelium, which is finally replaced by host epithelium (Fig. 12.1). Acute epithelial defects associated with inflammation may be a presenting sign of graft rejection in children [22].

12.5.2.2 Subepithelial Rejection

This is characterised by small, discrete subepithelial infiltrates (Krachmer spots), similar to those seen with Adenoviral epidemic keratoconjunctivitis, however, limited only to donor cornea (Fig. 12.2). These lesions are an early sign of rejection and can often be associated with endothelial rejection.

12.5.2.3 Stromal Rejection

Stromal rejection rarely occurs in isolation, and usually associated with neovascularisation. It presents with peripheral full-thickness haze or infiltrate along with circumlimbal injection in a previously clear graft. This is usually located at the graft host junction and can progress towards the central cornea. Stromal rejection can be seen after DALK with stromal oedema and neovascularisation (Fig. 12.3).

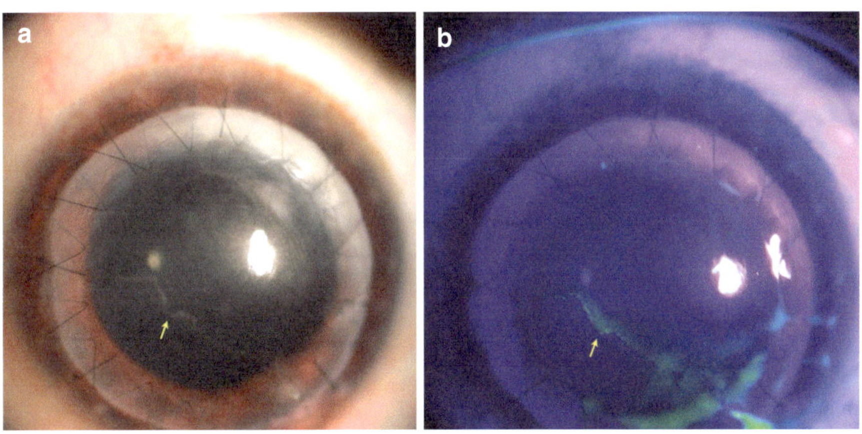

Fig. 12.1 Slit-lamp photograph showing acute epithelial rejection in a corneal graft. Note the elevated line of the opaque epithelium (arrow) (**a**), seen better under cobalt blue light using fluorescein dye (**b**)

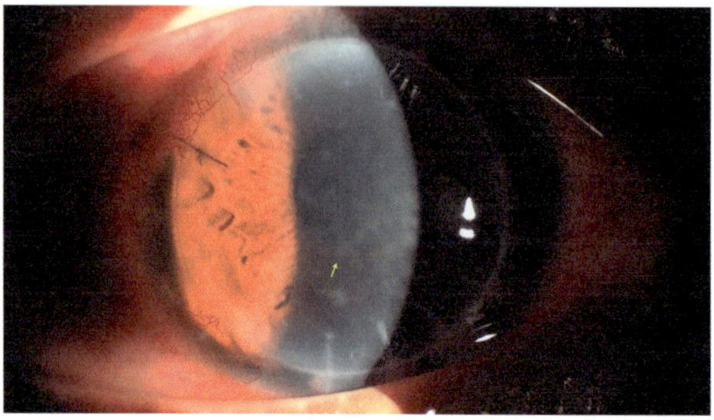

Fig. 12.2 Slit-lamp photograph showing acute epithelial rejection in a corneal graft with subepithelial infiltrates (Krachmer spots)

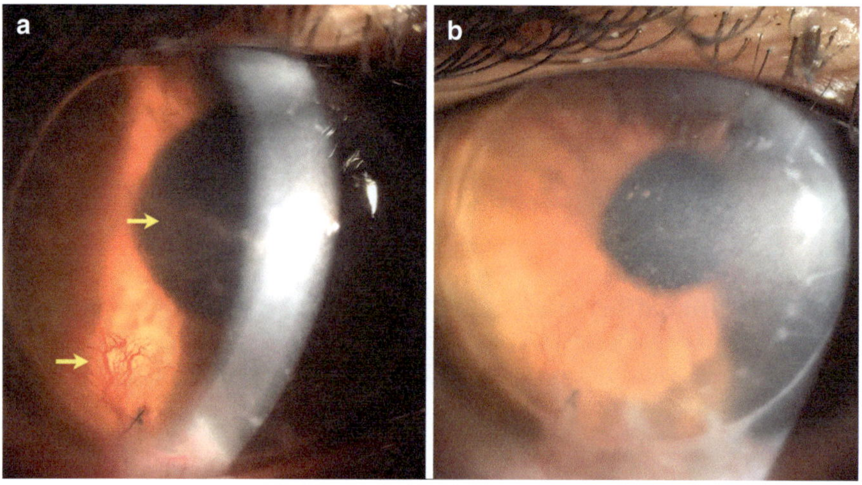

Fig. 12.3 Slit-lamp photograph showing (**a**) corneal vascularization and oedema along with keratic precipitates (KP) post DALK—stromal rejection (**b**) resolution of oedema and KP's after initiation of corticosteroid therapy

12.5.2.4 Endothelial Rejection

Endothelial rejection is the most common presentation in eyes post PK. It presents with mild to moderate anterior chamber reaction, in association with endothelial rejection line (Khodadoust line), which consists of mononuclear white cells that damage the endothelium (Fig 12.4a). Left untreated, this line progresses across the endothelial surface of the graft over several days. The donor cornea appears clear in front of this line and oedematous behind it. It can also present with scattered keratic precipitates, anterior chamber reaction and diffuse corneal oedema (Fig 12.4b). Endothelial rejection is an emergency situation that requires prompt treatment for the survival of the corneal graft. The clinical presentation is usually milder following endothelial keratoplasty procedures such as DSAEK or DMEK, with keratic precipitates occurring only on the transplanted endothelial layer (Table 12.1) [13, 23–29]. Graft oedema occurs secondary to endothelial dysfunction and anterior chamber inflammation; hence corneal pachymetry can be used to monitor onset or

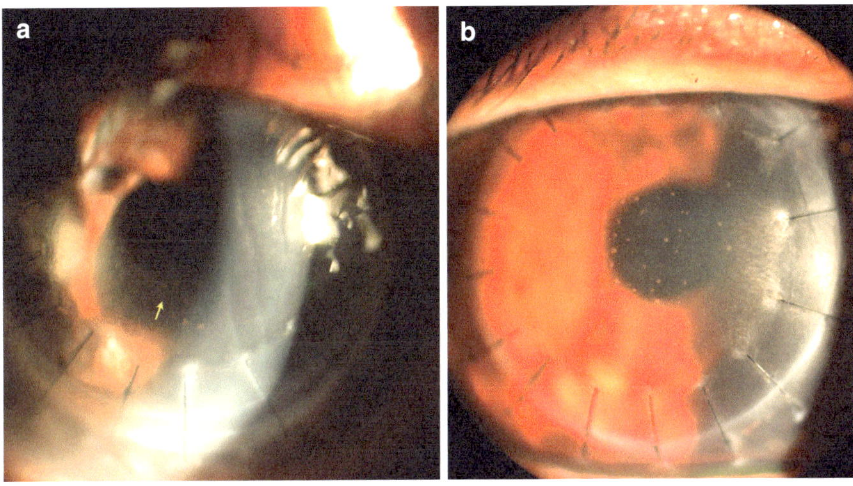

Fig. 12.4 Slit-lamp photograph showing acute endothelial rejection in a corneal graft. (**a**) shows the Khodadoust line of keratic precipitates (arrow) with oedema behind the line and clear cornea ahead of the rejection line, (**b**) diffuse keratic precipitates across the entire corneal graft

response to therapy of graft rejection. Change in endothelial cell morphology in eyes post-DMEK has been suggested as an early marker of rejection episodes and may prompt early intervention to prevent subsequent graft failure.

12.5.3 Differential Diagnosis

Various conditions can often make it difficult to diagnose graft rejection due to identical clinical presentations. Epithelial and subepithelial lesions can occur with adenoviral or Herpes simplex keratitis. Herpetic keratouveitis is most difficult to differentiate from endothelial rejection unless associated with dendriform epithelial lesion or endothelial keratic precipitates which extend beyond the donor graft. Low-grade infections can be associated with stromal haze or oedema, anterior chamber inflammation and keratic precipitates, which can be confused as graft rejection. Epithelial in growth can mimic an endothelial rejection line with overlying oedema; however, it is not associated with significant anterior chamber inflammation.

12.6 Treatment

Early initiation of intensive therapy greatly improves the chances of reversing the rejection episode and maintaining graft clarity. Clinical management usually depends on the type and severity of graft rejection (Fig. 12.5). Corticosteroid therapy using topical, periocular, or systemic administration is the mainstay of treatment for acute corneal allograft rejection [30].

Table 12.1 Overview of variable aspects of graft rejection seen in different types of lamellar keratoplasty

Types of Lamellar keratoplasty		Types of rejection	Commonest timing of occurrence of rejection	Risk of developing immune rejections	Factors associated with altered risk	Clinical course/picture	Outcomes in cases with immune rejections	Follow-up examination recommended
DALK		Epithelial, subepithelial, stromal	Within first post-operative year [23]	Can occur at a rate of approximately 8–10% [24, 25]	Absence of ACAID mechanisms	Depends on type of rejection (as elaborated in the text)	Good	–
Endothelial keratoplasty	DSAEK	Endothelial	Between 12 and 18 months [26]	Can occur at a rate of 8–14% within 2 years [13, 27, 28]	Reduced exposure of APCs (mainly located in anterior stroma) to donor antigens	Endothelial immune response is clinically more subtle than after PK	Good	At 1, 3, 6, 12, 18, and 24 months postoperatively and annually thereafter
				Risk is less in comparison to PK	Reduced Effective ACAID mechanism	Often with only focal precipitates		
					Absence of corneal sutures	Classical endothelial rejection lines are rare		
	DMEK	Endothelial	Within the first two post-operative years [27]	Can occur at a rate of 0.9% at 1 year to 2.3% at 4 years [27, 29]	Quantitatively less alloantigen in comparison to DSAEK too	Most episodes are asymptomatic	Good	At 1, 3, 6, 12, 18, and 24 months postoperatively and annually thereafter
				Risk is significantly lower than after PK or DSAEK		Clinically very subtle	Endothelial cell density seems to be stable after graft rejection episode subsides	
						Immune reactions may present with a classical Khodadoust line, but mostly show diffuse endothelial precipitates		

Epithelial and subepithelial rejections in isolation are usually self-limiting, and in symptomatic patients can be managed using topical corticosteroids (prednisolone acetate 1% or dexamethasone 0.1%) 4–6 times daily till resolution of rejection, followed by a gradual tapering of topical steroids [31]. Topical lubricants can be added for symptomatic relief as well.

Stromal rejection without endothelial involvement can be managed using topical corticosteroids using a similar regimen of four–six times daily. A close watch is essential during treatment to rule out any possibility of endothelial rejection.

Endothelial rejection has to be treated more aggressively as the damage to donor endothelium is usually irreversible. Corticosteroids therapy is the treatment of choice, including topical and systemic routes of administration.

- Topical corticosteroids (prednisolone acetate 1% or dexamethasone 0.1%) are usually started every hour while awake and as frequently as possible during the night, for the first 2–3 days, followed by every 2 h till signs of rejections start resolving. Subconjunctival injection of corticosteroids (0.5 mL of 4 mg/mL dexamethasone) can also be considered in non-compliant patients. Thereafter a gradual tapering over several weeks to few months is done depending on the original indication for corneal graft and response to therapy. Steroid ointment can be used at bedtime as the regimen is tapered. If no clinical response is seen after at least 4–6 weeks of intense topical therapy, it is likely that the graft has failed.
- Additional topical therapy would include cycloplegics (homatropine 2% or atropine 1% once or twice daily), intraocular pressure-lowering agents to maintain normal eye pressure. The benefit of using topical Cyclosporin 2% for acute rejection episodes is still unclear due to delayed onset of action.

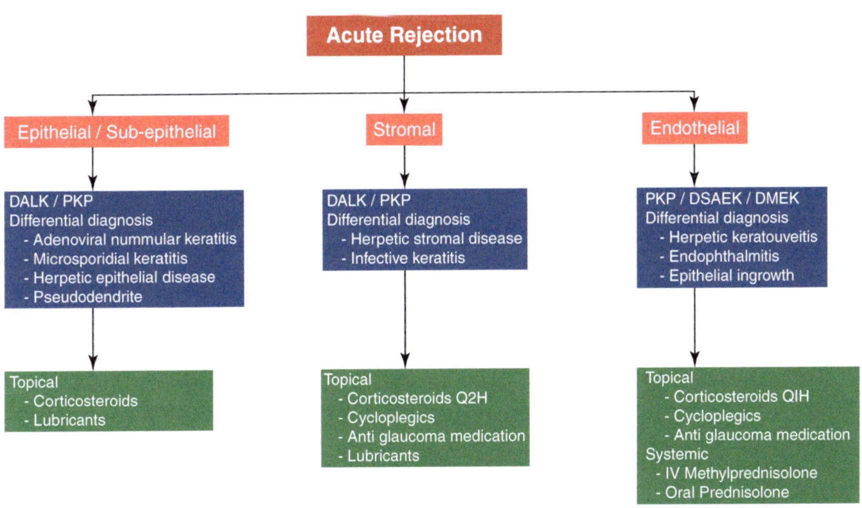

Fig. 12.5 Differentials to be considered and treatment options available for the episodes of acute graft rejection depending on the type of rejection

- Systemic administration of corticosteroids, especially pulsed intravenous (IV) steroid therapy, seems to be more effective compared to oral steroids in reversing endothelial rejection [32]. Improved graft survival rates have been noted with the use of pulsed steroids (IV administration of single dose of 500 mg Methylprednisolone) within 8 days of onset of rejection. The other advantages of pulsed steroid therapy being reduced risk of subsequent rejection episodes and avoiding prolonged administration of oral steroids. Alternatively IV dexamethasone (100 mg) can also be used and has been found to be as efficacious as Methylprednisolone (500 mg) in reversing endothelial rejection episodes [33]. Oral Prednisolone is usually started at a dosage of 60–80 mg daily for 1–2 weeks before tapering. If systemic corticosteroids are contraindicated, subconjunctival, or posterior sub tenon's injection of Triamcinolone acetonide injection in combination with topical steroids can be used for the treatment of endothelial rejection episode [34].
- Topical Cyclosporine A (CsA) has been used extensively for the management of graft rejection, however, majority of studies have failed to demonstrate any benefits regardless of the concentration used or duration of therapy [35, 36].

Intraocular pressure should be monitored closely and treated appropriately, as it can often be raised secondary to intraocular inflammation or used to frequent topical steroids. Chronic systemic use of corticosteroids can be associated with Diabetes, weight gain, osteoporosis, and hypertension, hence has to be used judiciously for long-term immunosuppression. Systemic immunosuppression using agents such as Cyclosporine [37], Mycophenolate mofetil, Tacrolimus, Azathioprine, in high-risk grafts can lead to improved graft survival but can be associated with side effects such as impaired renal or hepatic function and bone marrowsuppression.

12.6.1 Response to Treatment

Corneal thickness being a principal marker of endothelial function remains an important measure of response to treatment making pachymetry a useful tool for monitoring of same. Response to treatment in cases of endothelial rejection can be monitored by serial pachymetry along with improvement in other clinical parameters evaluated with slit lamp. Clinical features which need to be examined comprise of visual acuity, intraocular pressure, anterior chamber reaction and corneal clarity. They appear to be deranged during an episode of graft rejection, while showing remarkable improvement with response to treatment. Endothelial rejection usually presents with varying grades of corneal edema and anterior chamber inflammation, ranging from mild to marked. Appropriate and timely treatment improves the clinical parameters with subsequent quantified improvement in corneal thickness.

12.7 Prophylaxis

Topical steroids, either Prednisolone acetate 1% or Dexamethasone phosphate 0.1%, are the most commonly used medications for effective immune prophylaxis following resolution of a rejection episode. Difluprednate, a novel strong synthetic steroid, is now being considered in high-risk eyes [31]. Duration of therapy depends on the type of graft, with high-risk grafts often requiring maintenance dose for an indefinite period.

CsA is a macrolide agent with powerful immunosuppressive activity, which modulates T cell function. Calcineurin inhibition reduces the production and release of pro-inflammatory cytokines like IL-2, IL-4, and TNF-alpha, as well as the activity of CD4+ and CD8+ cells. Although systemic CsA is highly efficient in preventing immunological rejection in solid organ transplantation, it has had mixed results in high-risk corneal grafts. Long-term (more than 1 year). CsA therapy appears to improve graft survival over short-term therapy. Recommended systemic dosage is 15 mg/kg/day for 2 days followed by 7.5 mg/kg/day for 2 days, then adjusted to 2–3 mg/kg/day to maintain blood trough levels of 120–150 ng/mL for 6 months. Because of probable nephro- and hepato-toxicity, changes in glucose metabolism, hypertension, and gingival hyperplasia, the use of CSA is confined. Additionally, owing to its variable absorption, monitoring of liver function and renal function tests should be done regularly. Topical CsA usage (concentration varying from 0.05–2%) is indicated in cases of steroid-induced glaucoma, to reduce the usage of topical steroids for immune prophylaxis. In high-risk patients and in patients with steroid-induced elevated IOP, dosing frequency of five times a day is recommended both pre- and postoperatively. Tacrolimus 0.03% ointment has a beneficial effect on immune prophylaxis.

Other immunosuppressive agents which can be used in high-risk grafts for the prevention of rejection episodes include Azathioprine, Mycophenolate mofetil, Tacrolimus (FK-506), and Rapamycin (Sirolimus) [38]. Numerous studies have shown variable outcomes when used alone or in combination with steroids. Systemic monitoring is essential to monitor the side effects of these agents, which appears to limit their safe usage for long-term duration.

Azathioprine prevents cell replication by inhibiting purine synthesis during a specific phase of the cell cycle. It is effective in the early stages of rejection when given orally at a dose of 1–2 mg/kg/day in combination with topical corticosteroids, minimising the requirement for high-dose systemic corticosteroids and their accompanying systemic problems. During maintenance therapy, complete blood counts and liver function tests are mandatory. However, due to potential complications like bone marrow suppression, thrombocytopenia, leukopenia, hepatocellular necrosis, increased risk of neoplasia and alopecia, use of Azathioprine for prevention of corneal graft rejection is limited.

Mycophenolate mofetil (MMF) is a pro-drug of the active substance Mycophenolic acid (MPA). It is a potent inhibitor of Inosine monophosphate dehydrogenase and resultant selective inhibition of T and B lymphocyte proliferation. It is given in dose of 1.5–2 gm/day. Infection, anaemia, leukopenia, and gastrointestinal upset are the most commonly reported side effects. Blood cell counts must be monitored in order to diagnose any systemic infection timely. Tacrolimus (FK-506) is a more potent agent than CsA, which has a similar mechanism of action but fewer systemic side effects. At a dose of 0.16 mg/kg/day (2–12 mg daily), it is beneficial in preventing allograft rejection and in preventing rejection in high-risk corneal and limbal grafts. The main side effects associated with long-term usage are headache, malaise, gastrointestinal upset and renal toxicity.

Rapamycin being lipophilic in nature allows better corneal penetration and is more potent than CsA and FK-506. It inhibits immunophilic activity, interferes with IL-2 induced signals and suppresses T cell activation at the level of lymphokine production. It is given in dosage of 0.5–1 mg/kg/day to maintain a plasma level of 3–4 ng/mL.

Anti-VEGF drugs, particularly Bevacizumab (Avastin), have been utilised to minimise corneal neovascularization and increase graft life in high-risk transplants. Subconjunctival or intrastromal injections have been used to deliver it [39]. Although these medications have no role in the treatment of acute graft rejection, they can be used to minimise the overall risk of future episodes once the rejection episode has been resolved.

Newer evolving therapy includes targeted therapy using monoclonal antibodies against T cell antigens. Daclizumab and Basiliximab both target the IL-2 receptor on activated T cell to inhibit T cell proliferation [38]. Monoclonal antibodies in combination with CsA have shown to be effective to prevent immune rejection episodes and maintain clear grafts for up to 25 months [30].

Clinical observations show that penetrating keratoplasty without preceding restoration of limbal stem cell function increases the chances of graft rejection in patients with severe or complete LSCD [40, 41]. Outcome of acute graft rejection depends on the interval between the onset of the rejection episode and initiation of medical therapy. According to various research, reversibility percentages range from 63 to 92% [32, 42]. When compared to low-risk grafts, the associated high-risk factors also reduce recovery rates.

12.8 Prevention

The beneficial role of HLA & ABO matching is still not clear but it can be considered when dealing with a high-risk graft to improve graft survival, especially in a mono-ocular patient. Pre-operative use of corticosteroids, subconjunctival, or intrastromal anti-VEGF agents and fine-needle diathermy have been shown to be effective in reducing stromal vascularization. Immunomodulation to reduce the immunogenicity of corneas has been attempted by transfection of endothelial cells to over-express down-regulatory cytokines, such as IL-10 and IL-12 [43]. Usage of acellular glycerol-cryopreserved donor cornea for DALK can help avoid stromal and epithelial rejection compared to fresh corneal donor tissue in eyes with a high risk of rejection [44]. Another option is to use gamma-irradiated donor cornea for DALK in these situations [45]. Interrupted sutures using 10-0 monofilament nylon with burying of the knot on the donor side is the preferred suturing technique in high-risk cases.

12.9 Summary

Corneal graft rejection remains the most important factor limiting the successful outcome of corneal transplantation. The pathophysiology of corneal graft rejection is highly complex despite several advances being made in understanding the mechanisms involved. Pre-operative screening, choice of transplantation procedure including newer lamellar keratoplasty procedures, post-operative medications, and patient counselling for compliance with medications and follow-up visits, play a vital role is maintaining a clear corneal graft and avoiding rejection episodes. Identification of high-risk patients, attention to clinical risk factors, donor selection with HLA or ABO compatibility and gender match, especially in a mono-ocular patient can be considered preoperatively to reduce the risk of rejection. Early detection of rejection and aggressive therapy is vital, especially with high-risk grafts. Corticosteroids still remain the mainstay therapy for managing acute rejection episodes and post-operative immune prophylaxis. Other immunosuppressive therapyhas shown promise in immune prophylaxis and prevention of rejection episodes and needs further evaluation. Future development of targeted biologic therapy may provide new avenues in the treatment of acute graft rejection with minimal side effects and sustained therapeutic effects for graft survival.

Key Points

1. Corneal transplantation is one of the most frequently performed solid organ transplants with high success rates.
2. Immune privilege of the cornea is reduced in high-risk keratoplasty. Such cases require a combination of pre-operative planning, intra-operative surgical modifications and adequate post-operative immunosuppressive therapy for a successful outcome.
3. Topical corticosteroids remain the mainstay of treatment for prophylaxis and treatment of graft rejection. Pulsed therapy with IV Methylprednisolone is preferred over oral corticosteroids for reversing acute endothelial rejection.
4. Immunosuppressive therapy seems to be useful for high-risk grafts in combination with corticosteroids, however, frequent monitoring is necessary for systemic side effects.

References

1. Eye Bank Association of America. Eye banking statistical report. 2019. https://restoresight.org/wp-content/uploads/2020/04/2019-EBAA-Stat-Report-FINAL.pdf. Accessed 03 Sep 2020.
2. Tan DT, Dart JK, Holland EJ, Kinoshita S. Corneal transplantation. Lancet. 2012;379(9827):1749–61.
3. Yamada J, Streilein JW. Induction of anterior chamber-associated immune deviation by corneal allografts placed in the anterior chamber. Invest Ophthalmol Vis Sci. 1997;38(13):2833–43.
4. Faraj LA, Hashmani K, Khatib T, Al-Aqaba M, Dua HS. The changing face of corneal graft rejection. Br J Ophthalmol. 2012;96(8):1049–50.
5. Lam H, Dana MR. Corneal graft rejection. Int Ophthalmol Clin. 2009;49(1):31–41.
6. Panda A, Vanathi M, Kumar A, Dash Y, Priya S. Corneal graft rejection. Surv Ophthalmol. 2007;52(4):375–96.
7. The Australian Corneal Graft Registry. 1990 to 1992 report. Aust N Z J Ophthalmol. 1993;21(2 Suppl):1–48.
8. Alldredge OC, Krachmer JH. Clinical types of corneal transplant rejection. Their manifestations, frequency, preoperative correlates, and treatment. Arch Ophthalmol. 1981;99(4):599–604.
9. Maguire MG, Stark WJ, Gottsch JD, et al. Risk factors for corneal graft failure and rejection in the collaborative corneal transplantation studies. Collaborative Corneal Transplantation Studies Research Group. Ophthalmology. 1994;101(9):1536–47.
10. Thompson RW Jr, Price MO, Bowers PJ, Price FW Jr. Long-term graft survival after penetrating keratoplasty. Ophthalmology. 2003;110(7):1396–402.
11. Deng SX, Lee WB, Hammersmith KM, et al. Descemet membrane endothelial keratoplasty: safety and outcomes: a report by the American Academy of Ophthalmology. Ophthalmology. 2018;125(2):295–310.
12. Anshu A, Price MO, Price FW Jr. Risk of corneal transplant rejection significantly reduced with Descemet's membrane endothelial keratoplasty. Ophthalmology. 2012;119(3):536–40.
13. Price MO, Jordan CS, Moore G, Price FW Jr. Graft rejection episodes after Descemet stripping with endothelial keratoplasty: part two: the statistical analysis of probability and risk factors. Br J Ophthalmol. 2009;93(3):391–5.
14. Reinhart WJ, Musch DC, Jacobs DS, Lee WB, Kaufman SC, Shtein RM. Deep anterior lamellar keratoplasty as an alternative to penetrating keratoplasty a report by the American Academy of Ophthalmology. Ophthalmology. 2011;118(1):209–18.
15. Borderie VM, Guilbert E, Touzeau O, Laroche L. Graft rejection and graft failure after anterior lamellar versus penetrating keratoplasty. Am J Ophthalmol. 2011;151(6):1024–9.
16. Lomholt JA, Baggesen K, Ehlers N. Recurrence and rejection rates following corneal transplantation for herpes simplex keratitis. Acta Ophthalmol Scand. 1995;73(1):29–32.
17. Sharma N, Kandar AK, Singh TJ. Stromal rejection after big bubble deep anterior lamellar keratoplasty: case series and review of literature. Eye Contact Lens. 2013;39(2):194–8.
18. Fulton JC, Cohen EJ, Honig M, Rapuano CJ, Laibson PR. Pregnancy and corneal allograft rejection. Arch Ophthalmol. 1996;114(6):765.
19. Hopkinson CL, Romano V, Kaye RA, Steger B, Stewart RM, Tsagkataki M, Jones MN, Larkin DF, Kaye SB, National Health Service Blood Transplant Ocular Tissue Advisory Group and Contributing Ophthalmologists (OTAG Study 20). The influence of donor and recipient gender incompatibility on corneal transplant rejection and failure. Am J Transplant. 2017;17(1):210–7.
20. Küchle M, Cursiefen C, Nguyen NX, Langenbucher A, Seitz B, Wenkel H, Martus P, Naumann GO. Risk factors for corneal allograft rejection: intermediate results of a prospective normal-risk keratoplasty study. Graefes Arch Clin Exp Ophthalmol. 2002;240(7):580–4.
21. Price FW Jr, Price DA, Ngakeng V, Price MO. Survey of steroid usage patterns during and after low-risk penetrating keratoplasty. Cornea. 2009;28(8):865–70.
22. Stulting RD. Penetrating keratoplasty in children. In: Brightbill FS, editor. Corneal surgery: theory, technique, and tissue. 2nd ed. St Louis: Mosby; 1993. p. 374–85.

23. Giannaccare G, Weiss JS, Sapigni L, Bovone C, Mattioli L, Campos EC, Busin M. Immunologic Stromal Rejection After Deep Anterior Lamellar Keratoplasty With Grafts of a Larger Size (9 mm) for Various Stromal Diseases. Cornea. 2018 Aug;37(8):967–972.
24. Watson SL, Tuft SJ, Dart JK. Patterns of rejection after deep lamellar keratoplasty. Ophthalmology. 2006 Apr;113(4):556–60.
25. Watson SL, Ramsay A, Dart JK, Bunce C, Craig E. Comparison of deep lamellar keratoplasty and penetrating keratoplasty in patients with keratoconus. Ophthalmology. 2004;111(9):1676–82.
26. Li JY, Terry MA, Goshe J, Shamie N, Davis-Boozer D. Graft rejection after Descemet's stripping automated endothelial keratoplasty: graft survival and endothelial cell loss. Ophthalmology. 2012;119(1):90–4.
27. Allan BD, Terry MA, Price FW Jr, Price MO, Griffin NB, Claesson M. Corneal transplant rejection rate and severity after endothelial keratoplasty. Cornea. 2007;26(9):1039–42.
28. Sepsakos L, Shah K, Lindquist TP, Lee WB, Holland E. Rate of Rejection After Descemet Stripping Automated Endothelial Keratoplasty in Fuchs Dystrophy: Three-Year Follow-up. Cornea. 2016;35(12):1537–41.
29. Hos D, Tuac O, Schaub F, Stanzel TP, Schrittenlocher S, Hellmich M, Bachmann BO, Cursiefen C. Incidence and Clinical Course of Immune Reactions after Descemet Membrane Endothelial Keratoplasty: Retrospective Analysis of 1000 Consecutive Eyes. Ophthalmology. 2017;124(4):512–18.
30. Qazi Y, Hamrah P. Corneal allograft rejection: immunopathogenesis to therapeutics. J Clin Cell Immunol. 2013;2013(Suppl 9):006.
31. Kharod-Dholakia B, Randleman JB, Bromley JG, Stulting RD. Prevention and treatment of corneal graft rejection: current practice patterns of the Cornea Society (2011). Cornea. 2015;34(6):609–14.
32. Hill JC, Maske R, Watson P. Corticosteroids in corneal graft rejection. Oral versus single pulse therapy. Ophthalmology. 1991;98(3):329–33.
33. Tandon R, Verma K, Chawla B, et al. Intravenous dexamethasone vs methylprednisolone pulse therapy in the treatment of acute endothelial graft rejection. Eye (Lond). 2009;23(3):635–9.
34. Costa DC, de Castro RS, Kara-Jose N. Case-control study of subconjunctival triamcinolone acetonide injection vs intravenous methylprednisolone pulse in the treatment of endothelial corneal allograft rejection. Eye (Lond). 2009;23(3):708–14.
35. Poon A, Constantinou M, Lamoureux E, Taylor HR. Topical cyclosporin A in the treatment of acute graft rejection: a randomized controlled trial. Clin Exp Ophthalmol. 2008;36(5):415–21.
36. Ziaei M, Manzouri B. Topical cyclosporine in corneal transplantation. Cornea. 2015;34(1):110–5.
37. Hill JC. Systemic cyclosporine in high-risk keratoplasty. Short- versus long-term therapy. Ophthalmology. 1994;101(1):128–33.
38. Tabbara KF. Pharmacologic strategies in the prevention and treatment of corneal transplant rejection. Int Ophthalmol. 2008;28(3):223–32.
39. Fasciani R, Mosca L, Giannico MI, Ambrogio SA, Balestrazzi E. Subconjunctival and/or intrastromal bevacizumab injections as preconditioning therapy to promote corneal graft survival. Int Ophthalmol. 2015;35(2):221–7.
40. Gupta N, Farooqui JH, Patel N, Mathur U. Early results of penetrating keratoplasty in patients with unilateral chemical injury after simple limbal epithelial transplantation. Cornea. 2018;37(10):1249–54.
41. Sangwan VS, Matalia HP, Vemuganti GK, Ifthekar G, Fatima A, Singh S, Rao GN. Early results of penetrating keratoplasty after cultivated limbal epithelium transplantation. Arch Ophthalmol. 2005;123(3):334–40.
42. Hudde T, Minassian DC, Larkin DF. Randomised controlled trial of corticosteroid regimens in endothelial corneal allograft rejection. Br J Ophthalmol. 1999;83(12):1348–52.
43. Williams KA, Brereton HM, Coster DJ. Prospects for genetic modulation of corneal graft survival. Eye (Lond). 2009;23:1904–9.

44. Li J, Yu L, Deng Z, Wang L, Sun L, Ma H, Chen W. Deep anterior lamellar keratoplasty using acellular corneal tissue for prevention of allograft rejection in high-risk corneas. Am J Ophthalmol. 2011;152(5):762–70.e3.
45. Mathews PM, Fogla R, Samayoa E, VanCourt S, Akpek EK. Long-term clinical outcomes of keratoplasty using gamma-irradiated corneal lenticules. BMJ Open Ophthalmol. 2019;4(1):e000396.

13 Post-Surgical Corneal Wound Dehiscence

Saumya Yadav, Noopur Gupta, Neiwete Lomi,
and Radhika Tandon

13.1 Introduction

Partial or total separation of previously approximated wound edges can occur either spontaneously or more commonly following trauma. Cornea is exposed to the environment, and this makes it vulnerable to traumatic insults. A vascularity of the cornea is responsible for slow and ineffective healing and remodelling of corneal wounds [1, 2]. Most cases of corneal wound dehiscence occur within the first few weeks of surgery when healing is still in the early stages but can even occur decades after initial surgery [3, 4]. Any factor that contributes to poor wound healing can also cause wound dehiscence, e.g. ischemia, infection, glucocorticoid use, increased abdominal pressure, diabetes, malnutrition, smoking, radiation exposure and obesity [5, 6]. Early identification and re-suturing of dehiscence are important for preventing the progression of dehiscence and consequent complications. Complete wound dehiscence with herniation of intraocular contents is an undesirable event necessitating evisceration surgery.

13.2 Corneal Wound Healing

Corneal healing mechanisms are guided by complex molecular pathways and involve a complicated, dynamic process of cell death, migration, proliferation, differentiation and extracellular matrix remodelling [7]. Different cells of cornea, i.e. epithelial, stromal, and endothelial display similar and cell-specific healing processes. For the regeneration of epithelium, epithelial cells are repopulated by limbal stem cells. Corneal stroma, which constitutes more than 90% of corneal thickness and is the major contributor to corneal mechanical strength, heals by the

S. Yadav · N. Gupta · N. Lomi · R. Tandon (✉)
Dr Rajendra Prasad Centre for Ophthalmic Sciences, AIIMS, New Delhi, India

B. Sharma, J. S. Titiyal (eds.), *Corneal Emergencies*,
https://doi.org/10.1007/978-981-16-5876-1_13

transformation of keratocytes into fibroblasts and myofibroblasts. Endotheliumheals mainly by migration of residual endothelial cells with cell proliferation playing a minor role [7]. Bowman's layer cannot regenerate and once damaged results in the formation of scar. Any disruption of these healing mechanisms can lead to an inadequately healed wound with reduced tensile strength [2].

13.3 Wound Dehiscence Following Corneal Surgeries

13.3.1 Penetrating Keratoplasty

A full-thickness graft offers visual rehabilitation to patients with severe corneal blindness but leaves a structurally weak graft host junction. In literature, incidence of post-traumatic graft dehiscence is reported to range from 0.6%to 5.8% [8]. As corneal graft host junction never regains the tensile strength of the intact cornea and remains vulnerable even if the wound appears to be fully healed, patients with a full-thickness graft carry a life-long risk of graft dehiscence [9–11]. Although the maximum risk is in the early post-operative period wherein a blunt trauma to the globe can lead to graft dehiscence with sutures in situ, the longest case of post-traumatic graft dehiscence has been recorded to occur 33 years post-keratoplasty [4, 12].

13.3.1.1 Clinical Features

Patients commonly present to the ophthalmic emergency with complaints of sudden onset diminution of vision, pain, and/or bleeding and expulsion of intraocular contents in severe cases. A history of either a blunt force trauma (punch) to the face, being struck by an object, vigorous rubbing of eyes, finger trauma, fall or lifting of heavy objects can often be elicited. The dehiscence can be partial thickness or full thickness and can involve one or more quadrants.

13.3.1.2 Types of Graft Dehiscence

Post-PK graft dehiscence is of four main types: post-traumatic, suture-related, infectious keratitis related, and spontaneous wound dehiscence with post-traumatic cases being the most common type. Suture-related and spontaneous wound separations usually occur in the early post-operative period, when the wound healing is inadequate, either due to improper wound apposition or premature suture removal. Post-traumatic and infections related cases can occur any time after the surgery [13].

13.3.1.3 Predisposing Factors

Long-term steroid usage increased intraocular pressure, early suture removal and multiple grafts are the most important risk factors for graft dehiscence [4]. Post-keratoplasty patients are kept on topical steroid treatment for years, and sometimes for life; this weakens the graft host junction's integrity and puts it at risk of dehiscence, especially after suture removal. Uncontrolled high intraocular pressures post-PK either as a result of response to steroids or secondary angle closure can result in the separation of wound edges with intact sutures. Suturing techniques and suture materials can also play a role. Wound dehiscence is reported to be more common after removal of continuous suture than interrupted sutures [4, 14]. Nylon suture material is associated with lower tissue reactivity and thus makes the wound integrity weaker and more prone to separation compared to silk material [15].

13.3.1.4 Management

Management protocol to follow in a case of corneal wound dehiscence is outlined in Fig. 13.1. Surgical repair of the dehisced graft remains the only means to restore the globe's integrity. Depending upon the extent of wound disruption and graft status, either a prompt primary re-suturing of the corneal graft with anterior chamber reformation (Figs. 13.2 and 13.3) or graft exchange is done. Post-operatively, frequent instillation (2–4 hourly) of topical steroids is needed to curtail the risk of graft rejection. Secondary surgeries may be required to manage the complications.

13.3.1.5 Outcomes

Surgical restoration of the globe integrity within several hours of the event usually restores pre-dehiscence visual acuity in suture-related and spontaneous cases. Post-traumatic cases tend to have a poor prognosis wherein the force of trauma, involvement of intraocular structures, and extent of posterior segment injuries determine

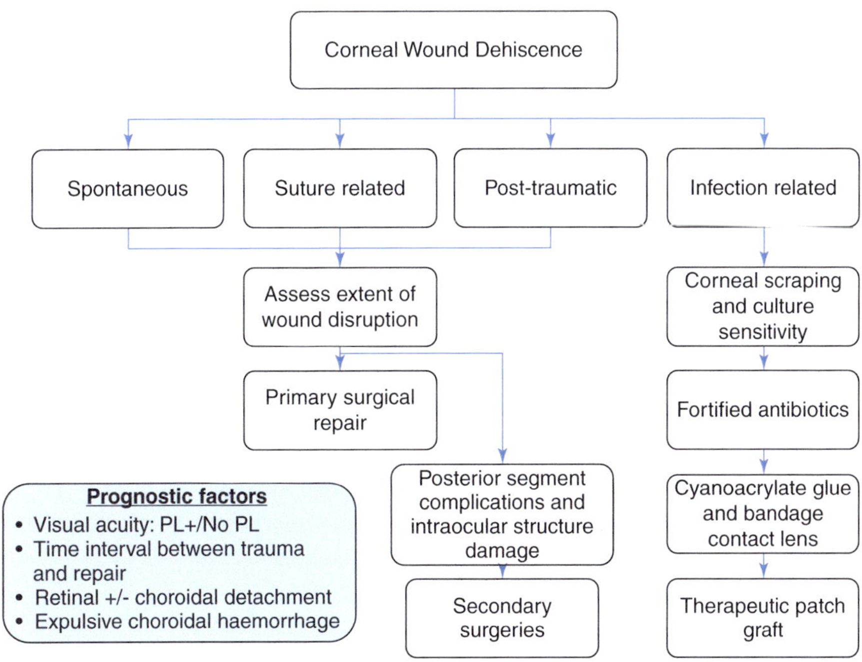

Fig. 13.1 Flowchart outlining the management protocol to be followed in a case of corneal wound dehiscence

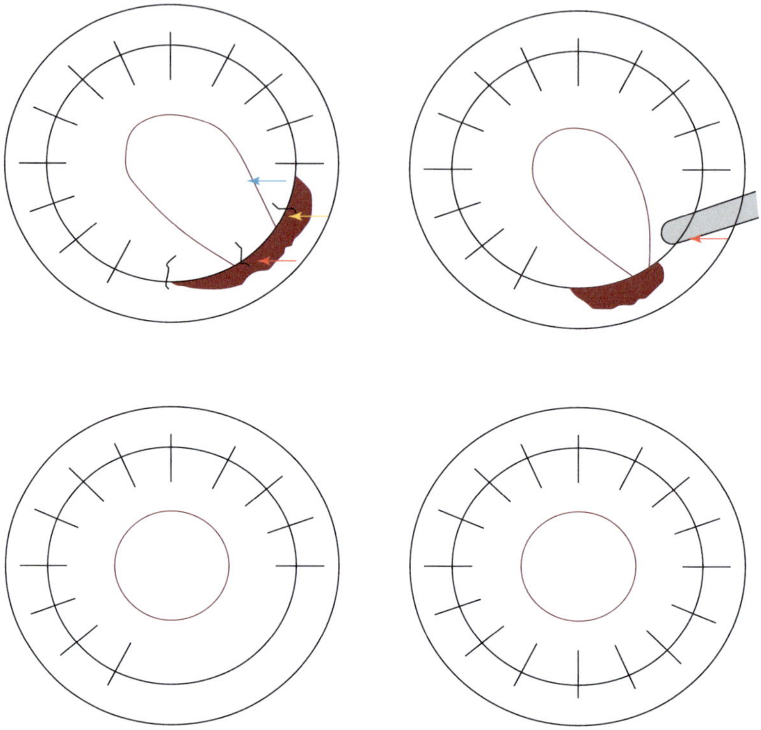

Fig. 13.2 Line diagram illustrating a case of graft dehiscence (upper left) extending up to 4 clock hours with uveal tissue prolapse (red arrow), the irregular pupil (blue arrow) and broken sutures (yellow arrow). An immediate surgical repair of the dehiscence includes reposition of prolapsed iris using an iris repositor (upper left). After ensuring a circular pupil with no incarceration of iris tissue in the wound (lower left), anterior chamber is formed, and wound is sutured (lower right)

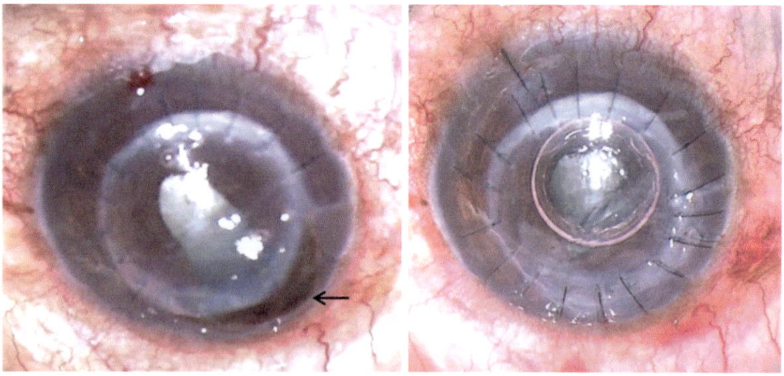

Fig. 13.3 Clinical picture of the left eye of a patient with post-traumatic dehiscence of a penetrating keratoplasty graft, extending 4 clock hours in infero-temporal quadrant, with uveal tissue prolapse and broken sutures (black arrow) (left). An immediate re-suturing of the graft was done to restore the globe integrity (right)

Table 13.1 Factors affecting final visual outcome in post-keratoplasty graft dehiscence

Prognostic factors for post-keratoplasty graft dehiscence
• Extent of injury • Time interval between injury and treatment initiation • Involvement of intraocular structures (e.g. irididodialysis, subluxation or expulsion of crystalline lens, and/or intraocular lens) • Posterior segment injuries (vitreous loss/haemorrhage, suprachoroidal hemorrhage, retinal detachment)

the final visual acuity obtained (Table 13.1) [4, 12, 16]. In such cases, an initial re-suturing of the graft with subsequent management of the complication is recommended. Corneal graft edema, graft rejection, failed graft, endophthalmitis can ensue and result in a grim prognosis [17, 18].

13.3.2 Lamellar Keratoplasty

Intact Descemet's membrane of the host in deep anterior lamellar keratoplasty (DALK) offers the advantage of reduced risk of graft rejection and greater biomechanical stability compared to full-thickness grafts. Compared to PK patients, DALK patients are less prone to develop full-thickness ruptures of graft host junction because of the reinforcement provided by the Descemet's membrane against the traumatic insults. Any separation of the wound, if noted, is managed along with the same guidelines as those for dehiscence of full-thickness grafts. Patients with lamellar grafts have less severe complications and better visual outcomes after dehiscence repair than those with full-thickness grafts [19, 20].

13.3.3 Repaired Corneal Perforation

Similar to graft host junction of penetrating keratoplasty, healed corneal scars of repaired perforations are inherently structurally weak. A repaired corneal wound is expected to obtain 80% of its original tensile strength over 2 years; with time, the scars become opaque and fibrotic but never regain the pre-injury tensile strength of normal cornea [2]. Improper wound apposition, poor suturing techniques, uveal tissue and vitreous incarceration in the wound, and epithelial ingrowth further weakens the tensile strength of corneal scars, which can reopen following a blunt force trauma to the eye.

13.3.3.1 Management

Immediate surgical repair of the wound with either reposition or excision of the prolapsed uveal tissue is recommended. Care should be exercised so as to remove any vitreous from the wound. Subsequent surgeries may be required to manage the resulting complications, e.g. secondary cataract removal, pars-plana vitrectomy for vitreous haemorrhage, vitreoretinal surgery for retinal detachment and trabeculectomy for secondary glaucoma.

13.3.4 Cataract Surgery

With the advent of modern minimally invasive cataract surgery, late dehiscence of cataract wounds have become a thing of the past and is mostly seen in the post-traumatic disruption of extracapsular cataract surgery (ECCE) incision wounds [21, 22]. A longer interval between surgery and trauma is reported to have a worse visual outcome, probably because greater traumatic force is required to cause the dehiscence of a wound, which is more structurally stable, causing more severe intraocular damage [23].

13.3.4.1 Predisposing Factors and Preventive Measures

Inadequate wound construction in phacoemulsification and SICS and incomplete wound closure in ECCE can lead to early wound leak. A large incision in the clear cornea, especially if not three planar self-sealing incision or an irregularly dissected tunnel, may not be self-sealing and may require sutures [21]. Excessive cautery and incarceration of iris or vitreous into the wound prevents adequate closure, promotes wound leak in early phases and results in the inadequately healed wound. Paediatric eye pose an additional challenge as reduced scleral rigidity of paediatric eyes increases chances of wound leak and inadequate wound healing due to poor apposition of edges, therefore incisions should always be sutured after paediatric lens aspiration.

13.3.4.2 Management

A shallow anterior chamber and hypotony on the first post-operative day should arouse suspicion of a wound leak due to inadequate wound closure, and the same should be confirmed on Seidel's test. Immediate suturing of such wounds is required in operation theatre settings to reduce the risk of infection. Before suturing, a wound sweep with a sponge or wet swab should be done to rule out any incarceration of vitreous. Any incarcerated iris should be reposited. Such cases of early wound leaks, if timely managed, generally have good outcomes. Post-traumatic cases are often associated with damage to intraocular structures and an inferior prognosis.

A cystoid cicatrix an untoward complication following a surgical incision at the limbus wherein dehiscence of the limbal wound occurs, and instead of a frank prolapse, the uveal tissue gets incarcerated in the dehisced wound, forming a dew-drop lesion (Fig. 13.4). Cystoid cicatrix can form a persistently filtering bleb resulting v chronic hypotony or can rupture following trauma requiring a tectonic patch graft [24].

13.3.5 Refractive Surgery

Radial keratotomy was a widely practiced refractive procedure before the advent of modern laser refractive surgeries. Unsutured incisions of radial keratotomy (RK) reduce ocular integrity permanently and are at a great risk of opening up with even minimal blunt force [25]. Several studies have documented that the radial

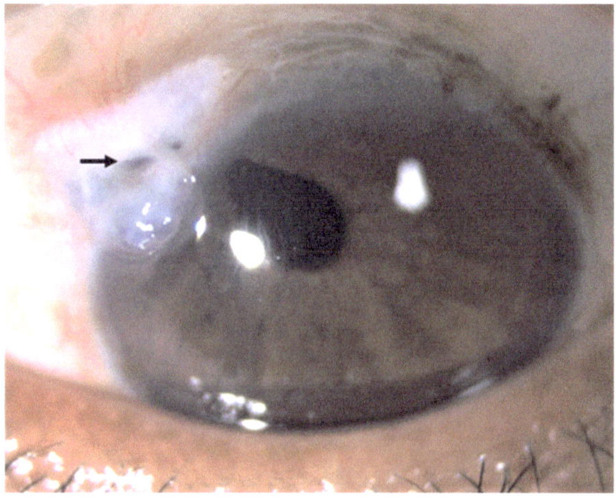

Fig. 13.4 Slit-lamp photograph of a case of cystoid cicatrix developed following trauma 3 weeks after phacoemulsification. Supero-temporal wound dehiscence (black arrow) with cystoid appearance can be seen, and irregularly up drawn pupil indicates incarceration of the iris tissue into the dehisced wound

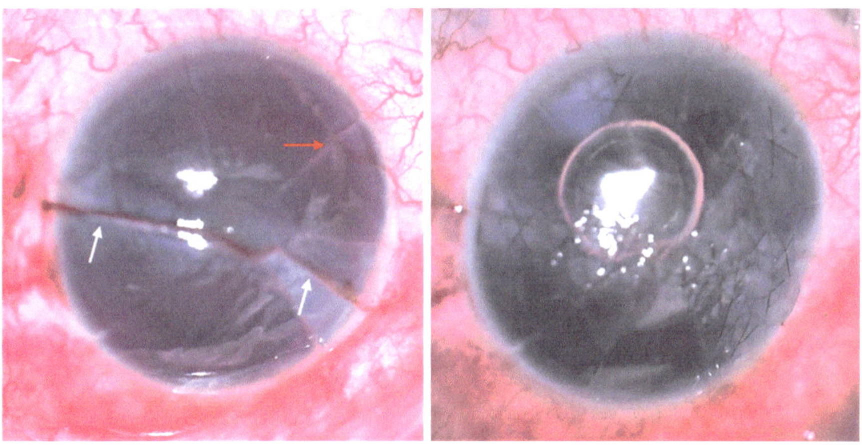

Fig. 13.5 Clinical photograph of post-traumatic rupture of radial keratotomy (RK) incisions (white arrows) extending from limbus to limbus (left). Partial dehiscence of incisions (red arrow) is also seen. Intraoperative photograph (right) shows repaired dehiscence of the RK incisions using cross sutures and formed anterior chamber with central air bubble (right)

keratotomy incisions indefinitely remain incompletely healed [26]. Because of the proximity of RK incisions to the visual axis, dehiscence along radial incisions tend to extend along the thin central corneas of these patients (Fig. 13.5) [27]. RK incisions also pose a challenge during other ocular surgeries and can open up while performing phacoemulsification or PK [28]. Because of the unpredictable refractive results, high rate of visual complications and aforementioned risks, RK is now considered an obsolete procedure.

Lasik in situ keratomileusis (LASIK) flap dislocations can occur any time after the surgery and have reported incidence of 1–2% [29]. Flapshifts in the early post-operative period (1 week) may result even due to minor trauma such as squeezing or rubbing of eyes. Relatively significant force is required for late flap dislocations. Traumatic flap dislocations have been reported to occur upto14 years post-surgery [29].

13.3.5.1 Risk Factors and Preventive Measures

As the majority of the cases of flap dislocation occur within the first 24 h following surgery, intraoperative and early post-operative care becomes of utmost importance. Poor intraoperative positioning and excessive irrigation of the flap can result in a poorly positioned flap in the early postoperative period and should be avoided. Adherence to the flap should be checked at the end of the procedure. Patients should be properly counselled regarding postoperative care. Avoidance of rubbing and squeezing of eyes should be emphasised. If necessary, use of eye shield for the first 24 h may be advised. Adequate lubricants should be prescribed in patients with dry eye.

13.3.5.2 Management

Dislocated LASIK flaps should be treated as an emergency and managed in the operating room. An immediate refloatation and repositioning of the flap with irrigation along with flattening of any associated folds is required to prevent the formation of fixed folds or epithelial ingrowth. In the event of a persistent fold, suturing of the flap may be required. A bandage contact lens may be placed to further reduce the chances of flap wrinkling [30]. In cases with rupture of multiple RK incisions, sometimes primary re-suturing of the incisions might not be feasible, and instead, an emergency penetrating keratoplasty needs to be planned. Therefore, access to an optical grade donor cornea should be ensured before taking such patients to the operation theatre.

13.4 Conclusion

Post-surgical wound dehiscence is an uncommon but serious complication following corneal surgeries. Depending upon its extent, wound disruption can cause severe irreversible damage to visual function. Importance of the prevention of ocular trauma must be emphasised to all patients undergoing ocular surgeries. Post RK/ keratoplasty/repaired corneal perforation patients should be advised to wear protective polycarbonate glasses or eye shields and avoid activities (e.g. contact sports) that pose a risk of ocular trauma. Intact corneal sutures, if are not inducing significant astigmatism, may be indefinitely left in situ, especially in patients at high risk of dehiscence.

Key Points

- Corneal wounds never regain their pre-incisional/injury tensile strength.
- Non-penetrating or small incision surgical techniques should be adopted to minimise the risk of wound dehiscence and severity of complications.

- Immediate surgical intervention and suturing of the wound are required to restore the globe integrity and prevent further damage.
- Patients undergoing corneal surgeries should be properly counselled to prevent ocular trauma and use protective eyewear.

References

1. Calkins JL, Hochheimer BF, Stark WJ. Corneal wound healing: holographic stress-test analysis. Invest Ophthalmol Vis Sci. 1981;21:322–34.
2. Gasset AR, Dohlman CH. The tensile strength of corneal wounds. Arch Ophthalmol. 1968;79:595–602.
3. Kartal B, Kandemir B, Set T, et al. Traumatic wound dehiscence after penetrating keratoplasty. Ulus Travma Acil Cerrahi Derg. 2014;20(3):181–8.
4. Das S, Whiting M, Taylor HR. Corneal wound dehiscence after penetrating keratoplasty. Cornea. 2007;26(5):526–9.
5. Bor E, Kremer I. Endophthalmitis and wound dehiscence following late removal of penetrating keratoplasty sutures. Ophthalmic Surg Lasers Imaging. 2011;42(3):234–40.
6. Whipple KM, Lee JE, Huang AS, Broun SI. Dehisced corneal button with no evidence of a ruptured globe. JAMA Ophthalmol. 2013;131(11):1434.
7. Ljubimov AV, Saghizadeh M. Progress in corneal wound healing. Prog Retin Eye Res. 2015;49:17–45.
8. Ma JF, Rapuano CJ, Hammersmith KM, Nagra PK, Dai Y, Azari AA. Outcomes of wound dehiscence post-penetrating keratoplasty. Cornea. 2016;35(6):778–83.
9. Lam FC, Rahman MQ, Ramaesh K. Traumatic wound dehiscence after penetrating keratoplasty-a cause for concern. Eye (Lond). 2007;21(9):1146–50.
10. Simonsen AH, Andreassen TT, Bendix K. The healing strength of corneal wounds in the human eye. Exp Eye Res. 1982;35(3):287–92.
11. Rehany U, Rumelt S. Ocular trauma following penetrating keratoplasty: incidence, outcome, and postoperative recommendations. Arch Ophthalmol. 1998;116(10):1282–6.
12. Tseng SH, Lin SC, Chen FK. Traumatic wound dehiscence after penetrating keratoplasty: clinical features and outcome in 21 cases. Cornea. 1999;18:553–8.
13. Renucci AM, Marangon FB, Culbertson WW. Wound dehiscence after penetrating keratoplasty: clinical characteristics of 51 cases treated at Bascom Palmer Eye Institute. Cornea. 2006;25(5):524–9.
14. Brown SL, Tragakis MP. Wound dehiscence with keratoplasty: complication of the continuous-suture technique. Am J Ophthalmol. 1971;72:115–6.
15. Stark WJ, Paton D, Maumenee MJ, et al. The results of 102 penetrating keratoplasties using 10-0 monofilament suture. Ophthalmic Surg. 1972;3:11–25.
16. Perry HD, Donnenfeld ED. Expulsive choroidal hemorrhage following suture removal after penetrating keratoplasty. Am J Ophthalmol. 1988;106:99–100.
17. Viestenz A, Schrader W, Küchle M, Walter S, Behrens-Baumann W. Management der Bulbusruptur [management of a ruptured globe]. Ophthalmologe. 2008;105(12):1163–75.
18. Kawashima M, Kawakita T, Shimmura S, Tsubota K, Shimazaki J. Characteristics of traumatic globe rupture after keratoplasty. Ophthalmology. 2009;116(11):2072–6.
19. Zarei-Ghanavati S, Zarei-Ghanavati M, Sheibani S. Traumatic wound dehiscence after deep anterior lamellar keratoplasty: protective role of intact descemet membrane after big-bubble technique. Cornea. 2010;29(2):220–1.
20. Sari ES, Koytak A, Kubaloglu A, et al. Traumatic wound dehiscence after deep anterior lamellar keratoplasty. Am J Ophthalmol. 2013;156(4):767–72.
21. Ernest PH, Lavery KT, Kiessling LA. Relative strength of scleral corneal and clear corneal incisions constructed in cadaver eyes. J Cataract Refract Surg. 1994;20:626–9.

22. Ernest PH, Kiessling LA, Lavery KT. Relative strength of cataract incisions in cadaver eyes. J Cataract Refract Surg. 1991;17:668–71.
23. Chowers I, Anteby I, Ever-Hadani P, Frucht-Pery J. Traumatic wound dehiscence after cataract extraction. J Cataract Refract Surg. 2001;27(8):1238–42.
24. Singh A, Sen S, Vanathi M, Tandon R. Corneal keloid with cystoid cicatrix: post-small-incision cataract surgery. Can J Ophthalmol. 2017;52(3):e93–5.
25. Girard LJ, Rodriguez J, Nino N, Wesson M. Delayed wound healing after radial keratotomy (letter). Am J Ophthalmol. 1985;99(4):485–6.
26. Binder PS, Waring GO III, Arrowsmith PN, Wang C. Histopathology of traumatic corneal rupture after radial keratotomy. Arch Ophthalmol. 1988;106(11):1584–90.
27. McNeill JI. Corneal incision dehiscence during penetrating keratoplasty nine years after radial keratotomy. J Cataract Refract Surg. 1993;19(4):542–3.
28. Freeman M, Kumar V, Ramanathan US, O'Neill E. Dehiscence of radial keratotomy incision during phacoemulsification. Eye (Lond). 2004;18(1):101–3.
29. Melki SA, Azar DT. LASIK complications. Surv Ophthalmol. 2001;46(2):95–116.
30. Shah DN, Melki S. Complications of femtosecond-assisted laser in-situ keratomileusis flaps. Semin Ophthalmol. 2014;29(5-6):363–75.

Contact Lens-Associated Emergencies 14

Vijay K. Sharma, Nidhi Kalra, and Rajesh Sinha

14.1 Introduction

Contact lenses have improved the quality of life of patients by virtue of their therapeutic, optical, and cosmetic attributes. In patients with keratoconus and irregular corneas such as post keratoplasty and trauma, contact lenses can correct refractive errors which are otherwise not correctable by glasses. The use of cosmetic contact lenses provides a better appearance. Other advantages of contact lenses include symptomatic improvement of dry eye patients as in Steven Johnson syndrome and Sjogren syndrome, promote healing among post anterior lamellar corneal transplants and persistent epithelial defects as well as providing less restriction in activities compared to glasses. Contact lenses have a significant global market share (approx. 12,476.3 million US dollars in 2020) with 6.7% growth rate. Cosmetic contact lenses, which were originally developed for disfiguring anomalies of cornea and iris, are frequently used for cosmetic enhancements by individuals without any ocular pathology. Scleral contact lenses have markedly improved patients with dry eyes symptomatically, and they are able to lead a productive social life.

Despite these numerous advantages, contact lenses can cause visually devastating complications [1–3]. Some of these complications require emergent care to salvage visual acuity and prevent further complications. This chapter intends to describe contact lens-related corneal emergencies, their causative factors, clinical features, diagnosis, and management.

V. K. Sharma
Command Hospital (EC), Kolkata, India

N. Kalra · R. Sinha (✉)
Rajendra Prasad Centre for Ophthalmic Sciences, All India Institute of Medical Sciences, New Delhi, India

B. Sharma, J. S. Titiyal (eds.), *Corneal Emergencies*,
https://doi.org/10.1007/978-981-16-5876-1_14

14.2 Pathogenesis of Contact Lens-Related Emergencies

Contact lens (CL) wear has diverse effects on the ocular surface and the tear film [4–12]. Etiological causes of various complications associated with contact lens usage can be classified as:

14.2.1 Hypoxia

Being avascular, the cornea derives most of its required oxygen from the atmosphere. Contact lenses with the physical potential of separating the ocular surface from direct contact with environmental oxygen, reduce oxygen availability to the cornea, a phenomenon that has long been thought to contribute to the risk of infection associated with soft contact lens wear. The phenomenon is more marked in extended wear contact lenses and while wearing them overnight.

14.2.2 Mechanical Factors

Mechanical factors can cause foreign body sensation, irritation and subsequent abrasion of the eye or lid due to improper fit, inappropriate design and lens material, and physical forces such as rapid decompression or high G-forces from acceleration. Additionally, debris, germs, and chemicals may become trapped, increasing the risk of keratitis. The majority of CL-related emergencies are caused by the risk factors listed above. Soft and rigid contact lenses are the most common types of contact lenses used. This distinction in structure also relates to the accompanying risk of infection. The soft lenses are more encased across the corneal surface, causing tear film stagnation and compartmentalization. Additionally, they cover the limbus and directly predispose corneal epithelial stem cells to lens-induced hypoxia, tear film disturbances, and mechanical effects.

Other factors have also been attributed to contact lenses-related adverse effects on the cornea. Despite the fact that silicone hydrogel lenses do not cause hypoxia, they do cause infections. This suggests that factors other than hypoxia, such as stagnation, compartmentalization, and reduced cell turnover, may play a role. For cytotoxic strains that normally cannot infect the cornea owing to blinking and shear stress that prevent sufficient contact time, contact lens wear can predispose to such infections due to stagnation even in the absence of hypoxia. For invasive bacteria, that are normally removed by sloughing after they invade surface cells, stagnation, decreased cell turnover and impaired shedding of sloughed-cell during contact lens wear remains an important predisposition. The high modulus of these lenses appears to be linked to an increased risk of mechanical complications such as mucin balls, superior epithelial arcuate lesions, giant papillary conjunctivitis, and inflammatory keratitis. Because of the prolonged wear durations and weaker protective mechanisms in an operated eye, complications are more common in aphakic eyes.

14.2.3 Immunological Factors

Mainly related to ocular allergies and can further be associated with lens intolerance.

14.2.4 Tear Film Abnormality

Contact lenses can cause tear film abnormalities due to the combined effect of mechanical and environmental factors such as low humidity or high airflow leading to derangement of the tear film and impaired lubrication of ocular surface subsequently to impaired removal of waste products and clearing of debris from the eye and epithelial desiccation.

14.3 Classification

Various corneal emergencies associated with contact lens usage can be classified as:

1. Contact lens-associated microbial keratitis (CLMK)
2. Contact lens-related peripheral ulcer (CLPU)
3. Contact Lens Adhesion Phenomenon or Binding
4. Sterile corneal infiltrates
5. Contact lens-associated red eyes (CLARE)
6. Corneal abrasion

Each corneal emergency is described below, with their incidence and association with various types of contact lenses summarized in Table 14.1 [13].

Table 14.1 Definition and incidence of common contact lens-related emergencies (Adapted from Alipour et al. [13])

Complication	Definition	Incidence	Type of lens
CLPU	Epithelial excavation and infiltration while Bowman's layer is intact	2–3%	
Bacterial keratitis	Active inflammation and infiltration of the cornea caused by bacteria such as *Pseudomonas* and *Staphylococcus epidermidis*	1.2–25.4%	SCL > RGP
Acanthamoeba keratitis	Active inflammation and infiltration of the cornea caused by *Acanthamoeba*	1–33 per million CL wearers	SCL > RGP
Fungal keratitis	Active inflammation and infiltration of the cornea caused by fungi such as *Fusarium*	<4.8% of CL-related keratitis	SCL > RGP
Corneal staining	Staining of the cornea after instillation of fluorescein in CL wearer	54%	RGP = SCL
Herpes reactivation		95% in CL users vs. 62% in non-CL users	All types

RGP rigid gas permeable, *SCL* soft contact lens, *CLPU* contact lens-related peripheral ulcer, *GPC* giant papillary conjunctivitis, *MRD* margin reflex distance, *CL* contact lens

14.4 Contact Lens Associated Microbial Keratitis

14.4.1 Acanthamoeba Keratitis

Acanthamoeba species is ubiquitous free-living protozoa found in soil and fresh water and causes severe sight-threatening protozoal infection of the cornea, i.e., *Acanthamoeba* keratitis. It was first time described in 1973 and has been implicated in sporadic epidemics around the world [14–22]. Since 2004, its incidence has increased by ten-folds.

Acanthamoeba keratitis is predominantly seen among contact lens wearers in developed countries, whereas in developing countries, contaminated water from ponds or lakes, sand, and mud are important predispositions. In USA, more than 85% of cases of acanthamoeba are seen among contact lens wearers [19]. It has an association with the use of tap water for handling and cleaning the lenses, showering and swimming with the lenses on, and usage of hard water and lime build-up in water lines. More than 80% of these are associated with soft contact lenses while 12% are seen with rigid gas permeable (RGP) lenses [18, 21].

Contact lens wear is the major risk factor for *Acanthamoeba* keratitis and should be suspected in patients with suspected corneal ulcers who are using contact lenses. The patient presents with severe pain, watering, photophobia, and discharge from the affected eye. Pain is the most important clinical presentation caused by radial peri-neuritis. Clinical picture varies with the stage of presentation. Early signs include epithelial defects with stromal infiltrate and lid edema. Radial peri-neuritis causes prominent corneal nerves. Classical ring-shaped infiltration or abscess is seen in advanced stages of the disease, which may also be associated with endothelial plaque and hypopyon. In the absence of appropriate and timely treatment, disease can rapidly progress with visual acuity decreasing to hand movement or light perception (Fig. 14.1).

Early suspicion and diagnosis of acanthamoeba keratitis is the key to favorable outcome. Delayed diagnosis results in deeper infiltration, rapid progression of vision loss, poor response to treatment and overall poor visual prognosis. In a case of suspicious acanthamoeba keratitis, recommended culture media (e.g., non-nutrient agar with *Escherichia coli* overlay or buffered charcoal-yeast extract agar) and staining techniques (e.g., calcofluor white, acridine orange, or indirect immunofluorescence antibody) should be performed as early as possible. Confocal scan gives a direct diagnosis based on the identification of acanthamoeba double-walled cyst or even trophozoites in the corneal stroma in vivo.

Acanthamoeba is highly resistant to antimicrobial treatment due to the presence of tough, double-walled cyst in the corneal stroma. It requires a combination therapy over a period extending from 6 to 12 months for eradication of trophozoite and cystic form of the parasite from the corneal stroma. Poly-hexamethylene biguanide (PHMB) 0.1% and Chlorhexidine 0.02% are the most frequently used combination therapy. Other medications, including neomycin, paromomycin, voriconazole, imidazole/triazole family drugs, have also been found to be effective in the management of acanthamoeba keratitis.

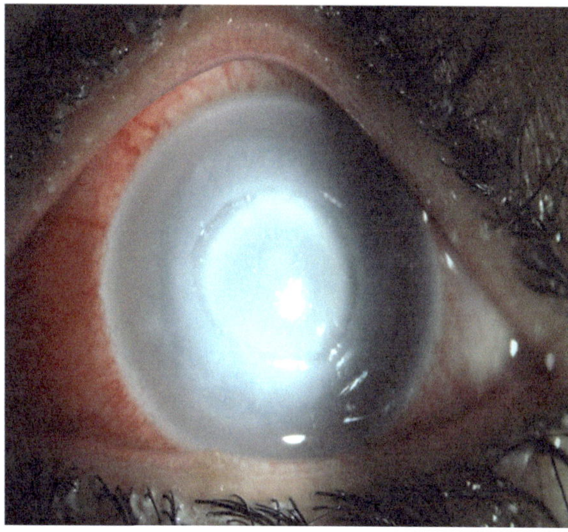

Fig. 14.1 Acanthamoeba keratitis

14.4.2 Pseudomonas Keratitis

Pseudomonas aeruginosa is the most common Gram-negative bacteria implicated in contact lens-induced keratitis. Infections due to *Pseudomonas* are particularly worrisome owing to rapid progression and potentially difficult treatment [23, 24]. Isolates from samples collected from pseudomonas corneal infections found two types of strains, i.e., invasive and cytotoxic. Corneal epithelial cells internalize invasive *Pseudomonas aeruginosa* strains. After epithelial cell invasion, they break out of the endocytic vacuole, replicate efficiently within the cytoplasm, travel from cell to cell, and eventually kill infected cells by apoptosis. In contrast, cytotoxic *P. aeruginosa* strains remain outside cells, and instead, they inject a toxin called Exo U that quickly kills cells by an undetermined mechanism. Cytotoxic strains tend to be more resistant to contact lens disinfectants. The differences between invasive and cytotoxic strains lie within the bacterial chromosome and translate into the secretion of different effector molecules into host cells and differences in the proteolytic modification of these effectors. Both invasion and cytotoxicity involve bacterial exploitation of host corneal cell surface molecules, cellular structures, and signal transduction pathways. Host protein tyrosine kinase activity is involved in both *P. aeruginosa* invasion and cytotoxicity, invasion involving Src family tyrosine kinases and other signaling molecules such as intracellular calcium-calmodulin and MEK-ERK signaling.

Pseudomonas keratitis presents as a rapidly evolving infection that may lead to perforation and loss of an eye, if left untreated. They can also be slow to progress or take an indolent course occasionally. The organism adheres to the wounded cornea with ensuing infection. Within an hour of this adherence to the injured epithelium, invasion into the stroma occurs. Thus, the infection heralds an epithelial defect, superficial edema, and stroma micro-infiltration as early as within 6 h after the

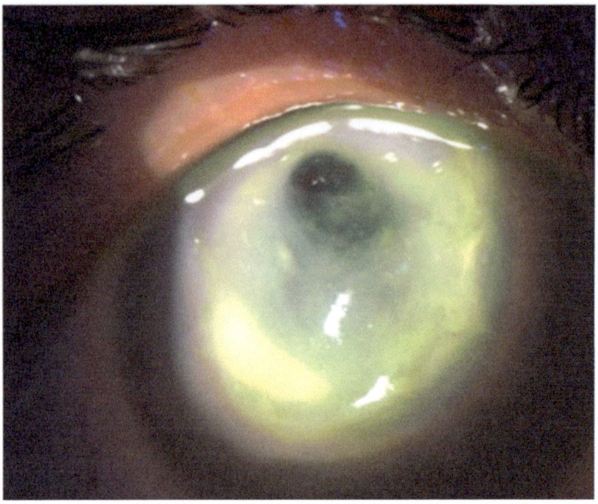

Fig. 14.2 Pseudomonas keratitis with perforation

trauma. The infiltration extends peripherally and deeply within 18–24 h in addition to evenly and concentrically across the entire corneal dimension. A characteristic feature of *Pseudomonas* ulcer is diffuse epithelial graying, which characteristically occurs away from the main site of epithelial and stromal infiltration. A ring ulcer often develops within a duration of 2–3 days in cases which does not receive timely treatment. The progressive untreated ulcer is associated with melting of the cornea and with greenish-yellow mucopurulent discharge, which is adherent to the ulcer. This leads to descemetocele formation and eventual perforation within 2–5 days of onset of infection. (Fig. 14.2).

Early diagnosis and definitive management are the keys to the successful management of pseudomonal keratitis. Sample should be collected by scraping the corneal ulcer, contact lenses, contact lens case and solution. Culture and sensitivity should be performed as standard protocol for the diagnosis of corneal ulcers. Fortified broad-spectrum antibiotics combination therapy should be used till specific culture reports are available. Subsequently, monotherapy or combination therapy with sensitive antibiotics is the mainstay for management.

14.4.3 Fungal Keratitis

In many developing countries like India and Nepal, fungal keratitis is seen frequently among contact lens wearers. Twenty-one percent of patients with fungal keratitis have a history of contact lens wear in these countries compared to 10% in developed countries. Common causes include *Aspergillus, Fusarium* and *Candida* [25, 26]. In 2006, a worldwide outbreak of Fusarium keratitis was seen with the contact lens solution *Renu Moisture Loc* [27]. This product was recalled from the market after the outbreak.

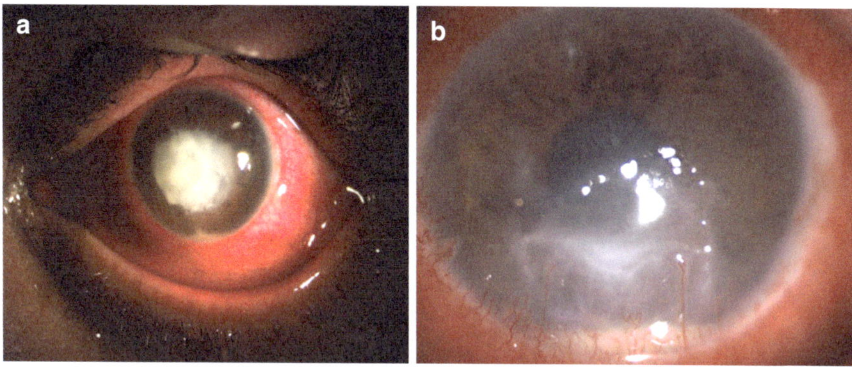

Fig. 14.3 Fungal Keratitis (**a**) central dry ulcer with sloughing (**b**) ulcer with convex hypopyon

The use of contact lenses is a significant risk factor for fungal keratitis. Extended wear hydrogel lenses are most commonly implicated. RGP lenses have shown a lesser incidence of fungal keratitis. It is characterized by grayish white infiltration with dry sloughing ulcers having feathery borders. Satellite lesions and endothelial plaques are not uncommon. A convex, immobile hypopyon is seen in the anterior chamber. (Fig. 14.3) The patient has relatively lesser symptoms, including pain, compared to signs. Rarely, a ring-shaped ulcer may also be seen. Staining and culture on fungal media clinch the diagnosis. Confocal microscopy can identify fungal hyphae and branching patterns. Topical antifungal medications commonly used in fungal keratitis include Natamycin 5%, Fluconazole 0.3%, Voriconazole 1%, and Amphotericin B 0.15–0.30%. The Mycotic Ulcer treatment trial found Natamycin to be more efficacious in the management of filamentous fungi than the azoles. Intrastromal and intracameral targeted therapy in addition to systemic antifungals may be administered in severe grades of corneal ulcer. In non-responding cases or cases with impending perforation, an urgent surgical intervention in the form of therapeutic keratoplasty is required.

14.5 Corneal Edema

It used to be a common feature in contact lens wearers with polymethyl methacrylate (PMMA) use. It is less frequently seen in rigid gas permeable lenses. Slit lamp aided clinical examination by sclerotic scatter, optical section, direct and indirect focal techniques is crucial in the diagnosis and further management. It is manifested by an increase in corneal thickness, as confirmed quantitatively by pachymeter with the variable extent of epithelial edema, increase in stromal thickness, corneal striae and Descemet's folds, polymegathism and decrease in the number of endothelial cells. (Fig. 14.4).

Causative factors comprise hypoxia, lack of adequate tear exchange, and pre-existing epithelial and endothelial pathology. Main symptoms associated with

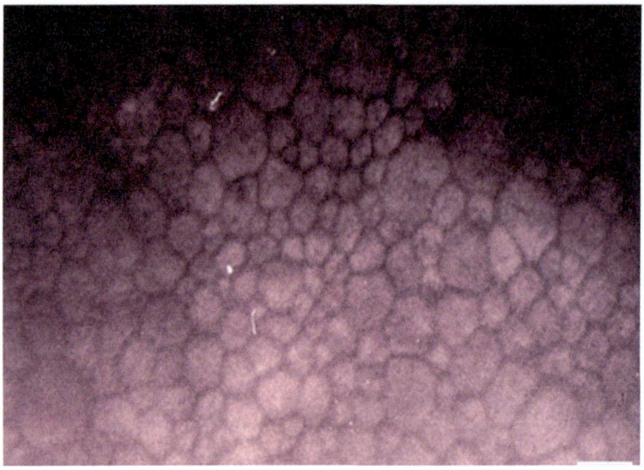

Fig. 14.4 Polymegathism seen on specular microscopy in a contact lens user

corneal edema comprise of pain if the epithelial bullae rupture, glare and drop in visual acuity.

It is prevented by pre-fit assessment of the endothelial function giving a proper fit, choosing highly oxygen permeable lens material and using the lens on daily wear basis rather than extended wear basis.

Occlusive problems can be prevented by

(a) Proper fit-ensuring tear exchange
(b) Choosing proper material with high DK value
(c) Using thinner and smaller lenses
(d) Proper blinking
(e) Avoiding hypoxic environment

Discontinuation of contact lens wear leads to the resolution of corneal edema in most cases.

14.6 Contact Lens-Related Peripheral Ulcer (CLPU)

CLPU is defined as epithelial excavation and infiltration with an intact Bowman's layer as opposed to breach in Bowman's membrane seen in corneal ulcer. It is commonly seen in extended wear lenses. CLPU mainly needs to be differentiated from microbial keratitis. Absence of lid edema focal conjunctival congestion, focal and localized corneal infiltration involving anterior stroma with typically clear cornea around the lesion are the diagnostic determinants in CLPU. The size of the lesion is almost always <2 mm and is located in the periphery or mid periphery.

CLPU presents as mild, localized conjunctival congestion with peripheral corneal infiltrates not extending beyond 1.5 mm from the limbus [28, 29]. They are round to oval in shape and grayish white in color. CLPU may not have epithelial defects, unlike corneal ulcers (Fig. 14.5). The attributable cause has been identified

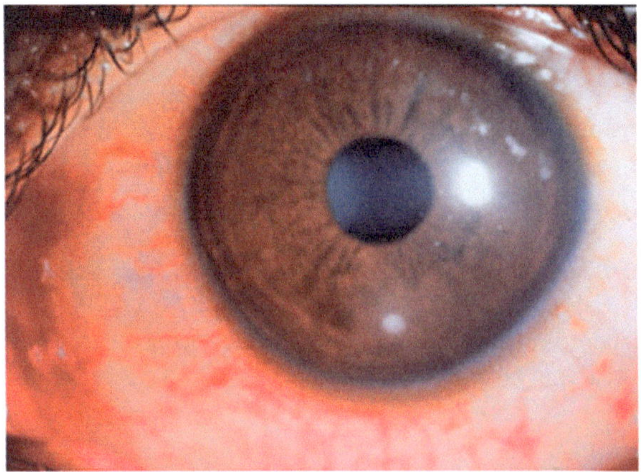

Fig. 14.5 Contact lens-related peripheral ulcer

Table 14.2 Differences between CLPU and Microbial keratitis

Sl. no	Features	CLPU	Microbial keratitis	Sterile corneal infiltrates
1	Pathogenesis	Inflammatory	Infectious	Immunological response
2	Size of lesion	<2 mm	>1 mm	<1 mm
3	Pain/redness/ photophobia	Mild to moderate	More severe	Less pain and photophobia
4	Visual acuity	Not affected	Affected	Not affected
5	Congestion	Superficial	Circumcorneal ciliary	Superficial
6	Location	Periphery	Paracentral or central	Peripheral, circumlimbal
7	Shape	Generally circular	Variable depending on the organism	Round, gray white lesions
8	Epithelium	Generally spared; negative Fluorescein staining	Significant epithelial damage Fluorescein staining of epithelial defect	Minimal epithelial damage
9	Stroma	Anterior stroma involved	Variable depth; can extend to deep stroma, even perforate	Minimal stromal involvement
10	Anterior chamber	Not involved	May have inflammation, hypopyon	Minimal to no anterior chamber reaction

to be the presence of bacteria such as *Staphylococcus aureus,* which release exotoxins. These toxins initiate inflammation which in the presence of corneal abrasions due to microtrauma by contact lenses, may lead to infiltration. CLPU typically regresses after discontinuation of contact lenses. Though sometimes steroid eye drops or NSAIDs eye drops may be required and can be given after ruling out microbial keratitis. (Table 14.2).

14.7 Contact Lens Adhesion Phenomenon or Binding

Contact lens adhesion phenomenon or binding is not uncommon in individuals using rigid extended wear contact lenses. There are few reports of adhesion phenomenon with rigid daily wear contact lenses.

14.7.1 Pathogenesis

There are multiple hypotheses concerning the etiology of RGP lens adherence, including lens suction, negative pressure effects, tear film mucus adhesion, etc. The most acceptable cause which explains the pathogenesis is the suction cup effect of the lens causing ring impression and subsequently leading to adherence to the cornea. The patient is usually unaware of this adhesion.

14.7.2 Clinical Features

Signs of adherence in patients, who are using RGP lenses, are as follows:

- Signs of tear deficiency as determined using sequential fluorescein staining
- Irregular retro lens debris ring, seen in most cases in midperiphery
- A corneal indentation ring adjacent to the edge of the contact lens
- Central corneal staining is often present after lens removal
- Peripheral arcuate staining is often seen outside the zone of adherence

14.7.3 Treatment

Management includes rehydration of eyes before removal of contact lenses, treatment of dry eyes and changes in the base curve of the contact lens.

14.8 Sterile Corneal Infiltrates

Corneal infiltrative events (CIEs) have shown to be of increasing incidence in the recent past among contact lens wearers. Sterile infiltrates are more common than microbial keratitis in contact lens wearers. They may be wary from isolated infiltrates to diffuse lesions with excessive inflammation. (Fig. 14.6) These are more common with extended wear hydrogel lenses. The basic pathophysiology is inflammation-induced accumulation of leukocytes in the corneal stroma. Known risk factors for CIEs include age <25 years, smoking, overnight contact lens wear, bacterial contamination on eyelids, and silicone hydrogel material [30]. Mild cases resolve without any significant effect on visual acuity, however, in severe cases involving deep stroma, they may lead to scarring and impaired visual acuity.

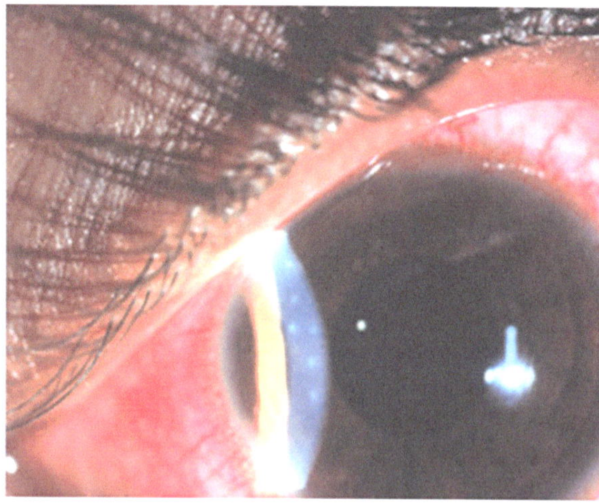

Fig. 14.6 Sterile corneal infiltrates

Sterile infiltrates are usually smaller, multiple, and arcuate shaped. The patient presents without significant pain, epithelial staining, or anterior chamber reaction. The most common symptoms are ocular discomfort, photophobia, and redness of the eyes.

Treatment of sterile corneal infiltrates involves topical corticosteroids in tapering doses along with lubricating eye drops and prophylactic antibiotic coverage.

14.9 Contact Lens-Induced Acute Red Eye-CLARE

Contact lens-induced acute red eye response is generally seen with extended wear lenses. This is clinically seen as severe unilateral congestion along with stromal infiltrates, but no epithelial involvement. CLARE is an inflammatory reaction of the cornea and conjunctiva most commonly attributed to prolonged contact lens wear. A typical patient may have history of sleeping with contact lenses. Pathophysiology of CLARE has been attributed to tight fit, and low oxygen permeability of extended wear contact lenses in addition to continuous wear hydrogel lenses. Deposits of denatured protein, calcium and lipids and mechanical trauma has been implicated in some cases. Additionally, colonization of the lens surface with Gram negative bacteria, like *H. influenza* and *Pseudomonas aeruginosa* have been reported leading to inflammatory response which is triggered by endotoxins released by the breakdown of bacterial cell walls [31–33].

14.9.1 Clinical Features

CLARE is typically characterized by sudden onset of pain in eyes, usually unilateral associated with photophobia, epiphora, and foreign body sensation. Visual acuity is usually unaffected.

Clinical signs include diffuse conjunctival and circumciliary congestion and stromal infiltrates generally seen in periphery and mid periphery. Corneal lesions do not typically stain with Fluorescein, due to the absence of epithelial involvement. Severe untreated cases of CLARE are associated with corneal edema, and anterior uveitis may also be present. Important differentials to be considered while evaluating such patients include sterile corneal infiltrates, CLPU, and microbial keratitis, while fluorescein staining remains the most important diagnostic test to differentiate between them.

14.9.2 Treatment

Treatment of CLARE essentially necessitates discontinuation of contact lens wear as the condition is often self-limiting in addition to ocular surface lubrication to relieve symptoms and promote healing.

Fluorescein staining of the lesion is an important guide to further treatment. If there is corneal staining associated with infiltrate, the diagnosis of microbial keratitis should be considered, and topical antibiotic should be initiated till the lesions heal. In severe cases with anterior uveitis, topical steroids, NSAIDS, and cycloplegic agents are warranted in tapering doses. After complete healing of lesions, lens wear can be resumed with optimal lens fit, material, and replacement schedule to prevent a recurrence. The infiltrates take days to weeks to resolve, depending on severity. However, recurrence of lesions has been reported in 50–70% of patients [34, 35]. Prevention is best achieved by advising the patients to discontinue lenses with symptoms of ocular discomfort and avoidance of prolonged wear or sleeping with worn lenses.

14.10 Corneal Abrasions

Abrasions can occur due to traumatic insertion or removal of lenses and by rubbing the eyes inadvertently during wear. Untreated abrasions can lead to microbial keratitis and, therefore, require prompt treatment in the form of discontinuation of lenses, prophylactic antibiotics and lubricants.

14.11 Conclusion

Contact lenses are associated with a host of complications, some of which are ocular emergencies. Knowledge of risk factors, signs, and symptoms, causative factors, pathogens and treatment regimes is essential for effective management.

It is, therefore, imperative to be aware of these emergencies so that prompt intervention can be initiated by the treating ophthalmologist. Preventive strategies and education regarding precautionary measures are important while managing such cases. Though smaller noninfective lesions are self-limiting and have a good visual prognosis, central, and large lesions should be treated as per the diagnostic scraping for the best chance of successful treatment.

Key Points

- Hypoxia, mechanical factors like stagnation, compartmentalization, reduced cell turnover and infections contribute to the pathogenesis of contact lens-associated corneal emergencies.
- Contact lens wear is the major risk factor for *Acanthamoeba* keratitis and should be suspected in patients with suspected corneal ulcers who are using contact lenses.
- Early diagnosis and definitive management are the keys to successful management of contact lens-associated infective keratitis. Sample should be collected by scraping the corneal ulcer, contact lenses, contact lens case and solution.
- Corneal edema, Contact Lens-Related Peripheral Ulcer (CLPU), Contact Lens Adhesion Phenomenon or Binding, Sterile Corneal Infiltrates, and Contact Lens-Induced Acute Red Eye (CLARE) are entities that presents as a corneal emergency with contact lens wear.
- Preventive strategies and education regarding contact lens wear and precautionary measures are important to prevent sight-threatening corneal emergencies associated with contact lens wear.

References

1. Dart JK, Stapleton F, Minassian D. Contact lenses and other risk factors in microbial keratitis. Lancet. 1991;338:650–3.
2. Poggio EC, Glynn RJ, Schein OD, et al. The incidence of ulcerative keratitis among users of daily - wears and extended - wear soft contact lenses. N Engl J Med. 1989;321:779–83.
3. Schein OD, Buehler PO, Stamler JF, et al. The impact of overnight wear on the risk of contact lens-associated ulcerative keratitis. Arch Ophthalmol. 1994;112:186–90.
4. Bruce AS, Brennan NA. Corneal pathophysiology with contact lens wear. Surv Opthalmol. 1990;35:25–58.
5. Madigan MC, Holden BA, Kwok LS. Extended wear of contact lenses can compromise corneal epithelial adhesion. Curr Eye Res. 1987;6:1257–60.
6. Holden BA, Sweeney DF, Vannas A, Nilsson KT, Efron N. Effects of long-term extended contact lens wear on the human cornea. Invest Opthalmol Vis Sci. 1985;26:1489–501.
7. Mac Rae SM, Matsuda M, Shellans S, Rich LF. The effect of hard and soft contact lenses on the corneal endothelium. Am J Opthalmol. 1986;102:50–7.
8. Aswad MI, John T, Barza M, Kenyon K, Baum J. Bacterial adherence to extended wear soft contact lenses. Ophthalmology. 1990;97:296–302.
9. Costerton JW, Irvin RT, Cheng KJ. The bacterial glycocalyx in nature and disease. Annu Rev Microbiol. 1981;35:299–324.
10. Elder MJ, Stapleton F, Evans E, Dart JK. Biofilm related infections in ophthalmology. Eye. 1995;9:105–9.
11. Sulsher MM, Myrvik QN, Lewis JC, Gristina AG. Extended wear lenses, biofilm and bacterial adhesion. Arch Ophthalmol. 1987;105:110–5.

12. Collinus MJ, Carney LG. Patient compliance and its influence on contact lens wearing problems. Am J Optom Physiol Optic. 1986;63:952–6.
13. Alipour F, Khaheshi S, Soleimanzadeh M, et al. Contact lens-related complications: a review. J Ophthalmic Vis Res. 2017;12:193–204.
14. Chun MW, Weissman BA. Compliance in contact lens care. Am J Optom Physiol Optic. 1987;64:274–6.
15. Donzis PB, Mondino BJ, Weissman BA, Bruckner DA. Microbial contamination of contact lens care systems. Am J Ophthalmol. 1987;104:325–33.
16. Bowden FW, Cohen EJ, Arentsen JJ, Laibson PR. Patterns of lens care practices and lens product contamination in contact lens associated microbial keratitis. CLAO. 1989;15(1):49–54.
17. Clark BJ, Harkins LS, Munro FA, Devonshire P. Microbial contamination of cases used for storing contact lenses. J Infect. 1994;28:293–304.
18. Devonshire P, Munro FA, Abernethy C, Clark BJ. Micorbial contamination of contact lens cases in thewest of Scotland. Br J Opthalmol. 1993;77:41–5.
19. Dart JK, Saw VP, Kilvington S. Acanthamoeba keratitis: diagnosis and treatment update 2009. Am J Ophthalmol. 2009;14:487–99.
20. Radford C, Minassian D, Dart J. Acanthamoeba keratitis in England and Wales: incidence, outcome, and risk factors. Br J Ophthalmol. 2002;86:536–42.
21. Dart J. Contamination of contact lens storage cases. Br J Ophthalmol. 1990;74:129–30.
22. Sweeney DF, Jalbert I, Covey M, Sankaridurg PR, Vajdic C, Holden BA, et al. Clinical characterization of corneal infiltrative events observed with soft contact lens wear. Cornea. 2003;22:435–42.
23. Alarcon I, Tam C, Mun JJ, LeDue J, Evans DJ, Fleiszig SM. Factors impacting corneal epithelial barrier function against Pseudomonas aeruginosa traversal. Invest Ophthalmol Vis Sci. 2011;52:1368–77.
24. Zaidi T, Mowrey-Mckee M, Pier GB. Hypoxia increases corneal cell expression of CFTR leading to increased Pseudomonas aeruginosa binding, internalization, and initiation of inflammation. Invest Ophthalmol Vis Sci. 2004;45:4066–74.
25. Alfonso EC, Cantu-Dibildox J, Munir WM, et al. Insurgence of fusarium keratitis associated with contact lens wear. Arch Ophthalmol. 2006;124:941–7.
26. Bernal MD, Acharya NR, Lietman TM, et al. Outbreak of fusarium keratitis in soft contact lens wearers in San Francisco. Arch Ophthalmol. 2006;124:1051–3.
27. Epstein AB. In the aftermath of the fusarium keratitis outbreak: what have we learned? Clin Ophthalmol. 2007;1(4):355–66.
28. Grant T, Chong MS, Vajdic C, Swarbrick HA, Gauthier C, Sweeney DF, et al. Contact lens induced peripheral ulcers during hydrogel contact lens wear. CLAO J. 1998;24:145–51.
29. Aasuri MK, Venkata N, Kumar VM. Differential diagnosis of microbial keratitis and contact lens-induced peripheral ulcer. Eye Contact Lens. 2003;29:S60–2.
30. Szczotka-Flynn L, Lass JH, Sethi A, Debanne S, Benetz BA, Albright M, Gillespie B, Kuo J, Jacobs MR, Rimm A. Risk factors for corneal infiltrative events during continuous wear of silicone hydrogel contact lenses. Invest Ophthalmol Vis Sci. 2010;51(11):5421–30.
31. Sankaridurg PR, Willcox MD, Sharma S, Gopinathan U, Janakiraman D, Hickson S, Vuppala N, Sweeney DF, Rao GN, Holden BA. Haemophilus influenzae adherent to contact lenses associated with production of acute ocular inflammation. J Clin Microbiol. 1996;34(10):2426–31.
32. Sankaridurg PR, Vuppala N, Sreedharan A, Vadlamudi J, Rao GN. Gram negative bacteria and contact lens induced acute red eye. Indian J Ophthalmol. 1996;44(1):29–32.
33. Holden BA, La Hood D, Grant T, Newton-Howes J, Baleriola-Lucas C, Willcox MD, Sweeney DF. Gram-negative bacteria can induce contact lens related acute red eye (CLARE) responses. CLAO J. 1996;22(1):47–52.
34. Robboy MW, Comstock TL, Kalsow CM. Contact lens-associated corneal infiltrates. Eye Contact Lens. 2003;29(3):146–54.
35. Sweeney DF, Grant T, Chong MS, et al. Recurrence of acute inflammatory conditions with hydrogel extended wear. Invest Opthalmol Vis Sci. 1993;34:S1008.

Peripheral Ulcerative Keratitis

15

Swapnali Sabhapandit, Priyanka Sudana,
and Somasheila I. Murthy

15.1 Introduction

Peripheral ulcerative keratitis (PUK) is an inflammatory disorder characterized by a crescentic epithelial breakdown in the peripheral part of the cornea; along with stromal necrosis, edema and subepithelial infiltrates at the edges. The condition may be unilateral or bilateral [1]. In some eyes, contiguous involvement of conjunctiva, episclera, sclera or uvea may be noted. The age of presentation is reported between 40 and 70 years but can occur in all age group and has a male preponderance [2].

The causes of PUK are multiple and include both ocular and systemic causes. Immune-mediated PUK has an association with collagen vascular disease in about 50% of patients [3]. The ophthalmologist may thereby be the first observer of this ocular manifestation of underlying systemic disease [1, 3]. As the associated systemic disease is severe and, if untreated, has a high rate of morbidity and mortality [4], the onus is on the ophthalmologist to promptly recognize and refer the patient to a physician for detecting and managing the systemic disease.

The estimated incidence of PUK as has been reported, ranges between 3 and 3.5/million/year [5]. Although rare, it is a blinding condition if not treated promptly. The most common disorders associated with PUK are systemic collagen vascular diseases, of which rheumatoid arthritis is the most common, accounting for 34% of noninfectious PUK cases. Approximately 50% of all noninfectious PUK cases have an associated collagen vascular disease [6]. Some cases of PUK show a rapidly

S. Sabhapandit
Department of Ophthalmology, Asian Institute of Gastroenterology, Gachibowli, Hyderabad, Telangana, India

P. Sudana · S. I. Murthy (✉)
Cornea and Anterior Segment Service, The Cornea Institute, L V Prasad Eye Institute, Hyderabad, Telangana, India
e-mail: smurthy@lvpei.org

B. Sharma, J. S. Titiyal (eds.), *Corneal Emergencies*,
https://doi.org/10.1007/978-981-16-5876-1_15

progressive course with early corneal perforation and other complications [6]. Hence emergency surgical treatment along with aggressive systemic therapy as well as looking for the primary systemic disease are needed for salvaging the eye and avoiding systemic morbidity. Timely ocular management can also help avoid chronic sequelae such as posterior or peripheral anterior synechiae, corneal scarring with high astigmatism, glaucoma and the risks associated with large keratoplasty.

In this chapter, the etiopathogenesis, clinical features and management of PUK in an emergency setting will be discussed.

15.2 Clinical Presentation

15.2.1 Symptoms

Patients present with foreign body sensation, pain, redness, and photophobia. The pain can range from chronic, low grade to severe pain if associated with scleritis [3] or if due to infectious causes [7]. Reduced visual acuity ranging from mild to moderate based on the presence of corneal edema and inflammation as well as intraocular inflammation; or due to induced astigmatism caused by peripheral thinning and ulceration is also noted.

15.2.2 Clinical Features

1. Epithelial defect, stromal infiltration and cellularity with thinning in the peripheral cornea (Figure 15.1a).
2. Progression occurring circumferentially, centrally and/or posteriorly (Figure 15.1b).
3. Associated conjunctival and/or episcleral congestion.
4. The interpalpebral peripheral cornea is most often involved first, followed by the inferior and the superior limbus.
5. Advanced stage with total involvement may result in a "contact lens" cornea, where there is a central opaque edematous island of cornea stroma whereas the peripheral 3–4 mm of the cornea would show healing with pannus and

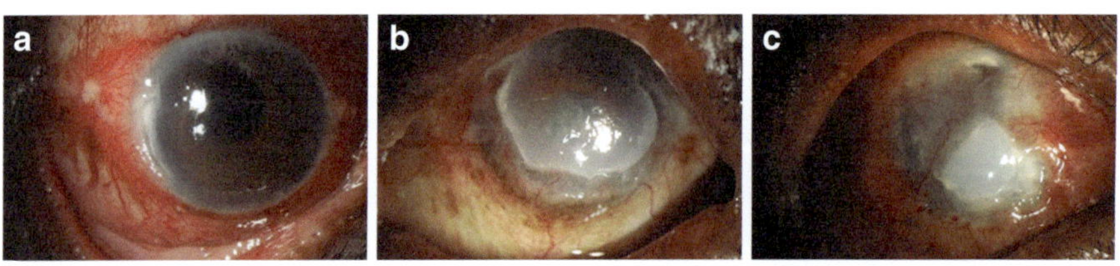

Fig. 15.1 (**a–c**): Peripheral ulcerative keratitis (PUK) at different stages: (**a**) starting with an epithelial defect, stromal ulceration and peripheral corneal thinning; (**b**) circumferential and central spread; (**c**) total corneal involvement with vascularization and scarring

vascularization (Figure 15.1c). End-stage disease is characterized by grossly thinned, scarred, and vascularized tissue [1].

15.3 Etiology and Pathogenesis

15.3.1 Etiology

There are several causes of PUK: both immune-mediated and infectious (both ocular and systemic). In addition, several conditions may present with a PUK-like picture that need to be distinguished. Table 15.1 enumerates the etiologies of PUK.

Table 15.1 Etiological causes in peripheral ulcerative keratitis

Etiology	
Immune-mediated: Ocular	Mooren's ulcer
Immune-mediated: Systemic Collagen vascular diseases:	a. Rheumatoid arthritis b. Granulomatosis polyangiitis c. Relapsing polychondritis d. Systemic lupus erythematosus e. Polyarteritis nodosa f. Behçet's disease g. Sarcoidosis h. Inflammatory bowel disease
Other systemic conditions	a. Acne rosacea b. Dry eye disorders: Sjogrens disease, Stevens-Johnson syndrome, Ocular Cicatricial Pemphigoid (OCP)
Infections: Ocular	a. Bacterial (*Staphylococcus, Streptococcus, Gonococcus, Moraxella, Hemophilus, Pesudomonas*sp) b. Viral (Herpes simplex, Herpes zoster) c. Amoebic (Acanthamoeba) d. Fungus
Infectious: Systemic	a. Tuberculosis b. Syphilis c. Acquired immunodeficiency syndrome (AIDS) d. Helminthiasis e. Varicella zoster f. Hepatitis
Conditions mimicking PUK:	a. Traumatic: chemical, thermal, radiation burn b. Abnormalities of eyelids or lashes: entropion, ectropion, cicatricial, exposure, trichiasis, lagophthalmos, incomplete blink c. Allograft reaction d. Neurologic:neurotrophic keratitis e. Contact lens-related infiltrative keratitis f. Marginal keratitis g. Ectatic conditions: Keratoglobus Terrien's marginal degeneration h. Malignancy: ocular surface squamous neoplasia (OSSN)

15.3.1.1 Mooren's Ulcer

The most common presentation of PUK is Mooren's ulcer. This is an idiopathic chronic serpiginous ulcer of the cornea, characterized by crescent-shaped peripheral corneal ulceration with what is classically described as overhanging (undermined) margins and cellular infiltration at the advancing edges. The other features include circumferential spread, no scleral involvement and absence of associated systemic disease [2].

15.3.1.2 Collagen Vascular Diseases

The second most common cause of immune-mediated PUK includes systemic collagen vascular diseases. For PUK associated with systemic collagen vascular disease, the patient may already have a known systemic disorder or may present for the first time to the ophthalmologist with undiagnosed systemic disease. Appropriate laboratory testing is necessary, based on history and physical examination. Rheumatoid arthritis (RA) is the most common systemic disease associated with PUK with an incidence of 30–42% [8]. It tends to occur late in the disease process and may indicate worsening of the disease. On the other hand, PUK in the setting of granulomatosis polyangiitis (GPA) (formerly known as Wegener's granulomatosis) can be an early phenomenon [9].

15.3.1.3 Infectious Causes

Infection is an important cause of peripheral corneal inflammation and has to be excluded by microbiological evaluation of corneal scraping sample [6]. The presence of severe symptomatology, with lid edema, purulent discharge, severely congested conjunctiva, rapid worsening, presence of dense infiltrate at the ulcer bed and presence of hypopyon should raise the suspicion of microbial infection.

15.3.2 Pathogenesis

PUK occurs due to an interplay of various factors:

15.3.2.1 Immune Complexes

The capillary vascular arcades and subconjunctival lymphatic network of the limbal area introduce antigens into the peripheral cornea for antigen-antibody reactions [1, 3, 8]. The classical pathway of complement cascade is triggered, leading to neutrophils and macrophages entry into the stroma, increased phagocytosis, the release of cytokines and proteolytic enzymes [3, 8]. All these factors cause corneal collagen loss and resultant stromal ulceration. A 66 K-Dalton protein autoantigen called cytokeratin-3 present in corneal epitheliumis over-expressed in GPA and RA. It can contribute to increased immune complex formation in the peripheral cornea [10].

15.3.2.2 Matrix Metalloproteinases (MMP)

These enzymes are released by conjunctival goblet cells, corneal keratocytes and lymphatics via activation of tumor necrosis factor-alpha (TNF-α) in the complement cascade [10]. MMPs digest the extracellular matrix of the peripheral cornea leading to stromal melt. MMPs are also released from tears [11].

15.4 Management

Depending on the severity at presentation and the etiology, the cases are managed medically or surgically.

15.4.1 Medical Management

Based on the cause of the PUK, various ocular and systemic investigations are indicated to rule out infectious pathology or immune-mediated disease. Table 15.2 lists the investigations in cases of PUK.

15.4.1.1 Infectious Causes

For cases that appear to be infiltrated, corneal scrapings are taken and subjected to microbiology. The therapy is started based on reports of the corneal smears. For Gram-positive organisms, 5% topical fortified cefazolin sodium is commenced every hour, and for Gram negatives, 0.3% ciprofloxacin hydrochloride or 0.3% tobramycin eye drops are used. If the smears are negative, empirical board spectrum antibiotics are used. In case of detection of fungal filaments, topical natamycin 5% is started every hour, and in the case of viral keratitis, antiviral eye ointment (3% acyclovir ointment five times a day) is started. Systemic antimicrobials (ciprofloxacin 500 mg twice a day, voriconazole tablets 200 mg twice a day and acyclovir tablets 400 mg five times a day) are prescribed as needed. Topical lubricating drops or gels promote re-epithelialization. Homatropine bromide 2% or Atropine sulfate

Table 15.2 Investigations in a case of peripheral ulcerative keratitis

Etiology	Investigations
Infectious	a. Microbiology: Smear—Gram's stain and potassium hydroxide (KOH) wet mount. Culture—Blood agar, Chocolate agar, Sabouraud dextrose agar, brain heart infusion broth, non-nutrient agar overlaid with Escherichia coli b. Polymerase chain reaction (PCR) for Herpes simplex virus antigen detection c. Tuberculin test with purified protein derivative, chest radiograph/ high-resolution CT to rule out tuberculosis in clinically suspected cases d. Hepatitis C detection, stool examination for helminthiasis
Noninfectious	a. Complete blood count (CBC) b. Rheumatoid factor c. Anti-cyclic citrullinated peptides (anti-CCP) d. Anti-Neutrophil Cytoplasmic Antigen (c and p) e. Erythrocyte sedimentation rate, C-reactive protein f. Anti-nuclear antibody

1% three times a day is started for cycloplegia and in cases of severe anterior uveitis and hypopyon.

15.4.1.2 Mooren's Ulcer

In Mooren's ulcer, a stepladder approach to treatment is followed to control inflammation, prevent tissue destruction and promote epithelialization [12], as noted in Table 15.3.

15.4.1.3 With Associated Systemic Disease

Peripheral ulcerative keratitis with the associated systemic disease can be life-threatening and often requires serological investigations for establishing the systemic association and may require prolonged immunosuppression. Such cases are better co-managed with the rheumatologist for systemic immunomodulation.

In RA with PUK, apart from oral corticosteroids, oral methotrexate (MTX) is used as a steroid-sparing agent and also for long-term control. Other immunomodulators which can be used are azathioprine (2 mg/kg/day), cyclophosphamide (2 mg/

Table 15.3 Step ladder therapy for Mooren's ulcer

Level	Drug	Indication
Level 1	Topical corticosteroids (Prednisolone acetate 1%)	Unilateral cases Less than two quadrants of peripheral corneal involvement Less than 50% stromal loss
Level 2	Topical corticosteroids + oral corticosteroids (1–1.5 mg/kg—Prednisolone)	Bilateral cases More than two quadrants of peripheral corneal involvement More than 50% stromal loss
Level 3	Oral methotrexate (7.5–25 mg/week) or azathioprine (2 mg/kg/day), mycophenolate mofetil (1 g twice daily), cyclosporine (2.5–5 mg/kg/day) or other immune-modulator used as steroid-sparing agent	Steroid intolerance/contraindication Young patients <40 years Requirement of long-term steroids, as steroid-sparing agents Requirement of additional immunomodulatory therapy Failure of level 2 therapy
Level 4	Intravenous (IV) methylprednisolone (single pulse 1 g)	Bilateral, single eyed More than three quadrants corneal involvement, >50% stromal loss, impending perforation Rapid progression and extensive damage
Level 5	IV methylprednisolone +IV cyclophosphamide (1 g pulse dose)	Bilateral, single eyed More than three quadrants corneal involvement, >50% stromal loss, impending perforation Perioperative for Keratoplasty
Level 6	Biologicals: adalimumab infusions, Rituximab infusion	Bilateral, single eyed More than three quadrants corneal involvement, >50% stromal loss, impending perforation, relentless progression, refractory to cyclophosphamide (CYP) or inability to induce remission with CYP

kg/day), mycophenolate mofetil (1 g twice daily), cyclosporine (2.5–5 mg/kg/day) and adalimumab (40 mg subcutaneously every other week). Disease-modifying antirheumatic drugs (DMARDs) such as sulfasalazine inhibit TNF-α and interleukins and reduce the production of matrix metalloproteinases, which would halt the progression of corneal stromal lysis in the treatment of PUK with systemic associations [13]. Because of the potential side effects of these treatments, regular laboratory investigations at periodic intervals including complete blood count, liver function test and renal function test is essential to monitor for side effects.

15.4.2 Surgical Management

15.4.2.1 Conjunctival Resection with Tissue Adhesive and Bandage Contact Lens Application

This time-tested technique is presumed to act by decreasing the influx of inflammatorycells, collagenases and proteinases and promotes resolution. The surgical technique involves gentle resection of the conjunctiva by performing a peritomy at least two clock hours on either side of the affected peripheral ulcer, and dissecting the conjunctiva from the limbus up to the bare sclera in a strip of about 3–4 mm. The bleeders are gently cauterized with sparing use of the cautery. The overhanging lip of the edematous, infiltrated cornea centrally is excised with the help of a Vanna's scissors. The base of the ulcer is debrided. Cyanoacrylate glue is applied to the peripheral ulcer with the help of a needle in one or two layers to form a thin layer (Figure 15.2a). Excess glue is trimmed, and a 14 mm bandage contact lens is placed. While the goal of surgical tectonic procedures in PUK is mainly to maintain the integrity of the globe, cyanoacrylate glue also acts as a limbal barrier to conjunctival derived inflammatory cytokines, thus helping in controlling the inflammation.

15.4.2.2 Management of Perforations <2 mm

Amniotic membrane graft (AMG) and tissue adhesives are indicated in the management of impending perforation and in perforations <2.0 mm.

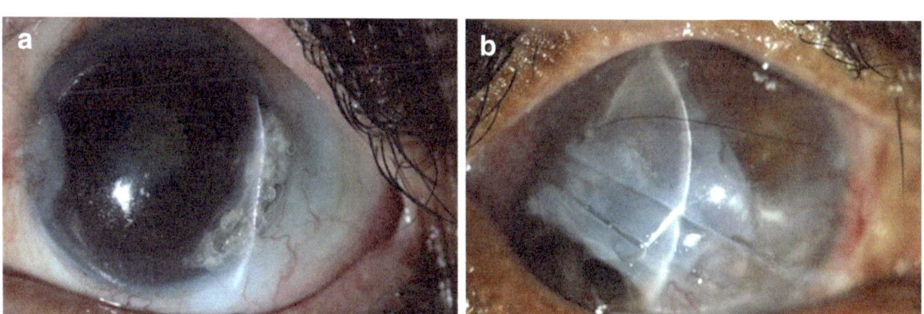

Fig. 15.2 (**a**) Conjunctival resection with cyanoacrylate glue and bandage contact lens application in a Mooren's ulcer (post-operative 1 month). (**b**) Multi-layered amniotic membrane graft in a case of large corneal perforation in recurrent peripheral ulcerative keratitis, involving the center

AMG helps in early epithelialization and nerve proliferation. It also suppresses cytokine expression in inflamed tissue and leads to apoptosis of inflammatory cells. [14, 15] However, the role of AMG in the healing cases of Mooren's ulcer is controversial [16, 17]. Multi-layered or rolled-up AMG can be used to seal <2 mm size corneal perforations and intensive follow-up and adjuvant therapy is necessary [16, 18].

15.4.2.3 Large Perforations

Several surgical techniques can be effectively employed to tackle corneal perforations larger than 2 mm.

Multi-Layered AMG

Multi-layered AMG (for perforations larger than 2 mm): the outcome of AMG in large perforations may not be satisfactory as the tectonic stability is not achieved [18]. It can be used as a temporary measure till a corneal graft is planned (Figure 15.2a).

Tenon's Patch Graft

Tenon's patch graft is commonly used in glaucoma surgery to seal leaking blebs or valves [19]. For PUK with 6 mm size perforation or less, tenon's capsule can be excised posterior to its limbal insertion in the inferonasal and inferotemporal quadrants. The size of the graft is taken slightly larger than the size of the corneal defect. The tenon's capsule is then firmly attached as a thin layer over the perforated area and adjoining de-epithelialized margin using tissue adhesive or sutures [20]. Advantages of this technique include the absence of graft rejection as it is an autologous tissue, and less antigenic surface for future corneal transplants. Tenon's tissue is easy to acquire as opposed to amniotic membrane or corneal tissue.

Patch Graft

This surgical modality includes smaller-sized grafts for lamellar or full-thickness keratoplasty, usually <6 mm in size, or free-hand, such as annual or banana-shaped grafts. Patch grafts an also be used as a temporizing method in perforated PUK till a penetrating keratoplasty (PK) could be planned. Various materials such as periosteum, donor cornea stromal cap which is not used during descemet stripping endothelial keratoplasty, unused sclerocorneal rims donor tissue used for penetrating keratoplasty or scleral tissue, glycerol preserved nonantigenic donor cornea, and even the lenticule obtained from small incision refractive lenticule extraction (SMILE) procedure have been used as patch graft [21–24]. Crescentic corneal or corneal scleral patch grafts are used in RA with melt (Figure 15.3a, b) and in advanced Mooren's ulcer to stabilize the condition with varying success. There are increased risks of graft opacification, graft melt, vascularization, persistent epithelial defects and the eventual need for PK in most cases [25]. The use of long-term immunosuppression can increase the success rate of these patch grafts.

Keratoplasty

Keratoplasty performed for PUK has the highest likelihood of failure and need for regraft [7]. Lamellar keratoplasty is done for large PUK without perforation with

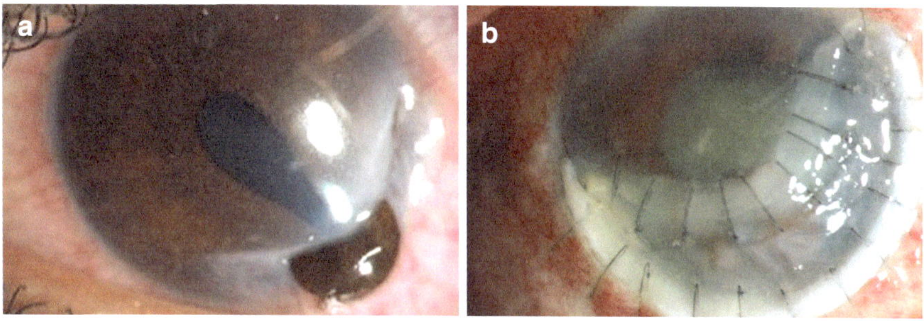

Fig. 15.3 Complication of peripheral ulcerative keratitis in a case of rheumatoid arthritis; (**a**) peripheral corneal perforation with surrounding stromal melt; (**b**) crescentic patch graft from donor sclerocorneal tissue is performed

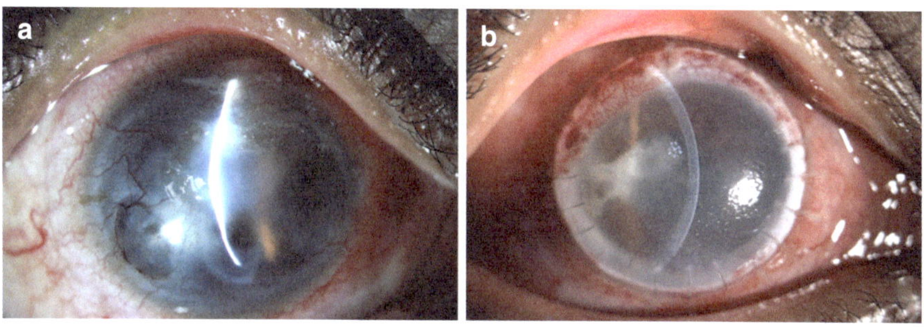

Fig. 15.4 Advanced Mooren's ulcer with peripheral sealed corneal perforation and island of stromal corneal tissue (**a**); stable disease and cataract on systemic immunosuppression (**b**); penetrating keratoplasty with cataract extraction done with immunosuppression continued after surgery

post-operative adequate immunosuppression [25]. Use of glycerol preserved donor cornea has been reported to have good outcome due to the absence of keratocytes, dendritic cells and other antigenic cells in the preserved tissue [26, 27]. PK is performed for extreme thinning for large perforations in PUK, mainly for tectonic stability [28–30]. It is important to control the inflammation by aggressive immunosuppression first before proceeding with PK. The use of perioperative intravenous methylprednisolone, or oral prednisolone has been advocated. Despite this, the survival and visual outcomes for emergency PK are not satisfactory in such an indication, with high changes of graft failure. (Figure 15.4a–c).

15.5 Differential Diagnosis

PUK can be confused with other clinical entities involving the peripheral cornea. However, there are relevant points that can differentiate among these pathological conditions [31]. Table 15.4 lists the differential diagnosis of various entities mimicking PUK. Figure 15.5 depicts a flow chart on the differential diagnosis and management in PUK.

Table 15.4 Differential diagnosis in peripheral ulcerative keratitis

	PUK	Terrien's marginal degeneration	Marginal keratitis	Pellucid marginal degeneration
Etiology	Autoimmunity to cornea antigens	Peripheral cornea degeneration	Hypersensitivity reaction against staphylococcal exotoxins	Ectatic cornea disorder
Laterality	Usually unilateral	Usually bilateral asymmetrical presentation	Usually bilateral	Usually bilateral
Clinical picture	Progressive painful stromal ulceration	Painless, intact epithelium, non-inflammatory stromal opacities due to lipid infiltrates	Lucid interval from limbus, epithelial defect less than the cornea infiltrate, coexisting chronic blepharitis	Noninflammatory, painless
Location	Interpalpebral cornea, later 360 degrees extension	Superior cornea/ inferior cornea (less common)	2, 4, 8, 10 clock hours	Inferior cornea

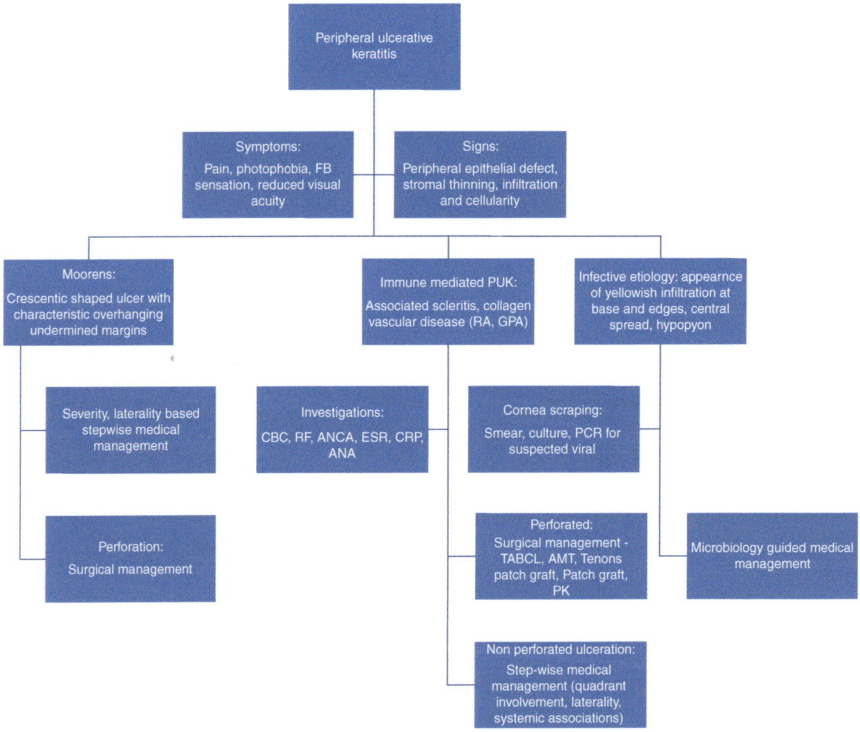

Fig. 15.5 Flow chart on differential diagnosis and management of cases of peripheral ulcerative keratitis presenting to the emergency clinic

15.6 Conclusion

PUK is a clinical diagnosis of corneal infectious and inflammatory diseases resulting in peripheral corneal ulceration and thinning. Inflammatory causes are usually autoimmune systemic diseases. The mainstay of treatment is to control inflammation with corticosteroids and immunosuppressive therapy to prevent progressive vision loss. Surgical management is for tectonic stability.

Key Points

- PUK is a rare entity, with potentially serious consequences for vision if left untreated.
- Immune-mediated conditions include Mooren's ulcer and systemic diseases such as RA and GPA, which have the highest association with PUK.
- The presentation could be the first sign of such a systemic disease and needs thorough investigations.
- Infectious keratitis, such as bacterial, fungal, and viral, can also present as PUK and need to be promptly identified.
- Medical management, after evaluating the cause, involves the use of topical and oral corticosteroids for immune-mediated conditions.
- Surgical management includes conjunctival resection and tissue adhesive application for smaller perforations and patch grafts with amniotic membrane, tenons, or corneal tissue for larger perforations.

Funding Support For Priyanka Sudana and Somasheila I Murthy from Hyderabad Eye Research Foundation.

References

1. Bartly J, Mondino BJ. Inflammatory diseases of the peripheral cornea. Ophthalmology. 1988;95:463–72.
2. Srinivasan M, Zegans ME, Zelefsky JR, Kundu A, Lietman T, Whitcher JP, Cunningham ET Jr. Clinical characteristics of Mooren's ulcer in South India. Br J Ophthalmol. 2007;91(5):570–5.
3. Tauber J, Sainz de la Maza M, Hoang-Xuan T, Foster CS. An analysis of therapeutic decision making regarding immunosuppressive chemotherapy for peripheral ulcerative keratitis. Cornea. 1990;9:66–73.
4. Foster CS, Forstot SL, Wilson LA. Mortality rate in rheumatoid arthritis patients developing necrotizing scleritis or peripheral ulcerative keratitis: effects of systemic immunosuppression. Ophthalmology. 1984;91:1253–63.
5. McKibbin M, Isaacs JD, Morrell AJ. Incidence of corneal melting in association with systemic disease in the Yorkshire region, 1995–7. Br J Ophthalmol. 1999;83:941–3.
6. Ladas JG, Mondino BJ. Systemic disorders associated with peripheral corneal ulceration. Curr Opin Ophthalmol. 2000;11:468–71.
7. Yagci A. Update on peripheral ulcerative keratitis. Clin Ophthalmol. 2012;6:747–54.
8. Shiuey Y, Foster CS. Peripheral ulcerative keratitis and collagen vascular disease. Int Ophthalmol Clin. 1998;38:21–32.

9. Bullen CL, Liesegang TJ, McDonald TJ, DeRemee RA. Ocular complications of Wegener's granulomatosis. Ophthalmology. 1983;90:279–90.
10. Reynolds I, Tullo AB, John SL, et al. Corneal epithelial-specific cytokeratin 3 is an autoantigen in Wegener's granulomatosis-associated peripheral ulcerative keratitis. Invest Ophthalmol Vis Sci. 1999;40:2147–51.
11. Smith VA, Hoh HB, Easty DL. Role of ocular metalloproteinases in peripheral ulcerative keratitis. Br J Ophthalmol. 1999;83:1376–83.
12. Ashar JN, Mathur A, Sangwan VS. Immunosuppression for Mooren's ulcer: evaluation of the stepladder approach--topical, oral and intravenous immunosuppressive agents. Br J Ophthalmol. 2013;97(11):1391–4.
13. Cao Y, Zhang W, Wu J, Zhang H, Zhou H. Peripheral ulcerative keratitis associated with autoimmune disease: pathogenesis and treatment. J Ophthalmol. 2017;2017:7298026.
14. Solomon A, Rosenblatt M, Monroy D, et al. Suppression of interleukin 1 and interleukin 1 in human limbal epithelial cells cultured on the amniotic membrane stromal matrix. Br J Ophthalmol. 2001;85:444–9.
15. Touhami A, Grueterich M, Tseng SCG. The role of NGF signaling in human limbal epithelium expanded by amniotic membrane culture. Invest Ophthalmol Vis Sci. 2002;43:987–94.
16. Ngan ND, Chau HT. Amniotic membrane transplantation for Mooren's ulcer. Clin Exp Ophthalmol. 2011;13(5):386–92.
17. Schallenberg M, Westekemper H, Steuhl KP, Meller D. Amniotic membrane transplantation ineffective as additional therapy in patients with aggressive Mooren's ulcer. BMC Ophthalmol. 2013;13:81.
18. Liu J, Li L, Li X. Effectiveness of cryopreserved amniotic membrane transplantation in corneal ulceration: a meta-analysis. Cornea. 2019;38(4):454–62.
19. Morris DA, Ramocki JM, Shin DH, Glover BK, Kim YY. Use of autologous Tenon's capsule and scleral patch grafts for repair of excessively draining fistulas with leaking filtering blebs. J Glaucoma. 1998;7:417–9.
20. Korah S, Selvin SS, Pradhan ZS, Jacob P, Kuriakose T. Tenons patch graft in the management of large corneal perforations. Cornea. 2016;35:696–9.
21. Portnoy SL, Insler MS, Kaufman HE. Surgical management of corneal ulceration and perforation. Surv Ophthalmol. 1989;34(1):47–58.
22. Kaz Soong H, Farjo AA, Katz D. Lamellar corneal patch grafts in the management of corneal melting. Cornea. 2000;19(2):126–34.
23. Lin H-C, Lee Y-S, Chia J-H. Management of rheumatoid arthritis-related peripheral ulcerative keratitis using glycerol-preserved corneas. Asia-Pac J Ophthalmol. 2013;2:291–4.
24. Yang J, Li Y, Liu X-W. A novel tectonic keratoplasty with femtosecond laser intrastromal lenticule for corneal ulcer and perforation. Chin Med J. 2016;129:1817–21.
25. Liu J, Shi W, Li S. Modified lamellar keratoplasty and immunosuppressive therapy guided by in vivo confocal microscopy for perforated Mooren's ulcer. Br J Ophthalmol. 2015;99:778–83.
26. Li J, Yu L, Deng Z, et al. Deep anterior lamellar keratoplasty using acellular corneal tissue for prevention of allograft rejection in high-risk corneas. Am J Ophthalmol. 2011;152(5):762–770.e3.
27. Gao H, Wang X, Echegaray JJ, et al. Partial lamellar keratoplasty for peripheral corneal disease using a graft from the glycerin-preserved corneoscleral rim. Graefes Arch Clin Exp Ophthalmol. 2014;252:963–8.
28. Alhassan MB, Rabiu M, Agbabiaka IO. Interventions for Mooren's ulcer. Cochrane Database Syst Rev. 2014;(1):CD006131.
29. Palay DA, Stulting RD, Waring GO, et al. Penetrating keratoplasty in patients with rheumatoid arthritis. Ophthalmology. 1992;99(4):622–7.
30. Tobias R, Berthold S, Achim L, et al. Visual acuity and astigmatism after eccentric penetrating keratoplasty - a retrospective study on 117 patients. Klin Monatsbl Augenheilkd. 2002;219:40–5.
31. Lohchab M, Prakash G, Arora T, Maharana P, Jhanji V, Sharma N, Vajpayee RB. Surgical management of peripheral corneal thinning disorders. Surv Ophthalmol. 2019;64(1):67–78.

16 Emergencies Associated with Advanced Corneal Ectasias

Ritu Arora and Nikhil Gotmare

16.1 Introduction

Corneal ectasia is a term to describe a group of disorders characterized by progressive thinning, bulging, and distortion of the cornea. Keratoconus, Pellucid marginal degeneration (PMD), Terrien's marginal degeneration (TMD), keratoglobus, and ectasias occurring after corneal refractive surgery (Photorefractive keratectomy, Radial Keratotomy and LASIK) or Penetrating keratoplasty (PKP) are the most prevalent corneal ectatic disorders seen in clinical practice (PKP) [1].

In the instance of keratoconus, the term advanced corneal ectasia (ACE) is clearly defined, but there are no defining criteria for other conditions like PMD or TMD. According to the classification proposed by Krumeich et al., an eye with advanced keratoconus has a keratometry reading (K) of >55.00 D, unmeasurable refraction, central corneal scarring, and corneal thickness <200 μm at the thinnest point [2].

For other disorders, advanced ectasia might be defined as the stage at which standard interventions are no longer sufficient to treat the underlying problem [3]. Acute corneal hydrops and corneal perforations are two ACE-related emergencies.

16.2 Acute Corneal Hydrops

16.2.1 Introduction

Acute hydrops occurs when Descemet's membrane is stretched beyond its elastic breaking point. Due to aqueous leakage into the corneal stroma and epithelium,

R. Arora (✉) · N. Gotmare
Guru Nanak Eye Center, Maulana Azad Medical College, New Delhi, India

B. Sharma, J. S. Titiyal (eds.), *Corneal Emergencies*,
https://doi.org/10.1007/978-981-16-5876-1_16

such a rupture causes abrupt, severe corneal edema. Although it was first identified in keratoconus [4], it has now been seen in various other corneal ectasias such PMD [5], keratoglobus [6], and TMD [7]. It is also seen in keratectasia after surgeries, such as laser-assisted in situ keratomileusis [8], radial keratotomy [9], deep anterior lamellar keratoplasty (DALK) [10], and penetrating keratoplasty [11, 12]. There have been cases of corneal hydrops following keratoplasty done for Keratoconus, usually after 15–20 years.

Corneal hydrops (CH) occur in approximately 2.5–3% of eyes with KC [4, 13, 14]. The majority of cases are seen in the second or third decade. There is a male gender preponderance, however, bilateral cases are infrequent [4, 13, 14]. No racial predisposition has been reported so far [4, 13, 14].

16.2.2 Predisposing Factors

Early onset, eye rubbing, vernal keratoconjunctivitis (VKC), atopy, and Down's syndrome are several of the risk factors linked to an increased risk of CH [14–16]. Eye rubbing appears to be the most significant risk factor, with the trauma associated with intense eye rubbing possibly serving as an inciting factor [14].

16.2.3 Pathogenesis

Acute hydrops develop with the tear and subsequent breach of DM, causing the margins to roll, thus allowing aqueous from the anterior chamber to seep into the corneal stroma. The build-up of aqueous causes the collagen lamellae to separate and the creation of large fluid-filled stromal pockets [4, 17]. Meanwhile, as a part of the reparative process, the adjacent endothelium grows over the defect, causing a partial seal so that the seepage is prevented with subsequent resolution of stromal edema. According to various studies, the resolution of corneal edema may occur any time between 5 and 36 weeks [4, 13, 14].

16.2.4 Clinical Characteristics

Acute hydrops is characterized by significantly diminished visual acuity, severe photophobia, and pain [4]. A visible "white spot" over the cornea may also be noticed by the patient. A history of forceful eye rubbing or coughing is frequently present [4, 13–15].

Slit-lamp examination reveals stromal and epithelial microcystic edema, intrastromal cysts/clefts, and conjunctival hyperemia in most cases (Fig. 16.1a, b).

Corneal edema can be graded according to its extent;

Grade I = within a circle of 3-mm diameter.

Grade II = within a circle of 3–5-mm diameter.

Grade III = larger than circle of 5 mm in diameter [4, 18].

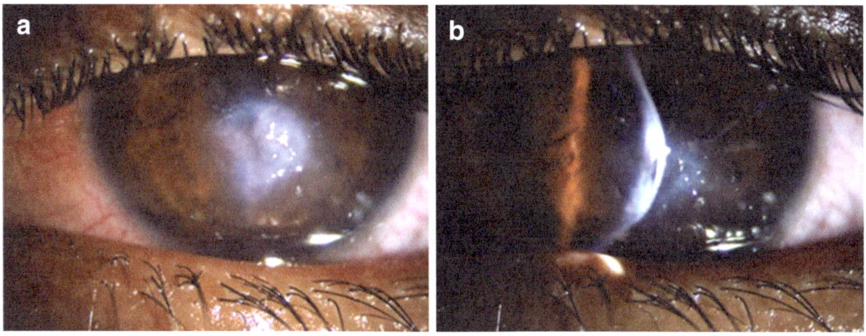

Fig. 16.1 Slit-lamp examination in a case of hydrops showing (**a**). Stromal edema (**b**). Rupture in Descemet's membrane and cleft

Time for resolution of edema and subsequent final BCVA achieved are inversely related to the area of involvement [4, 14, 18, 19]. Not uncommonly diagnosis of corneal opacity is made.

16.2.5 Investigations

The diagnosis is usually based on the patient's medical history and the results of slit-lamp examination. Investigations are required to assess the size and extent of edema and DM tear, which aids in the formulation of a treatment strategy, the monitoring of treatment response, and the identification of any complications. Ultrasound biomicroscopy (UBM) and anterior segment optical coherence tomography (ASOCT) are the two investigative techniques [4, 17, 20] (Fig. 16.2a, b).

16.2.6 Management

Acute CH can be treated conservatively or surgically, with the latter usually involving intracameral injection of air or gas [4, 19]. PKP compressive sutures with gas injection [21], cyanoacrylate tissue adhesive with BCL [22], and amniotic membrane transplantation (AMT) with cauterization are other surgical modalities that are useful in special circumstances [23].

A standard of care for the management of corneal hydrops, employing either topical ophthalmic medications or surgical intervention in the form of an intraocular injection, has yet to be established. A logical approach to treatment is to reduce the patient's symptoms and expedite corneal healing.

16.2.6.1 Conservative Approach

The goal of medical treatment is to provide symptomatic relief until the condition improves on its own. It includes topical lubricants, antibiotics (prevent secondary infection), cycloplegics (to reduce pain and photophobia), hypertonic saline eye

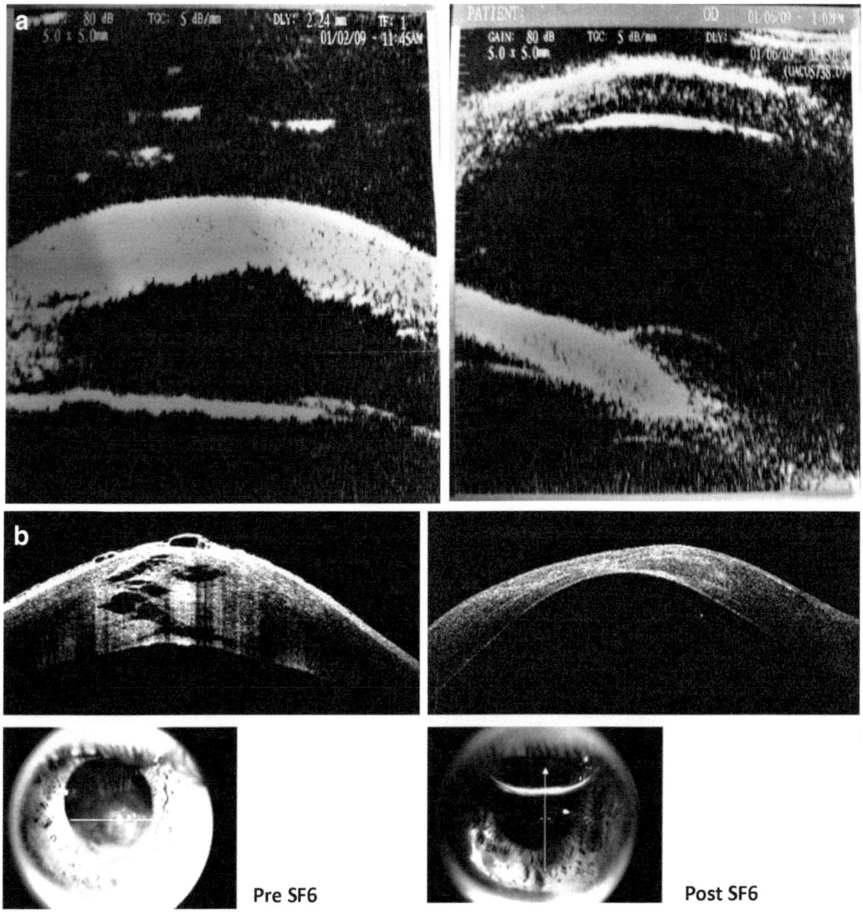

Fig. 16.2 (**a**) Ultrasound biomicroscopy in a case with hydrops at presentation and after SF6 injection. (**b**) ASOCT of the same patient as in Fig. 16.1, a. pre SF6 injection (Marked thickening of the cornea with multiple empty spaces as fluid clefts) b. post-SF 6 injection (Restoration to normal corneal thickness and disappearance of clefts)

drops (help draw fluid), anti-glaucoma medications (topical 0.5% Timolol maleate) (to lessen the hydrodynamic force on the posterior cornea), and topical steroids or nonsteroidal anti-inflammatory drugs (NSAIDs) [4, 13–15, 19]. Patching may be resorted to in cases with extremely thin corneas. The final best-corrected visual acuity (BCVA) is found to be comparable to surgery. A BCL may be used to provide pain relief till the edema resolves, or the patient becomes comfortable [4, 13–15, 19].

16.2.6.2 Intracameral Air/Gas Injection

Intracameral air/gas injection shortens the period of persistence of corneal edema in CH. Various agents used include air [24], 20% sulfur hexafluoride (SF6) [25], 14% perfluoropropane (C3F8) [13]. These agents have a tamponade action, which inhibits aqueous from penetrating the stroma, as well as unrolling the ruptured DM's torn ends [4, 13, 19].

Because air lasts for a shorter period of time, repeat injections may be necessary [4]. SF6, on the other hand, has a longer half-life than air (about 2 weeks), so repeat injections may be necessary [4]. C3F8 is the most long-acting of the three, and a single injection is generally sufficient [4, 13]. However, because the gas persists in the anterior chamber for a longer period, there is a chance of development of secondary glaucoma, which may lead to permanent blindness. Furthermore, the gas is toxic to the endothelium, which could lead to corneal decompensation and future corneal opacities. However, the use of a non-expansile concentration of perfluoropropane gas for successful reattachment of Descemet's membrane tear after complicated cataract surgery has been described as a safe and effective method [13]. The absorption of SF6 injection from the anterior chamber takes 2 weeks. The corneal endothelium remains unaffected. Nonetheless, it is regarded safer than C3F8 because it expands twofold in 24–48 h [25].

There are different techniques for injecting air or gas.

Procedure

Preoperative pupillary constriction by topical application of 2% pilocarpine nitrate eye drops at 15–20 min intervals 1 h before surgery to avoid intraoperative injury to the lens; anterior chamber (AC) paracentesis under aseptic conditions with a 26/27 gage needle or alternately a limbal paracentesis; aspiration of 0.1 mL of aqueous humor and injection of air/gas (14% non-expansile concentration of C3F8, 20% non-expansile concentration of SF6, sterile air) enough to fill two-thirds of the AC [4, 13, 19, 24, 25].

Postoperatively, a supine position is advised to the patient at least for 48 h or until the beginning of the resolution of corneal edema, topical antibiotics, hypertonic saline, and steroids are given. Anti-glaucoma treatment may have to be given to avoid any rise of intraocular pressure (IOP), acetazolamide tablets 250 mg 3 times daily for 3 days is given. In case of persistence of edema, repeat injections can be given [4, 13, 19]. Various studies have recommended repeat injections for the complete resolution of edema [24, 25].

Miyata et al. reported that repeat air injections resulted in an average resolution time of 20.1 ± 9.0 days, while Panda et al. reported that corneal edema resolves in 4 weeks with intracameral SF6. Various complications associated with intracameral substitutes are elevation of IOP, infection, endothelial damage, and intrastromal migration of gas.

16.2.6.3 Compressive Sutures

Compressive sutures along with gas injection have been tried in severe cases with wide separation of the DM edges and multiple stromal clefts [4, 21].

Compression sutures are applied for large gaping Descemet membrane tears or if edema persists after gas injection alone. Application of compressive sutures helps to bring the gaping edges closer and hastens the resolution of the edema [21].

Procedure: After injection of gas bubble in the anterior chamber, which delineates the Descemet tear or stromal cleft, 2–5 full-thickness sutures with 10-0 nylon are applied across the tear, starting from about 1 to 2 mm from its edges. The patient is kept in the supine position for 3 days.

Adding compression sutures is observed to reduce the recovery time significantly, especially in the presence of stromal clefts, and also to prevent repeated gas injections [21].

16.2.6.4 PKP

PKP is required rarely in cases of persistent edema, perforation, large DM tear, large intrastromal cyst, and corneal neovascularization [4, 19]. Results of PKP being guarded with increased inflammation in the immediate postoperative period.

16.2.6.5 Cyanoacrylate Tissue Adhesive with BCL

Cyanoacrylate tissue adhesive with BCL can be done in cases of small perforation with fistula formation [4, 22].

16.2.6.6 AMT with Cauterization

AMT with cauterization has been tried in persistent hydrops in mentally retarded patients as a quick and effective treatment with good results [4, 23].

Cauterization coupled with stromal puncture allows the excess fluid from the stroma to evaporate but leaves a thermally injured epithelium and stroma. Amniotic membrane (AM) strongly reduces inflammation, vascularization, and scarring, which could explain the improvement of corneal clarity without intense scarring, even in previously significantly edematous areas that received many cautery applications.

Procedure: 15–32 cautery applications (500 kHz) are performed to the entire oedematous area with continual saline irrigation to the point of mild whitening of the treated patches using diathermy. At the point of maximum edema, a 24-gage disposable needle is used to penetrate the stroma. Following cauterization, preserved human AM is applied to the cornea with the epithelial side facing outward and fixed to the eye with interrupted 10-0 nylon sutures, covering the entire coagulated area with a small margin of clear tissue before applying BCL. One patient was reported to have developed superficial vascularization that increased over time as a complication of this procedure.

16.2.6.7 ASOCT Guided Intrastromal Fluid Drainage with Air Tamponade

It can be done when there is extensive corneal edema with the presence of multiple stromal fluid pockets. Depending on the location of fluid pockets as detected by preoperative ASOCT, numerous corneal stromal venting incisions are made to drain the collected fluid in addition to anterior chamber air tamponade. This technique was found to reduce the duration of morbidity and avoid potential complications associated with repeat gas injections [26].

16.2.6.8 Microscope-OCT-Guided Puncture and Intrastromal Fluid Pockets Drainage with Gas Tamponade

Recently a novel technique consists of the MI-OCT-guided puncture and drainage of intrastromal fluid pockets combined with anterior chamber sulfur hexafluoride-fill, and compression pre-descemetic sutures using a commercially available MI-OCT has been described in small corneal defects. There was the fast resolution of corneal edema and reattachment of DM to the corneal stroma. Corneal thickness decreases with quick recovery of visual acuity [27].

Approach to Management

Topical treatment for corneal hydrops can take 2–4 months to resolve completely, whereas a surgical method can shorten the duration. While surgical intervention provides a rapid response, topical treatment is less intrusive and has fewer risks. The final visual result will be similar to either method. Perhaps the most successful treatment technique should be determined by the size, location, and amount of edema. If the hydrops is off-center and the patient's complaints are minor, topical treatment may be sufficient. Conversely, if the edema is large in diameter and central, and central scarring affecting visual acuity status post healing is a concern, referral to a cornea specialist for surgical intervention may be warranted.

16.2.7 Outcome

Hydrops leaves a scar on the cornea and renders it a flatter contour. Because the cone in KC normally does not involve the central area, VA may improve after the hydrops has healed [4, 13, 14, 19]. Corneal flattening can also help contact lenses fit better [4, 13, 14, 19].

16.2.8 Acute Corneal Hydrops with Microbial Keratitis

Acute corneal hydrops may rarely be complicated with superimposed infection leading to microbial keratitis. Breaks in Descemet membrane, stromal edema, disrupted stromal lamellae, epithelial bullae and their subsequent rupture is a cause of compromised mechanical barrier which can lead to the development of epithelial defect and secondary infection. The infection may rapidly spread throughout the cornea and can be a cause of scarring, neovascularization, and loss of vision, necessitating subsequent keratoplasty. Additionally, eye rubbing and concurrent use of topical steroids are contributory factors. Thus, prophylactic topical antibiotics should always be considered when treating acute corneal hydrops.

16.2.8.1 Diagnosis

The patient usually presents with onset of severe pain, photophobia, mucopurulent discharge, and diminution of vision. Corneal scrapings should be obtained for

Gram, Giemsa, and potassium hydroxide smear and for culture and sensitivity in addition to B-scan ultrasonography to rule out posterior segment involvement.

16.2.8.2 Treatment

The management of corneal hydrops with coexistent microbial keratitis is similar to infective keratitis. Broad-spectrum antibiotics should be started to be later reviewed as per the sensitivity reports. Treatment can be initiated with fortified cefazolin sulfate 5% eye drops and tobramycin 1.3% eyedrops alternated every hour, homatropine 2% eyedrops four times a day, anti-glaucoma drugs, and artificial tears every 4 h remain conventional treatments. Topical steroids need to be discontinued till complete healing of the epithelial defect.

16.3 Corneal Perforation

16.3.1 Introduction

Corneal perforation is full-thickness defect in the cornea. Although rare, spontaneous corneal perforation in KC and PMD [28, 29] can occur. In all these cases, perforation is preceded by hydrops [22]. Globe rupture has also been reported in advanced Terrien's marginal degeneration following eye rubbing in a young male [30].

Corneal stromal loss is thought to be caused by an imbalance in corneal homeostasis in TMD, with spontaneous perforation occurring in 9% of cases [31]. Early diagnosis and close observation are essential in TMD to prevent ocular injuries spontaneously or following trivial trauma.

Corneal tear or globe rupture in keratoglobus can occur either spontaneously or following trivial trauma. Cameron et al. had reported that 7/11 patients (9 eyes) having keratoglobus with blue sclera with connective tissue disorder, had a rupture either spontaneously or secondary to trivial trauma [32].

16.3.2 Clinical Features

In most cases, the presence of a corneal perforation is unambiguous.

Visual impairment, mild pain, and leakage that may be mistaken for tears are common symptoms. A perforation site, as well as shallowing or flattening of the anterior chamber, are classic indicators. Some perforations, however, do not appear to leak. The Seidel test can be useful in these situations. The eye is injected with concentrated fluorescein (in the form of drops or a dye strip). Dilution of the green fluorescein by aqueous leakage is seen as blue fluid pouring down the eye on slit-lamp examination with cobalt blue light. Another tell-tale sign of corneal perforation is a brown pigment from the iris in the wound itself.

16.3.3 Management

Management Options include the application of cyanoacrylate tissue adhesive with bandage contact lens, patch grafts and lamellar or penetrating keratoplasty [22, 28, 29, 33].

16.3.3.1 Cyanoacrylate Tissue Adhesive with Bandage Contact Lens (BCL)

It is indicated as the primary modality of treatment when perforation size is <2 mm in diameter. Conservative management of hydrops with bandage lens therapy has the advantage of corneal flattening and reduced astigmatism after the resolution, as well as the avoidance of surgical risks. A trial of bandage lens therapy is recommended before surgical intervention in individuals with hydrops and perforation because of the potential advantages and avoidance of risk [34].

Technique: The area of perforation is dried using a merocele sponge, and cyanoacrylate glue is applied over the area, followed by the application of a BCL. Because glue expands when it polymerizes, it is important to underfill the defect. Too much glue will result in an elevated mass, which is irritating for the patient and hinders contact lenses from fitting properly.

16.3.3.2 Patch Graft

Done for a small perforation outside the visual axis, preferably 3 mm in diameter or smaller.

16.3.3.3 Lamellar Transplant

It is indicated if the perforation is >2 mm, entails partial stromal loss or if the patient is intolerant to the gluing procedure. A layer-by-layer dissection is performed, peeling away the layers of cornea from the healthy cornea to the perforated area, followed by donor lamellar graft transplantation and suturing.

16.3.3.4 Penetrating Keratoplasty

Essential for treating large perforations or when a lamellar transplant would require cutting or suturing through visual axis. A full-thickness corneal trephination is done, and donor cornea is secured on host bed using sutures.

16.4 Rehabilitative Procedures

Once the CH or perforation resolves, the other visual rehabilitative procedures like contact lens fitting, keratoplasties are done. Deep anterior lamellar keratoplasty using the layer-by-layer technique and avoiding big bubble formation has been shown to give good results.

16.4.1 Nonsurgical Management

16.4.1.1 Optical Correction

Spectacle correction has a very limited role in ACE. However, patients who are intolerant to contact lenses and do not want to undergo surgery may be prescribed spectacles.

16.4.1.2 Contact Lenses

Newer-generation lenses such as Rose K lenses (Menicon), scleral lenses, Prosthetic Replacement of the Ocular Surface Ecosystem (PROSE; BostonSight), and the Boston Ocular Surface Prosthesis (BOSP; BostonSight) have shown promise in ACE in early studies [35]. These lenses, which provide improved visual acuity and stability, may be an alternative for patients who have failed to respond to other treatments.

16.4.2 Surgical Management

Most cases of ACE require surgery for visual rehabilitation and for improving corneal strength.

Challenges in Surgical Management of ACE

Because the paracentral and peripheral corneas are involved, a big graft with a closer proximity to the limbus is necessary, which increases the risk of graft rejection; extreme corneal thinning makes suturing difficult and increases the risk of intraoperative Descemet membrane rupture.

16.4.2.1 Intrastromal Corneal Ring Segment (ICRS)

ICRS implantation is a method of improving contact lens tolerance and BCVA for patients with corneal ectasia and a clear cornea. Intacs SK (Addition Technology) was recently developed for severe keratoconus, with good results and no noticeable concerns. Long-term results and their relevance in indications other than keratoconus, however, need to be confirmed [1, 36].

16.4.2.2 Large-Diameter PKP

Is performed in ACE with a caveat to include the thinned-out corneal periphery. The increased likelihood of rejection due to closeness to the limbus and severe postoperative astigmatism associated with a decentred graft are also issues with such grafts [1, 37].

16.4.2.3 Lamellar Keratoplasty (LK)

Crescentic LK, compressive C-shaped LK, and modified deep LK are variations in LK that have been reported for treating ACE. A match-and-patch lamellar graft method is used in most cases. The recipient bed is then sutured with a lamellar donor that is 0.25–0.50 mm undersized. Ectasia is flattened and reduced as a result [1, 38].

16.4.2.4 LK with PKP

This combination procedure combines the advantages of a lamellar graft and a full-thickness graft. A large-diameter lamellar graft can provide tectonic support to the weakened peripheral host cornea, and a central small-diameter, full-thickness graft can provide excellent visual outcomes [1].

16.4.2.5 Simultaneous Peripheral Crescentic LK and Central PKP

LK and PKP are done in a single step. The LK procedure is performed first to restore normal thickness to the peripherally thinned cornea and to allow for adequate edge-to-edge apposition during the PKP procedure, which is done subsequently [39]. The benefit of this method is that it eliminates the requirement for two donor corneas, as would be the case with sequential LK and PKP.

16.4.2.6 Tectonic LK Followed by Secondary PKP

A tectonic LK is performed in this method, and secondary PKP is performed in a second surgical session, usually 6 months later [40].

16.4.2.7 Tuck-in Lamellar Keratoplasty (TILK)

TILK is an LK technique designed for eyes with severe peripheral corneal thinning disorders such PMD, keratoglobus, post-PKP ectasia, and eyes with both keratoconus and PMD [41, 42].

16.4.2.8 Wedge Resection

This technique is useful When ectasia is limited to a small sector of the corneal periphery [43, 44]. It is advantageous over a corneal graft by ways of preservation of the natural core cornea, the absence of graft rejection or interface haze improved wound strength, and faster visual rehabilitation [43, 44]. However, because of the constant tension at the sutured site, unstable postoperative astigmatism remains a concern.

16.5 Conclusion

Acute corneal hydrops and corneal perforations are emergencies encountered in ACE. Newer diagnostic modalities like ultrasound biomicroscopy, ASOCT, and confocal microscopy are helpful in diagnosis and planning of treatment. In comparison to medical treatment alone, management with interventions such as intracameral air/gas injection reduces the length of symptoms and the risk of consequences.

16.6 Recommendations

Acute corneal hydrops and corneal perforation are emergent presentations of keratoconus and other ectatic conditions. Intracameral air/gas injections are useful in severe cases in reducing morbidity and also the risk of complications such as corneal neovascularization.

Key Points

- Advanced corneal ectasia (ACE) occurs in keratoconus, pellucid marginal degeneration, Terrien's marginal degeneration, keratoglobus, and post-LASIK keratectasia.
- Management of ACE is challenging. All efforts to be made to manage keratectasias to prevent the development of emergent situations like Corneal hydrops and perforations.
- Intracameral gas/air decreases the duration of corneal edema, other symptoms and corneal neovascularization once corneal hydrops develops. Less severe cases with the total size of corneal edema <3 mm may be just managed conservatively, and else there is no resolution.

References

1. Maharana PK, Dubey A, Jhanji V, Sharma N, Das S, Vajpayee RB. Management of advanced corneal ectasias. Br J Ophthalmol. 2015;100(1):34–40.
2. Ishii R, Kamiya K, Igarashi A, et al. Correlation of corneal elevation with severity of keratoconus by means of anterior and posterior topographic analysis. Cornea. 2012;31:253–8.
3. Maharana PK, Dubey A, Jhanji V, Sharma N, Das S, Vajpayee RB. The ABCs of ACEs. Cataract & Refractive Surgery Today Europe; 2017. p. 23–6.
4. Tuft SJ, Gregory WM, Buckley RJ. Acute corneal hydrops in keratoconus. Ophthalmology. 1994;101:1738–44.
5. Carter JB, Jones DB, Wilhelmus KR. Acute hydrops in pellucid marginal corneal degeneration. Am J Ophthalmol. 1989;107:167–70.
6. McClellan KA, Billson FA. Acute hydrops in keratoglobus. Arch Ophthalmol. 1987;105:1432–3.
7. Ashenhurst M, Slomovic A. Corneal hydrops in Terrien's marginal degeneration: an unusual complication. Can J Ophthalmol. 1987;22:328–30.
8. Chen CL, Tai MC, Chen JT, et al. Acute corneal hydrops with perforation after LASIK-associated keratectasia. Clin Exp Ophthalmol. 2007;35:62–5.
9. Sharma N, Sachdev R, Jindal A, Titiyal JS. Acute hydrops in keratectasia after radial keratotomy. Eye Contact Lens. 2010;36:185–7.
10. Javadi MA, Feizi S, Kanavi MR, et al. Acute hydrops after deep anterior lamellar keratoplasty in a patient with keratoconus. Cornea. 2011;30:591–4.
11. Ezra DG, Mehta JS, Allan BD. Late corneal hydrops after penetrating keratoplasty for keratoconus. Cornea. 2007;26:639–40.
12. Oshida T, Fushimi N, Sakimoto T, Sawa M. Acute hydrops in a host cornea after penetrating keratoplasty for keratoconus. Jpn J Ophthalmol. 2011;55:418–9.
13. Basu S, Vaddavalli PK, Ramappa M, Shah S, Murthy SI, Sangwan VS. Intracameral perfluoropropane gas in the treatment of acute corneal hydrops. Ophthalmology. 2011;118:934–9.
14. Grewal S, Laibson PR, Cohen EJ, Rapuano CJ. Acute hydrops in the corneal ectasias: associated factors and outcomes. Trans Am Ophthalmol Soc. 1999;97:187–203.
15. Sharma R, Titiyal JS, Prakash G, Sharma N, Tandon R, Vajpayee RB. Clinical profile and risk factors for keratoplasty and development of hydrops in north Indian patients with keratoconus. Cornea. 2009;28:367–70.
16. Stoiber J, Muss W, Ruckhofer J, Grabner G. Acute keratoconus with perforation in a patient with Down's syndrome. Br J Ophthalmol. 2003;87:120.
17. Sharma N, Mannan R, Jhanji V, Agarwal T, Pruthi A, Titiyal JS, et al. Ultrasound biomicroscopy-guided assessment of acute corneal hydrops. Ophthalmology. 2011;118:2166–71.

18. Akova YA, Dabil H, Kavalcioglu O, Duman S. Clinical features and keratoplasty results in keratoconus complicated by acute hydrops. Ocul Immunol Inflamm. 2000;8:101–9.
19. Sharma N, Maharana PK, Jhanji V, Vajpayee RB. Management of acute corneal hydrops in ectatic corneal disorders. Curr Opin Ophthalmol. 2012;23:317–23.
20. Basu S, Vaddavalli PK, Vemuganti GK, Ali MH, Murthy SI. Anterior segment optical coherence tomography features of acute corneal hydrops. Cornea. 2012;31:479–85.
21. Rajaraman R, Singh S, Raghavan A, Karkhanis A. Efficacy and safety of intracameral perfluoropropane (C3F8) tamponade and compression sutures for the management of acute corneal hydrops. Cornea. 2009;28:317–20.
22. Aldave AJ, Mabon M, Hollander DA, McLeod SD, Spencer WH, Abbott RL. Spontaneous corneal hydrops and perforation in keratoconus and pellucid marginal degeneration. Cornea. 2003;22:169–74.
23. Wylegala E, Tarnawska D. Amniotic membrane transplantation with cauterization for keratoconus complicated by persistent hydrops in mentally retarded patients. Ophthalmology. 2006;113:561–4.
24. Miyata K, Tsuji H, Tanabe T, Mimura Y, Amano S, Oshika T. Intracameral air injection for acute hydrops in keratoconus. Am J Ophthalmol. 2002;133:750–2.
25. Panda A, Aggarwal A, Madhavi P, Wagh VB, Dada T, Kumar A, et al. Management of acute corneal hydrops secondary to keratoconus with intracameral injection of sulfur hexafluoride (SF6). Cornea. 2007;26:1067–9.
26. Vajpayee RB, Maharana PK, Kaweri L, Sharma N, Jhanji V. Intrastromal fluid drainage with air tamponade: anterior segment optical coherence tomography guided technique for the management of acute corneal hydrops. Br J Ophthalmol. 2013;97(7):834–6.
27. Siebelmann S, Händel A, Matthaei M, Bachmann B, Cursiefen C. Microscope-integrated optical coherence tomography-guided drainage of acute corneal hydrops in keratoconus combined with suturing and gas-aided reattachment of descemet membrane. Cornea. 2019;38(8):1058–61.
28. Lucarelli MJ, Gendelman DS, Talamo JH. Hydrops and spontaneous perforation in pellucid marginal corneal degeneration. Cornea. 1997;16:232–4.
29. Orlin SE, Sulewski ME. Spontaneous corneal perforation in pellucid marginal degeneration. CLAO J. 1998;24:186–7.
30. Khurana S, Gupta PC, Kumar A, Ram J. Globe rupture following eye rubbing in a case of Terrien's marginal degeneration in a young male. Indian J Ophthalmol. 2020;68:2493–4.
31. Srinivasan S, Murphy CC, Fisher AC, Freeman LB, Kaye SB. Terrien marginal degeneration presenting with spontaneous corneal perforation. Cornea. 2006;25:977–80.
32. Cameron JA, Cotter JB, Risco JM, Alvarez H. Epikeratoplasty for keratoglobus associated with blue sclera. Ophthalmology. 1991;98:446–52.
33. Akpek EK, Altan-Yaycioglu R, Gottsch JD, et al. Spontaneous corneal perforation in a patient with unusual unilateral pellucid marginal degeneration. J Cataract Refract Surg. 2001;27:1698–700.
34. Forooghian F, Assaad D, Dixon WS. Successful conservative management of hydrops with perforation in pellucid marginal degeneration. Can J Ophthalmol. 2006;41:74–7.
35. Velazquez FFJ. Kerasoft IC compared to Rose-K in the management of corneal ectasias. Cont Lens Anterior Eye. 2012;35:175–9.
36. Lee JC, Chiu GB, Bach D, et al. Functional and visual improvement with prosthetic replacement of the ocular surface ecosystem scleral lenses for irregular corneas. Cornea. 2013;32:1540–3.
37. Speaker MG, Arentsen JJ, Laibson PR. Long-term survival of large diameter penetrating keratoplasties for keratoconus and pellucid marginal degeneration. Acta Ophthalmol Suppl. 1989;192:17–9.
38. Cheng CL, Theng JT, Tan DT. Compressive C-shaped lamellar keratoplasty: a surgical alternative for the management of severe astigmatism from peripheral corneal degeneration. Ophthalmology. 2005;112:425–30.
39. Rasheed K, Rabinowitz YS. Surgical treatment of advanced pellucid marginal degeneration. Ophthalmology. 2000;107:1836–40.

40. Lake D, Hamada S, Khan S, et al. Deep anterior lamellar keratoplasty over penetrating keratoplasty for host rim thinning and ectasia. Cornea. 2009;28:489–92.
41. Kaushal S, Jhanji V, Sharma N, et al. "Tuck in" lamellar keratoplasty (TILK) for corneal ectasias involving corneal periphery. Br J Ophthalmol. 2008;92(2):286–90.
42. Vajpayee RB, Jhanji V, Beltz J, et al. "Tuck in" lamellar keratoplasty for tectonic management of post keratoplasty corneal ectasia with peripheral corneal involvement. Cornea. 2011;30:171–4.
43. Busin M, Kerdraon Y, Scorcia V, et al. Combined wedge resection and beveled penetrating relaxing incisions for the treatment of pellucid marginal corneal degeneration. Cornea. 2008;27:595–600.
44. Maccheron LJ, Daya SM. Wedge resection and lamellar dissection for pellucid marginal degeneration. Cornea. 2012;31:708–15.

Stevens–Johnson Syndrome 17

Margaret C. Pollard, Laura M. Le,
and Deepinder K. Dhaliwal

17.1 History and Classification

In 1922, Stevens and Johnson reported two young boys with mucous membrane inflammation, conjunctivitis, stomatitis, and fever; this report was the first publication describing Stevens–Johnson Syndrome (SJS). The term toxic epidermal necrolysis was first introduced in 1956. Based on core differences in demographics, associated diseases, causes, and severity, erythema multiforme major (EMM) is now classified as a distinct disease entity from SJS/TEN [4]. Current classification of these bullous dermatosis conditions fall under five categories, in order of increasing severity: erythema multiforme major, SJS, SJS/TEN overlap, TEN with spots, and TEN without spots. SJS involves <10% body surface area, TEN involves >30% body surface area, and SJS/TEN overlap describes the continuum between 10 and 30% body surface area. Differing from EM, the distribution of SJS and TEN lesions is widespread, with common localization on the head and trunk, and typical ocular involvement. Cause is another key distinguishing factor, as the herpes simplex virus is a common cause of EM, while medications typically cause SJS and TEN [1].

M. C. Pollard
Maine Eye Center, Portland, ME, USA
e-mail: mpollard@maineeyecenter.com

L. M. Le · D. K. Dhaliwal (✉)
Department of Ophthalmology, University of Pittsburgh School of Medicine, Pittsburgh, PA, USA
e-mail: lelm@upmc.edu; dhaliwaldk@upmc.edu

B. Sharma, J. S. Titiyal (eds.), *Corneal Emergencies*,
https://doi.org/10.1007/978-981-16-5876-1_17

Table 17.1 Common medications associated with SJS

Category	Drugs
Aromatic Anticonvulsants	Carbamazepine, lamotrigine, phenobarbital, phenytoin, oxcarbazepine
Antibiotic	Beta-lactam antibiotics (aminopenicillins and cephalosporins), quinolones (ciprofloxacin), clarithromycin
Antiviral agents	Nevirapine
Sulfonamides	Dapsone, sulfasalazine, sulfamethoxazole
Others	Allopurinol, NSAIDs, COX-II inhibitors, strontium ranelate

17.2 Etiologies

SJS is thought to be an autoimmune response to environmental medications or infection, though the pathogenesis is still not fully understood. SJS most commonly arises as a severe adverse reaction to sulfonamides antibiotics, followed by analgesics, nonsteroidal anti-inflammatory drugs (NSAIDs), psycho epileptics, and anti-gout drugs, with highest risk of disease being during the first 2 months of treatment (Table 17.1). *Mycoplasma pneumoniae* is the most common infectious agent associated with SJS. Other pathogens associated with SJS include the *Yersinia* species, and *Herpes* virus [5, 6].

17.3 Pathogenesis

The high SJS recurrence rate in certain individuals has suggested a potential genetic predisposition and susceptibility. Mutations in human leukocyte antigen (HLA) and metabolic genetic elements (cytochrome P450) have been associated with drug-induced SJS [5].

It is thought that drug metabolites initiate an immune response in susceptible individuals. Fas–Fas ligand interactions, immune cell activation (MHC class I and T cell receptors), and cytokine release all are thought to play a role. The end result is an overwhelming inflammatory cascade resulting in keratinocyte apoptosis, blistering, and systemic inflammation [7].

17.4 Clinical Features

17.4.1 Systemic

SJS symptoms typically present 4–21 days after offending drug use. One to three days prior to mucocutaneous lesion development, a prodromal period is marked by non-specific lymphadenopathy and influenza-like symptoms, including fever, malaise, myalgia, and arthralgia. Early indicators of SJS are photophobia, conjunctivitis, dysphagia, skin tenderness, stomatitis, mucositis, and blistering [8].

Cutaneous lesions then present on the face and thorax, spreading diffusely in a symmetrical distribution. These lesions are characterized as irregular, coalescing, red macules with purpuric centers that develop into urticarial plaques, bullae, or vesicles. The lesions consist of a vesicular, purpuric, or necrotic core with surrounding erythema; ultimately progressing to the sloughing of skin and a positive Nikolsky sign, the dislodgement of intact superficial epidermis with lateral finger pressure. The esophagus, upper airway, genitalia, and tracheobronchial tree may be affected, as any mucosal surface can be involved. Severe cases can be life threatening with acute renal failure, severe pulmonary involvement, hepatic dysfunction, sepsis, gastrointestinal bleeding, and secondary infections [9].

17.4.2 Acute Ocular

A large majority of patients with SJS/TEN will develop ocular manifestations. Acute ocular involvement is reported to occur in 50–88% of SJS/TEN cases [10–12]. In the acute phase of SJS, there is rapid onset keratinocyte apoptosis and secondary effects of inflammation, causing ocular surface epithelium degradation. The acute phase of SJS has been defined as the first 2–6 weeks. However, it is most prudent to consider the acute phase as beginning with the onset of signs and ending with resolution of skin and mucosal ulcerations [12].

Early eye involvement can be highly variable. Mild cases present as conjunctivitis and self-limited hyperemia and localized epithelial defects on the bulbar or palpebral conjunctiva. Severe cases can present as total sloughing of the entire ocular surface epithelium. Symptoms of pain and photophobia are more pronounced with more severe findings.

Pathology involves the entire ocular surface epithelium, including the (a) conjunctiva, (b) eyelid skin and margins, (c) lacrimal gland and accessory glands, and (d) cornea (Figs. 17.1 and 17.2).

(A) *Lid Margins and Eyelid*

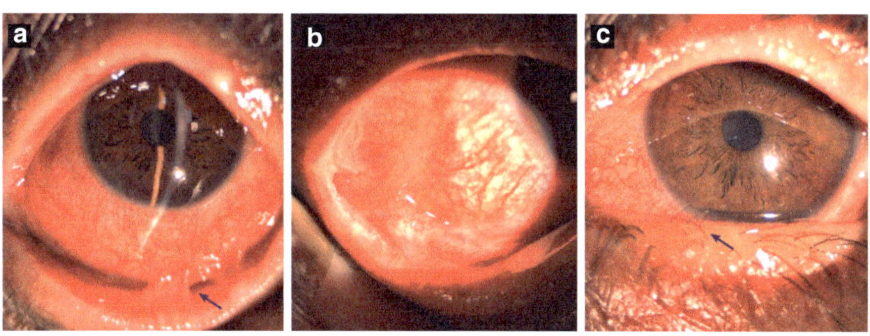

Fig. 17.1 (**a–c**) Slit lamp picture showing subacute SJS with intense conjunctival hyperemia and formation of symblepharon; Conjunctival necrosis and pseudo membranes; and trichiatic eye lashes

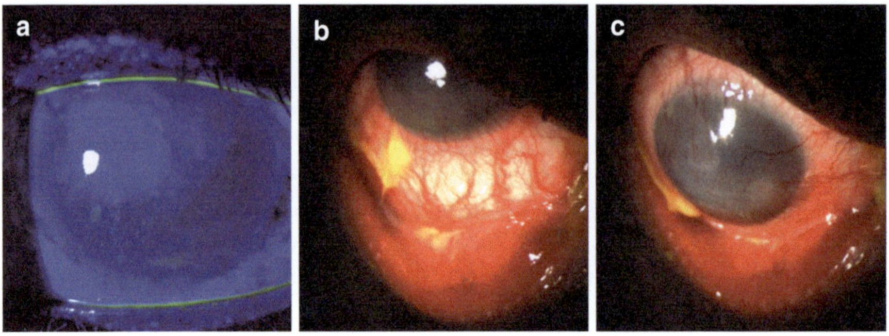

Fig. 17.2 (**a**–**c**) Slit lamp picture showing acute SJS with epithelial defects in conjunctiva and cornea. Also seen is the formation of conjunctival pseudo-membrane and conjunctivalization of cornea

The eyelids and eyelashes lose their normal architecture from tissue contracture and cicatricial changes, resulting in cicatricial entropion, trichiasis and distichiasis (Fig. 17.1c). The sites of tarsal and bulbar conjunctival acute-stage ulceration highly correlate with the development of late-stage posterior lid margin keratinization. Meibomian gland destruction and keratinization of the lid margins further create irregularities that propagate chronic ocular surface damage from blink-related trauma.

(B) *Lacrimal and Accessory Glands*

In the acute phase, intense and diffuse inflammation can destroy conjunctival goblet cells, accessory lacrimal glands, and the main lacrimal gland's secretory ductules. Inflammation in the lacrimal gland and scarring of the lacrimal ducts lead to reduced aqueous tear production and dysfunctional tear film.

(C) *Conjunctiva*

At initial presentation, bilateral conjunctival hyperemia is the most common ocular finding. Though typically bilateral, findings can be asymmetric. Conjunctivitis can occur before, simultaneous to or after systemic skin eruptions. Conjunctival epithelial defects on the bulbar or palpebral conjunctiva can be localized. However, severe cases are manifested by diffuse conjunctival sloughing of the bulbar and tarsal conjunctiva. Pseudomembranes or true membranes can form. Symblepharon formation and foreshortening of fornix can develop rapidly from adhesion of de-epithelialized tarsal and bulbar conjunctiva. Normal conjunctival mucosa becomes replaced with cicatricial epithelium and scar tissue. Tarsal conjunctival scarring, when present is typically seen within weeks of onset (Fig. 17.1a, b)

(D) *Cornea*

The cornea can acutely develop corneal epithelial defects that can lead to corneal ulceration, infection, and can ultimately lead to corneal perforation. Corneal limbal stem cell destruction is a dreaded complication, leading to corneal neovascularization, conjunctivalization of the cornea, and vision loss. Corneal limbal stem cell deficiency is especially difficult to treat in the setting of SJS and makes future corneal transplantation higher risk for failure [1, 12–14] (Fig. 17.2a–c).

17.5 Medical Management

17.5.1 Systemic Therapy

The only systemic intervention with evidence-based benefit on mortality is supportive care. Supportive care in an intensive care unit equipped to manage burn patients is preferred. These patients are often critically ill; fluid balance, respiratory function, and nutrition must be closely monitored.

The use of systemic corticosteroids, steroid sparing immunotherapy, and intravenous immunoglobulin has been reported both in the acute and chronic phase for systemic and ocular inflammation. Though immune modulators help reduce ocular and systemic inflammation, their role remains controversial. Lack of controlled trials evaluating their effectiveness, short-term and long-term side effects, and possible increased risk of infection must be considered [15, 16].

17.5.2 Ocular Examination and Classification

The skin and systemic involvement in SJS/TEN does not always correlate to the severity of eye involvement. Within the initial few days of SJS onset, there can be rapid eye inflammation progression. Any patient with SJS/TEN should be immediately evaluated by an ophthalmologist at their initial presentation, since timing of intervention is critical. Any patient with ophthalmic manifestations should have daily evaluations by an ophthalmologist since the severity can change quickly [17]. Daily exams should continue until it is clear that no worsening is evident. Hospital staff should be educated regarding the need for prompt ophthalmology evaluation in SJS/TEN patients. Evaluating ophthalmologists should be knowledgeable regarding indications for therapies, including amniotic membrane transplantation.

Daily examination by an ophthalmologist is of crucial importance. Examinations are typically done at the bedside given patients' critically ill status. Evaluating the extent of sloughing and symblepharon should start with a physiologic saline rinse to remove debris, followed by examination with fluorescein and a hand-held ophthalmoscope with blue-light filter. Emphasis is placed on examination of the fornices and tarsal conjunctiva, and to quantify degree of epithelial sloughing. To detect early symblepharon formation, fornices should be examined carefully, with lid retraction or eversion if necessary.

Quickly identifying inflammation and epithelial sloughing is crucial to minimizing long-term ophthalmologic complications, such as symblepharon formation and scarring. Gregory et al. proposed a grading scheme and associated treatment guideline for acute SJS and TEN in 2016 based on a prospective case series of 79 consecutive patients [18]. Mild cases are classified as conjunctival hyperemia with no staining of the conjunctiva, cornea, or lid margin. Moderate cases have discrete areas of conjunctival staining <1 cm, no corneal epithelial defect and epithelial sloughing involving <1/3 lid margin. Severe cases have at least one of the following: (1) corneal epithelial defect, (2) any bulbar or palpebral conjunctival staining >1 cm in largest diameter, (3) staining of >1/3 of at least 1 lid margin. Extremely severe is multiple areas of severe involvement (Table 17.2). This grading system provides a clinically relevant guideline to direct management based on measurements that can be made at the patient's bedside.

A flow diagram of recommended medical treatments for corresponding SJS ocular manifestations has been adapted (Fig. 17.3).

17.5.3 Acute Topical Therapy

Conventional medical therapy consists of ocular lubrication, sterile saline rinses, symblepharon prevention, anti-inflammatories, and antibiotic prophylaxis. Medical therapy alone may be appropriate in mild and moderate disease that is not progressive. Topical medications have no proven benefit and there is a lack of published cases and evidence-based guidelines in this regard. Still, medical therapy is thought to play a role and is prudent to institute. Cycloplegics or bandage contact lenses do not play a role in treatment.

Table 17.2 Ophthalmologic grading criteria and treatment recommendations for acute Stevens–Johnson syndrome (adapted from: Gregory DG. New grading system and treatment guidelines for the acute ocular manifestations of Stevens-Johnson syndrome. Ophthalmology. 2016;123(8):1653–1658)

Staining location and treatment recommendations	Severity of eye involvement			
	Mild	Moderate	Severe	Extremely severe
Lid margin	No stain	Stain <1/3 of lid margin length	Stain >1/3 of lid margin length on at least 1 lid	Stain >1/3 of lid margin length on more than 1 lid
Cornea	No stain	No stain	Any epithelial defect more than punctate staining	Any epithelial defect more than punctate staining
Conjunctiva (bulbar and palpebral)	Hyperemia, without stain	Stain <1 cm in greatest diameter	Stain >1 cm	Multiple areas of stain >1 cm
Treatment recommendations	Medical	Medical and close observation	Medical and urgent AMT	Medical and urgent AMT (may require repeat AMT)

AMT amniotic membrane transplantation

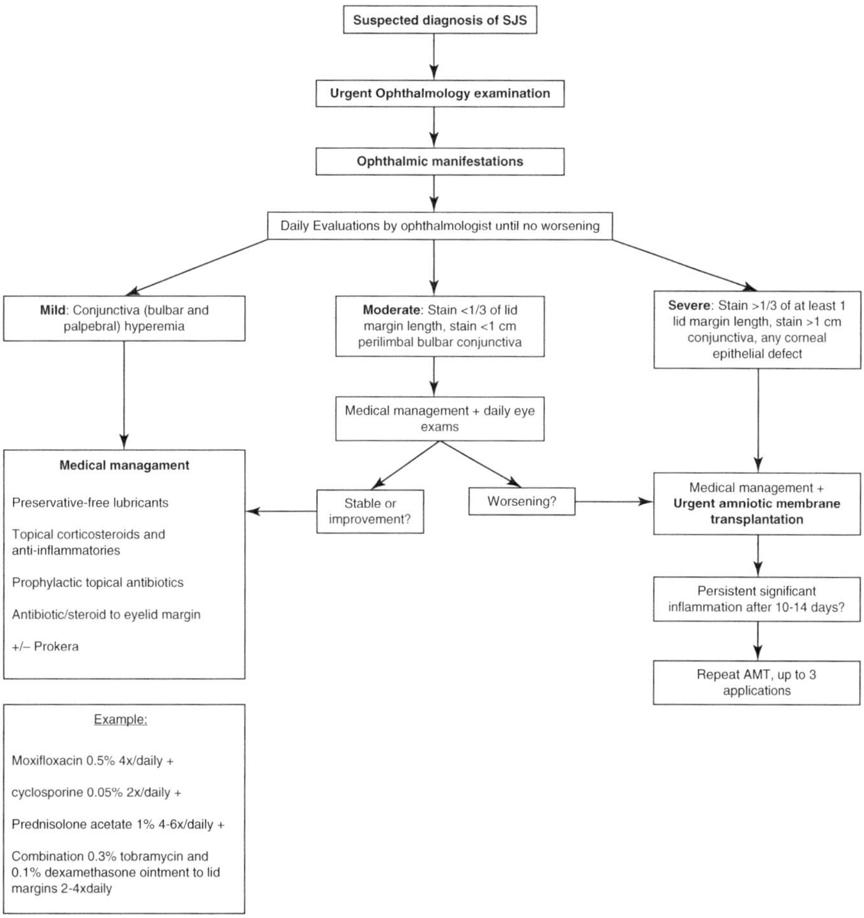

Fig. 17.3 Treatment algorithm for acute management of SJS ocular manifestations

17.5.3.1 Ocular Lubricants

Preservative-free lubricants 4–6 times daily during the acute stage may help rinse inflammatory substances and lubricate the ocular surface.

17.5.3.2 Topical Anti-Inflammatories

During the acute phase, topical corticosteroids can minimize surface ocular damage; the frequency of dosing can vary. There are no evidence-based dosing schedules or durations for topical treatment; however, a schedule of prednisolone acetate 1% 4–6 times daily is common. Dexamethasone 1% drops twice daily is an alternative. Combination tobramycin 0.3% plus dexamethasone 0.1% ointment (TobraDex; Alcon), dexamethasone or fluorometholone ointment should be applied to the lid margins 2–4 times daily. Several case reports have suggested topical cyclosporine's beneficial lessening of acute ophthalmic complications for TEN patients. Topical cyclosporine 0.05% is administered twice daily and can be continued long-term. Steroids are continued until ocular surface inflammation appears resolved, then can be tapered.

17.5.3.3 Topical Antibiotics

Prophylactic topical antibiotics to patients with ocular involvement decreases the risk of further ocular infection [13]. Moxifloxacin 0.5% achieves high conjunctival, corneal, and tear film concentration in comparison to other fluoroquinolone drops as well as having a preservative-free formulation [17]. Typical dosing is 3–4 times daily. Application of combination antibiotic/steroid ointment to the eyelid margins is often used as above.

17.5.3.4 Prokera and Symblepharon Preventative Measures

Prokera (Biotissue, Miami, FL) is an amniotic membrane fixed on a polycarbonate ring that is placed over corneal and perilimbal regions, acting as a biological contact lens. At the ocular surface, Prokera facilitates re-epithelialization through the amniotic membrane's anti-inflammatory effects. Despite some noted good outcomes of acute SJS/TEN cases treated with Prokera [19], Prokera alone does not treat eyelid margin and tarsal conjunctiva involvement. It may be appropriate in cases with isolated perilimbal bulbar conjunctival staining and may be used in conjunction with amniotic membrane transplantation to the eyelids. If severe tarsal and eyelid margin involvement is present, ocular surface reconstruction with large sheets of amniotic membrane is needed [18].

Symblepharon preventative measures include symblepharon rings in conjunction with amniotic membrane. The amniotic membrane separates deepithelialized palpebral conjunctiva and bulbar conjunctiva from becoming apposed and adherent, and the symblepharon ring keeps the fornices formed. Symblepharon rings alone are not sufficient in preventing lid scarring. A combination of subconjunctival triamcinolone (Kenalog 20 mg) injections, symblepharon rings, and a Prokera (Biotissue, Miami, Florida, USA) has been described [20], however this may only be useful in a small subset of patients. More commonly, a symblepharon ring is placed at the time of amniotic membrane transplantation and removed once the membrane has dissolved. Symblepharon ring can be obtained commercially or formed and custom fit to the fornices individually using IV tubing and connected with a variety of plastic tubing connectors.

Previously "sweeping the fornices" with a glass rod has been emphasized as a method to prevent symblepharon formation. Though mechanical lysis of symblepharon may have a role, it is more important to control the inflammation that leads to symblepharon formation. Mechanical lysis can be performed to aid in examination and implementation of additional therapy, but this should not be considered a standalone treatment modality.

17.6 Acute Surgical Management

17.6.1 Background

In 2002, the first report of successful use of amniotic membrane transplantation (AMT) as a therapy for acute ocular SJS/TEN was published [3]. Since then, many case series have followed, with growing evidence from case control and small randomized studies supporting AMT's role for prevention of severe ocular scarring and subsequent long-term morbidity [21, 22]. Amniotic membrane is the placental innermost layer of fetal membranes, composed of a single layer of epithelial cells fixed to a thick basement membrane with an avascular stromal matrix. It has anti-inflammatory and anti-scarring effects [23].

Early intervention is critical in preventing ocular surface scarring and damage, as there is a limited window of opportunity within the first week of symptom onset to make a difference with AMT [17]. AMT should be done as early as possible within the first week of symptom onset.

Prior to 2016, there were no clear guidelines or treatment algorithm for when AMT is indicated and when medical management alone may be sufficient. Based on Gregory's proposed guidelines, indications for AMT are severe eye involvement; any corneal epithelial defect, any bulbar or palpebral conjunctival staining >1 cm in largest diameter, or staining of >1/3 of at least 1 lid margin. Patients with mild and moderate involvement may be treated with medical management; however, in equivocal moderate cases, the general rule is to err on the side of treatment with AMT [18].

17.6.2 Amniotic Membrane Transplantation

AMT can be done at bedside under local anesthesia and/or conscious sedation if the patient's status allows and depending on the complexity of suturing required (Fig. 17.4). In other cases, intervention under general anesthesia in the operating room may be required, especially in the pediatric population. SJS/TEN patients are critically ill and often undergoing life support measures.

17.6.2.1 Technique

A sterile saline rinse is performed to remove mucous debris and necrotic tissue from the ocular surface and lid margin. Eyelashes are trimmed to better appose membrane to the meibomian glands. Antibiotic drops can be administered. Given the inflamed state of the ocular surface, standard povidone-iodine prep is generally not used.

There are multiple techniques for amniotic membrane transplantation and the surgical technique below is adapted from multiple surgeons [12, 24, 25].

With the stromal side down, cryopreserved amniotic membrane (typically 5 cm × 10cm) is partially peeled away from its carrier paper. The membrane is

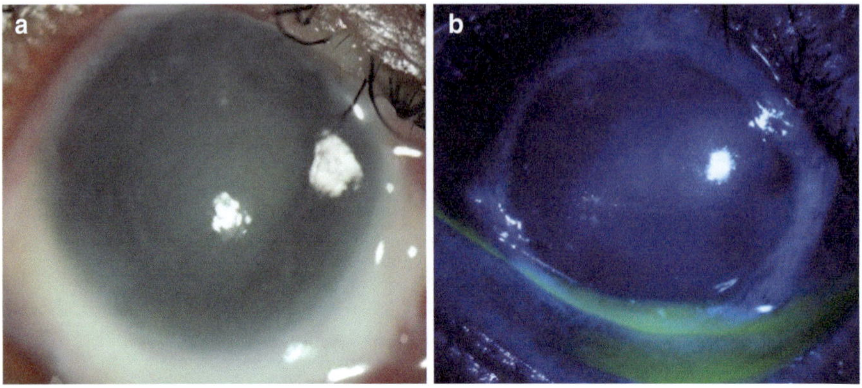

Fig. 17.4 (**a**, **b**) Slit lamp picture showing Amniotic membrane transplantation done in acute SJS (Image courtesy Prof Namrata Sharma; RP Centre for Ophthalmic Sciences AIIMS New Delhi)

positioned on the upper eyelid and may be sutured in place with running 8-0 nylon suture or in an interrupted fashion with bolsters. Generally, nonabsorbable suture is preferred as it incites less inflammatory reaction. The membrane is then removed from the nitrocellulose paper after it is attached superiorly. A blunt, 19-gauge cannula or muscle hook is used to sweep and flatten the membrane from the center to the edges; the membrane can be rewetted if it becomes dry and should not be grasped or handled with toothed forceps. The upper eyelid is then retracted, which aids in pushing the membrane into the upper fornix. A double-armed 6-0 polypropylene suture can be passed through the membrane full-thickness deep into the fornix and out through the eyelid skin, with twin passes 1 cm apart and tied over plastic bolsters. A symblepharon ring is then placed over the membrane and into the upper fornix to position the membrane in the fornix. The ring-membrane complex is placed in the lower fornix as the lower eyelid is retracted. The inferior forniceal sutures are placed in a similar fashion as superiorly. The membrane is then positioned over the lower eyelid margin and secured to the external lower eyelid using running or interrupted nonabsorbable suture. Finally, excess membrane can be trimmed. If there is no corneal involvement, the membrane over the cornea can be excised. In some cases, running perilimbal nylon suture is used to secure the membrane over the cornea. Antibiotic or combination antibiotic-steroid ointment can be applied to the eyelid and/or over the ocular surface at the end of the procedure.

17.6.2.2 Postoperative Management

Daily ophthalmic examinations are recommended following amniotic membrane transplantation. Topical antibiotics, steroid, and cyclosporine drops are used post-procedure and combination antibiotic-steroid ointment is applied to the eyelid margins as described in medical management (Sect. 17.5.3). Daily sterile saline rinses aid in removal of mucous and necrotic debris. Within 7–10 days, the membrane degrades. Degrading membranes can resemble mucopurulent discharge and careful examination for corneal infiltrate or superinfection must be performed. Sutures and bolsters are removed after 10–14 days.

Systemic and skin lesions typically improve first, so patients may be discharged from the hospital with membranes and symblepharon rings in place. Frequent outpatient checks are necessary.

17.6.2.3 Repeat AMT Applications

Persistent severe inflammation after initial AMT can be retreated multiple times with repeat AMT using the same surgical technique, with up to three membrane applications [18]. Once the initial membrane is degraded and the sutures and bolsters are removed 10–14 days after application, the degree of inflammation is then reassessed. If there is still significant inflammation, repeat treatment should be done immediately.

17.7 Chronic Management

Management of chronic SJS is very challenging. Goals of treatment are to restore the ocular surface, optimize tear function, and restore forniceal and eyelid anatomy [1].

17.7.1 Ocular Surface

Frequent preservative-free artificial tear supplementation should be used. Autologous serum tears help maintain the ocular surface. Mucolytic agents such as N-acetylcysteine can control filamentary keratitis. Specialized scleral contact lenses can improve vision quality and symptoms, as well as protect the cornea from eyelid scarring.

17.7.2 Eyelid and Forniceal Management

Eyelash dysfunction (trichiasis and distichiasis) is treated with epilation, electrolysis, cryotherapy, or surgically. Cicactricial lid changes can be repaired surgically, typically in conjunction with mucous membrane grafting.

17.8 Conclusions

SJS/TEN is a disease that has the potential for severe, chronic eyelid and conjunctival scarring, debilitating eye pain, and corneal neovascularization. Chronic sequelae are very difficult to manage and can lead to significant vision loss. The key to prevention of chronic sequelae is early recognition of severe cases and intervention within the first week of illness. Ophthalmologists must be actively and immediately involved in the acute management of SJS/TEN patients, as treatment of chronic surface ocular damage becomes progressively more difficult. Though medical management and Prokera may be sufficient for SJS/TEN patients with mild inflammation limited to the perilimbal bulbar conjunctiva, Prokera alone is not sufficient for cases of severe, eyelid and tarsal conjunctival sloughing. Amniotic membrane transplantation covering the eyelid margins and palpebral conjunctiva must be performed, with symblepharon rings and deep forniceal sutures over bolsters used to maintain the fornices. The persistence of significant inflammation after AMT justifies multiple membrane applications. Early intervention has been shown to preserve vision and improve long-term symptoms.

Key Points

- Ophthalmologists must be actively and immediately involved in the acute management of SJS/TEN patients.
- The key to prevention of chronic sequelae is early recognition of severe cases and intervention with amniotic membrane transplantation covering the eyelid margins and conjunctiva within the first week of onset.
- A sense of urgency is necessary in the treatment of this disease.

References

1. Gregory GG, Holland EJ, Mannis MJ. Cornea: erythema multiforme, Stevens-Johnson syndrome and toxic epidermal necrolysis. 4th ed. Elsevier; 2016. p. 558–72.
2. Pleyer U, Haberle H, Baatz H, et al. Acute manifestations of oculo-muco-cutaneous disorders: erythema multiforme major, Stevens–Johnson syndrome, and toxic epidermal necrolysis. In: Pleyer U, Hartmann C, Sterry W, editors. Oculodermal diseases. Buren: Aeolus Press; 1997. p. 169–91.
3. John T, Foulks GN, John ME, Cheng K, Hu D. Amniotic membrane in the surgical management of acute toxic epidermal necrolysis. Ophthalmology. 2002;109(2):351–60.
4. Heng YK, Lee HY, Roujeau JC. Epidermal necrolysis: 60 years of errors and advances. Br J Dermatol. 2015;173(5):1250–4.
5. Lin CC, Chen CB, Wang CW, Hung SI, Chung WH. Stevens-Johnson syndrome and toxic epidermal necrolysis: risk factors, causality assessment and potential prevention strategies. Expert Rev Clin Immunol. 2020;16(4):373–87.
6. Roujeau JC, Kelly JP, Naldi L, et al. Medication use and the risk of Stevens-Johnson syndrome or toxic epidermal necrolysis. N Engl J Med. 1995;333:1600–7.
7. Eginli A, Shah K, Watkins C, Krishnaswamy G. Stevens-Johnson syndrome and toxic epidermal necrolysis. Ann Allergy Asthma Immunol. 2017;118(2):143–7.
8. Roujeau JC, Stern RS. Severe adverse cutaneous reactions to drugs. N Engl J Med. 1994;331(19):1272–85.
9. Schwartz RA, McDonough PH, Lee BW. Toxic epidermal necrolysis: part I. introduction, history, classification, clinical features, systemic manifestations, etiology, and immunopathogenesis. J Am Acad Dermatol. 2013;69(2):173.e1–186.
10. Power WJ, Ghoraishi M, Merayo-Lloves J, et al. Analysis of the acute ophthalmic manifestations of the erythema multiforme/Stevens-Johnson syndrome/toxic epidermal necrolysis disease spectrum. Ophthalmology. 1995;102:1669–76.

11. Chang Y, Huang F, Tseng S, et al. Erythema multiforme, Stevens Johnson syndrome, and toxic epidermal necrolysis: acute ocular manifestations, causes, and management. Cornea. 2007;26:123–9.
12. Kohanim S, Palioura S, Saeed HN, et al. Acute and chronic ophthalmic involvement in Stevens-Johnson syndrome/toxic epidermal necrolysis - a comprehensive review and guide to therapy. II. Ophthalmic disease. Ocul Surf. 2016;14(2):168–88.
13. Gregory DG. The ophthalmologic management of acute Stevens-Johnson syndrome. Ocul Surf. 2008;6(2):87–95.
14. Di Pascuale MA, Espana EM, Liu DT, et al. Correlation of corneal complications with eyelid cicatricial pathologies in patients with Stevens-Johnson syndrome and toxic epidermal necrolysis syndrome. Ophthalmology. 2005;112:904–12.
15. Schneck J, Fagot JP, Sekula P, Sassolas B, Roujeau JC, Mockenhaupt M. Effects of treatments on the mortality of Stevens-Johnson syndrome and toxic epidermal necrolysis: a retrospective study on patients included in the prospective EuroSCAR study. J Am Acad Dermatol. 2008;58(1):33–40.
16. De Rojas MV, Dart JK, Saw VP. The natural history of Stevens–Johnson syndrome: patterns of chronic ocular disease and the role systemic immunosuppressive therapy. Br J Ophthalmol. 2007;91:1048–53.
17. Ciralsky JB, Sippel KC, Gregory DG. Current ophthalmologic treatment strategies for acute and chronic Stevens-Johnson syndrome and toxic epidermal necrolysis. Curr Opin Ophthalmol. 2013;24(4):321–8.
18. Gregory DG. New grading system and treatment guidelines for the acute ocular manifestations of Stevens-Johnson syndrome. Ophthalmology. 2016;123(8):1653–8.
19. Kolomeyer AM, Do BK, Tu Y, Chu DS. Placement of ProKera in the management of ocular manifestations of acute Stevens-Johnson syndrome in an outpatient. Eye Contact Lens. 2013;39(3):e7–e11.
20. Hsu M, Jayaram A, Verner R, Lin A, Bouchard C. Indications and outcomes of amniotic membrane transplantation in the management of acute Stevens-Johnson syndrome and toxic epidermal necrolysis: a case-control study. Cornea. 2012;31(12):1394–402.
21. Sharma N, Thenarasun SA, Kaur M, et al. Adjuvant role of amniotic membrane transplantation in acute ocular Stevens-Johnson syndrome: a randomized control trial. Ophthalmology. 2016;123(3):484–91.
22. Ma KN, Thanos A, Chodosh J, Shah AS, Mantagos IS. A novel technique for amniotic membrane transplantation in patients with acute Stevens-Johnson syndrome. Ocul Surf. 2016;14(1):31–6.
23. Tseng SC. Acute management of Stevens-Johnson syndrome and toxic epidermal necrolysis to minimize ocular seque. Am J Ophthalmol. 2009;147(6):949–51.
24. Kobayashi A, Yoshita T, Sugiyama K, et al. Amniotic membrane transplantation in acute phase of toxic epidermal necrolysis with severe corneal involvement. Ophthalmology. 2006;113:126–32.
25. Gregory DG. Treatment of acute Stevens-Johnson syndrome and toxic epidermal necrolysis using amniotic membrane: a review of 10 consecutive cases. Ophthalmology. 2011;118(5):908–14.

Corneal Emergencies Associated with Other Intraocular Surgeries

18

Manpreet Kaur, Sridevi Nair, and Jeewan S. Titiyal

18.1 Introduction

Ophthalmic surgeries have become increasingly safe over the decades with advancing technology, evolving surgical techniques, and advances in surgical training. Cornea-related complications may be observed in association with any intraocular surgery, including phacoemulsification, glaucoma surgeries, strabismus surgeries, lid and oculoplasty surgeries, and vitreoretinal surgeries. Majority of the corneal complications are minor and self-resolving in nature, including superficial abrasions and epithelial defects. Corneal emergencies after other intraocular surgeries are rare; however, timely diagnosis and management is imperative to prevent irreversible sequelae including corneal decompensation and scarring. We herein describe the corneal emergencies that may be observed after other intraocular surgeries, associated risk factors, their diagnosis, management, and preventive measures.

18.2 Corneal Emergencies in Cataract Surgery

Cataract surgery is one of the most commonly performed ophthalmic surgeries. Minor complications such as postoperative corneal edema, corneal abrasions, and epithelial defects are commonly observed especially with inexperienced surgeons. Rarely, corneal emergencies that require urgent management may occur, including acute corneal clouding, Descemet membrane detachment, toxic anterior segment syndrome with corneal endothelial toxicity, and clear corneal incision-related complications. It is imperative to recognize these complications and institute

M. Kaur (✉) · S. Nair · J. S. Titiyal
Cornea, Cataract and Refractive Surgery Services, Dr. Rajendra Prasad Centre for Ophthalmic Sciences, All India Institute of Medical Sciences, New Delhi, India

B. Sharma, J. S. Titiyal (eds.), *Corneal Emergencies*,
https://doi.org/10.1007/978-981-16-5876-1_18

appropriate treatment at the earliest to prevent sight-threatening visual and anatomical sequelae.

18.2.1 Descemet Membrane Tears and Detachment

Descemet membrane detachment (DMD) and tears may occur after any intraocular surgery but are most commonly associated with phacoemulsification (Fig. 18.1a). Incision-site DMD has been reported in 25–82% of cases undergoing phacoemulsification [1–3].

18.2.1.1 Predisposing Factors

Various instrument-related factors, surgeon factors, ocular and systemic co-morbidities predispose to the formation of wound-site DMD [4, 5]. Use of blunt keratomes to make the corneal incisions results in a ragged morphology of the incision and predisposes to DMD. Excessive surgical manipulations, prolonged phacoemulsification time, increased ultrasound energy, repeated entry into the anterior chamber with instruments or phacoemulsification probe, and surgeon inexperience increase the likelihood of developing DMD. Ocular pathologies including Fuchs' endothelial dystrophy, corneal scars, corneal injuries, and healed keratitis can lead to the formation of DMD during an otherwise uneventful cataract surgery. Old age and deep-set eyes with narrow palpebral fissures are risk factors for development of wound-site DMD.

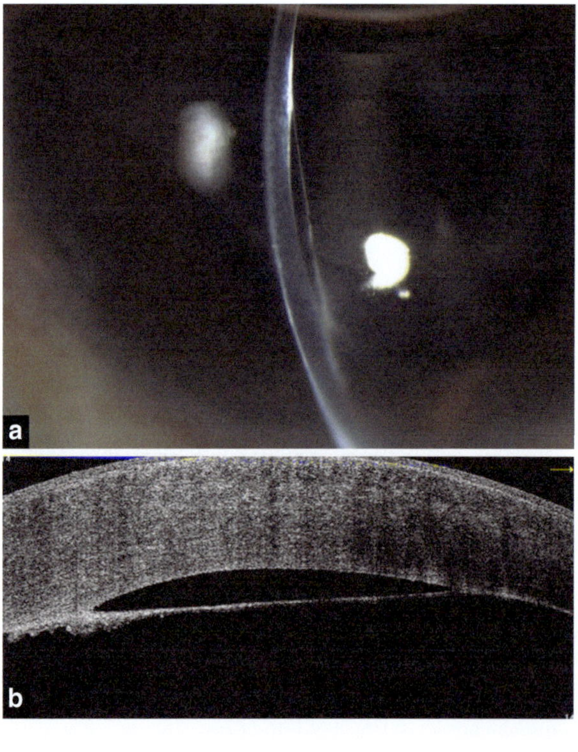

Fig. 18.1 Descemet Membrane Detachment (DMD) observed after phacoemulsification. (**a**) Slit-lamp examination showing Descemet membrane detachment involving the visual axis. (**b**) Anterior segment OCT can be used to assess the height and extent of DMD

18.2.1.2 Diagnosis

Intraoperatively, DMD may be directly visualized under the operating microscope. Intraoperative optical coherence tomography (iOCT) helps in the diagnosis and management of on-table DMD by providing a real-time visualization of the corneal ultrastructure even in the presence of overlying stromal edema.

Postoperatively, slit-lamp biomicroscopy can help visualize the detached Descemet membrane. Anterior segment optical coherence tomography (ASOCT) is a useful adjunct to monitor the location and extent of DMD and the effect of treatment (Fig. 18.1b). Ultrasound biomicroscopy (UBM) helps in the visualization of DMD in hazy corneas and guides surgical management; however, it is technician-dependent and time consuming as compared with ASOCT.

18.2.1.3 Management

Various classification systems have been proposed to differentiate different types of DMD and help in decision-making regarding management [5]. Mackool et al. classified DMD as planar or non-planar, based on the height of separation of the DM from stroma [6]. Kumar et al. developed the HELP algorithm for classification and management of DMD based on ASOCT, wherein DMD was classified based on the height, extend, chord length, and relation to pupil [7].

The management of DMD may be conservative or surgical based on the morphological characteristics of DMD and involvement of the visual axis (Fig. 18.2).

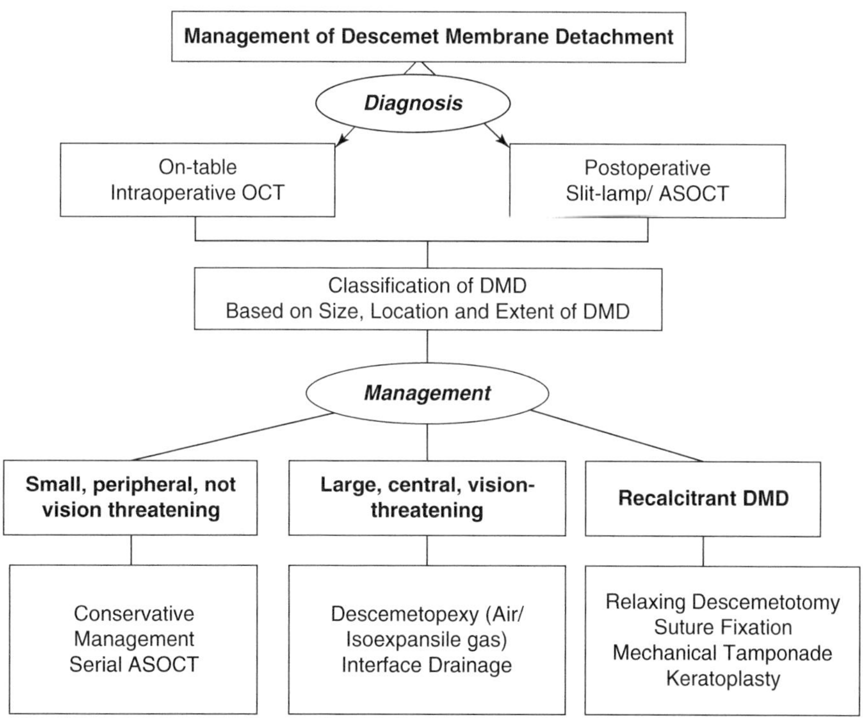

Fig. 18.2 Management algorithm for Descemet membrane detachment

Conservative management is advocated for small peripheral DMD localized to the incision-site, with <1 mm separation of the DM from the stroma. Descemetopexy is the gold standard for management of large DMDs involving the visual axis or cases not responding to conservative management [5]. Descemetopexy refers to the intracameral injection of air or isoexpansile gases (SF6 or C3F8) to tamponade the detached DM and promote its re-attachment. Gas or air is injected via a cannula through an anterior chamber paracentesis incision or directly using a 26/30 G needle while ensuring that the site of entry is located opposite to the area of DMD. A single continuous bubble is injected intracamerally after decompressing the anterior chamber by releasing some aqueous. The aim of descemtopexy is to fill at least 2/3rds of the AC with the gas or air bubble, approximately 8 mm in diameter and providing adequate tamponade to the involved area with DMD. Postoperatively, a supine position is advocated to facilitate the appropriate positioning and tamponade effect of the air/gas bubble [5]. Interface drainage of fluid may be required in large DMDs. A relaxing descemetotomy may be performed in taut DMDs to release the traction. In cases with bullous DMD refractory to pneumatic descemetopexy, performing an adjunctive relaxing descemetotomy can promote DM re-attachment by facilitating the drainage of the supra-descemetic fluid. A keratome may be used to incise the Descemet membrane while performing a descemetotomy. Rarely, persistent cases may require mechanical tamponade using OVDs or suture-fixation of DM. Suture fixation of DMD is performed by passing a full-thickness transcorneal 10-0 nylon suture which hitches the Descemet to the cornea [5]. Patients undergoing mechanical tamponade with OVDs are at a risk for postoperative intraocular pressure (IOP) spikes and should be prescribed prophylactic anti-glaucoma medications. Endothelial keratoplasty is reserved for cases of recalcitrant DMD with significant endothelial cell loss, whereas a full-thickness keratoplasty may be required in cases of long-standing DMD with stromal scarring.

18.2.1.4 Prevention

DMD may be prevented by using sharp non-reusable surgical keratomes and proper incision construction. Femtosecond laser assisted cataract surgery (FLACS) is associated with superior wound construction and decreased incision-site DMD as compared with conventional phacoemulsification. Increasing surgeon experience and skills helps to minimize the incidence of postoperative DMD.

18.2.2 Acute Corneal Clouding

Acute corneal clouding during phacoemulsification precludes intraoperative visualization and requires urgent management in order to allow the surgery to progress and prevent complications.

18.2.2.1 Predisposing Factors

Intracameral injection of the wrong concentration of drug, contaminated or wrong solution may result in acute toxicity to the corneal endothelium with immediate clouding. Acute clouding of the cornea has been reported after injection of an inappropriate mixture of Miochol as well as after accidental substitution of BSS by distilled water. Inadvertent intrastromal injection of trypan blue dye can lead to corneal staining and clouding [8].

18.2.2.2 Diagnosis

Acute clouding or staining of the cornea may be visualized directly under the operating microscope with an impairment of visualization of the anterior segment structures. Anterior segment optical coherence tomography (ASOCT) can help to monitor the corneal thickness and rule out any Descemet membrane detachment postoperatively [9].

18.2.2.3 Management

Immediate intracameral lavage with BSS is indicated in cases of acute corneal clouding due to the instillation of wrong solutions or drugs. Surgery should be abandoned in cases with persistent clouding and impaired visualization. Inadvertent trypan blue staining of the corneal stroma may spontaneously resolve over time with conservative management alone [8, 9].

18.2.2.4 Prevention

Proper labeling of all intraocular medications and solutions and good communication between the members of the surgical team can help minimize wrong intracameral injections. Good depth perception, surgical training, and use of sharp keratomes to make corneal incisions can help prevent inadvertent intrastromal injections of dye or BSS [8, 9].

18.2.3 Corneal Endothelial Toxicity and Toxic Anterior Segment Syndrome

Toxic anterior segment syndrome (TASS) refers to acute-onset postoperative sterile anterior segment inflammation that often results in corneal endothelial toxicity and decompensation. It is a rare complication with an incidence of 0.22% reported in large case series and is most commonly observed after phacoemulsification (Fig. 18.3) [10].

18.2.3.1 Predisposing Factors

TASS results from a toxic insult to the anterior segment structures and may be associated with inappropriate pH, osmolality, concentration and chemical composition of intraocular solutions, preservatives, intraocular medications, intraocular lenses, and ophthalmic viscosurgical devices (OVDs) [11]. Improper cleaning of ophthalmic instruments is most commonly implicated in TASS, which may lead to the introduction of bacterial endotoxins, detergents, denatured OVDs, and other impurities into the eye [10–12].

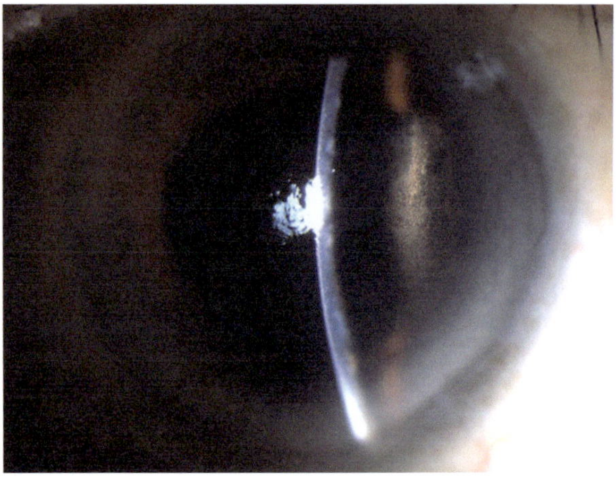

Fig. 18.3 Post-surgical toxic anterior segment syndrome (TASS) with limbus to limbus microcystic edema, Descemet membrane folds, iris pigments on endothelium, and iris chafing

18.2.3.2 Diagnosis

The diagnosis of TASS is established clinically based on the classical presentation of limbus to limbus corneal edema with severe anterior segment inflammation, presenting within 12–48 h of an uneventful cataract surgery. Severe fibrinous reaction may be observed in the anterior chamber with extensive pigment dispersion [11]. A hypopyon may be seen in severe cases.

Infectious endophthalmitis is the most important differential diagnosis and should be ruled out before starting treatment. In contrast to TASS, endophthalmitis usually presents 2–7 days after surgery, often associated with pain, significant vitritis is present and culture of vitreous may be positive. TASS has a more acute presentation with absence of vitritis and is always culture negative.

18.2.3.3 Management

TASS is a corneal emergency as a delay in diagnosis and timely institution of appropriate management may result in irreversible endothelial toxicity, corneal decompensation, and stromal scarring. Topical steroids are the mainstay of management and frequent round the clock instillation is recommended in the initial period. A potent steroid such as 1% prednisolone acetate or dexamethasone 0.1% may be used. The steroids are gradually tapered once the inflammation subsides. Fluctuations in IOP may occur and anti-glaucoma therapy is required to manage IOP spikes.

Endothelial or full-thickness keratoplasty may be required in cases with significant endothelial cell loss and corneal decompensation.

18.2.3.4 Prevention

Preservative free medications and intraocular irrigating solutions should be used. Training of the surgical staff and promoting awareness can help to prevent outbreaks of TASS. The most important preventive measure is proper cleaning and sterilization of the surgical instruments. Various guidelines have been formulated for instrument cleaning and sterilization by international ophthalmological societies which may be followed to minimize the incidence of intraocular contamination and TASS [13].

18.2.4 Clear-Corneal Incision Related Complications

Clear corneal incisions made during phacoemulsification may be associated with various complications that require emergent management to maintain the integrity of the wound and intraocular stability. Wound burns with contraction of the incision may be observed, making it difficult to adequately seal the incision at the end of surgery. Pre-existing corneal scars or radial keratotomy incisions may dehisce during phacoemulsification. In addition, clear-corneal incision-related infections have been reported [14, 15].

18.2.4.1 Predisposing Factors

Wound burn and incision contracture are observed due to thermal damage of the cornea and shrinkage of collagen fibers, which results from use of excessive ultrasound energy, prolonged phacoemulsification times, inadequate flow of fluid through the sleeve, tight incisions and kinking of the sleeve [16].

Improper incision construction and excessive intraocular manipulations leading to wound distortion can complicate effective wound-sealing after phacoemulsification. Multiple deep RK incisions are prone to rupture or dehiscence during phacoemulsification.

Incision-related infections are rare after cataract surgery, and predisposing factors include ocular co-morbidities such as an obstructed nasolacrimal duct, systemic co-morbidities including diabetes mellitus and immunosuppression, environmental contamination by fungal spores, and iatrogenic factors including inadequate instrument sterilization [15].

18.2.4.2 Diagnosis

Wound burn with incision contracture is diagnosed by the presence of a white coagulated wound with fish-mouthing, wound leak, and an unstable anterior chamber.

Dehiscence or rupture of RK incisions can be directly visualized under the operating microscope with irrigating fluids and/or aqueous leaking from the involved site.

Leaky wound can be diagnosed by the inability to form the anterior chamber after hydrating the wound. Aqueous may be seen leaking from the clear corneal incision, and a fluorescein stain may be applied on the surface of the wound to confirm the diagnosis.

Corneal infiltrates at the wound-site with anterior chamber reaction is observed in incision-related infections. Corneal scraping is performed to obtain infective material for definitive microbiological diagnosis.

18.2.4.3 Management

Wound burns, leaky wounds, and ruptured RK incisions need to be sutured to restore the anatomical integrity of the eye. Multiple interrupted 10-0 MFN sutures are required in cases with incision contracture due to wound burns. Use of tissue adhesives to seal the wound and bandage contact lens in the postoperative period are useful adjuncts in difficult cases. Ruptured RK incision should be repaired by placing 10-0 MFN interrupted sutures oriented perpendicular to the RK incision before proceeding with the cataract surgery.

Wound-site infection should be managed along the lines of infective keratitis with intensive broad-spectrum fortified topical antibiotics and cycloplegics. The antibiotic therapy should be tailored to the specific micro-organism based on the culture and sensitivity reports.

18.2.4.4 Prevention

Proper incision construction with sharp keratomes and avoiding instrument-incision mismatch helps prevent wound-related complications and wound leak. Adequate flow of irrigating solutions via the phacoemulsification sleeves to cool the ultrasound probe helps minimize heat build-up and protects against thermal burns.

Ocular and systemic co-morbidities must be adequately managed in the preoperative period to prevent wound-site infections. Proper incision construction and well-sealed wounds help to prevent ingress of contaminated material in the postoperative period and protect against localized infection. Instrument sterilization protocols must be adhered to strictly. A clear corneal incision should be avoided in challenging cases such as cataract with prior RK, iridofundal colobomas, and limbal stem cell deficiency and a posterior limbal or scleral incision may be preferred in these cases.

18.3 Corneal Emergencies in Glaucoma Surgeries

All glaucoma surgeries including canaloplasty, trabeculectomy, and glaucoma drainage devices may adversely affect the cornea. Corneal complications after glaucoma surgeries range from mild epithelial abrasions and transient postoperative edema to sight-threatening complications including corneal-tube touch, endothelial decompensation, and Descemet membrane detachment. Glaucoma drainage devices are associated with the highest incidence of post-surgical corneal complications. An urgent management is often required to prevent permanent visual loss and restore anatomical integrity.

18.3.1 Descemet Membrane Detachment

DMD is a relatively rare but sight-threatening complication that may be observed after various glaucoma surgeries, including canaloplasty, trabeculectomy, and implantation of glaucoma drainage devices [17–21]. It is more commonly reported after canaloplasty as compared with trabeculectomy. A meta-analysis of 28 studies reported DMD in 3.1% cases undergoing canaloplasty, with no report of DMD in cases undergoing trabeculectomy [18]. Jaramillo et al. observed DMD in7.4% of cases after canaloplasty; of these, 58% were hemorrhagic DMDs, majority were located in inferior quadrant and 83% were <3 mm in size sparing the visual axis [17].

18.3.1.1 Predisposing Factors

Predisposing factors for the development of DMD after glaucoma surgeries include anatomical factors such as a shallow anterior chamber or weak adhesions between the DM and stroma due to genetic predisposition. Iatrogenic factors for DMD include the use of blunt microkeratomes, shelved incisions, inadvertent intrastromal injection of saline or OVDs leading to a separation of the DM from the stroma or accidental insertion of surgical instruments in the potential space between the stroma and the DM [6, 21].

During canaloplasty, excessive OVD injection may gain access to the pre-descemetic space due to a weakness in the canal wall in the inferior quadrant, leading to characteristic inferior DMDs [17]. Intracorneal hemorrhage during visco-dilation of the Schlemm's canal may lead to the development of hemorrhagic DMD [17].

18.3.1.2 Diagnosis

It may be difficult to establish a timely diagnosis of DMD as corneal edema is frequently observed in the postoperative period after glaucoma surgeries, and there is a low index of suspicion.

Anterior segment optical coherence tomography (ASOCT) is an excellent non-invasive investigative modality that can help to establish the diagnosis of DMD after glaucoma surgeries even in the presence of significant corneal edema. Confocal microscopy is a useful adjunct to assess the corneal ultrastructural changes due to DMD and loss of endothelial cells [21]. Ultrasound biomicroscopy (UBM) may also be used to establish the diagnosis of DMD [21].

18.3.1.3 Management

Timely diagnosis and management of DMD is an emergency as untreated or mismanaged cases may progress to corneal scarring, endothelial decompensation, and loss of vision. The management is based on the size, location, and extent of DMD. Small planar DMDs of <3 mm size located peripherally may be managed conservatively by observation alone. Surgical management including descemetopexy or suture-fixation is often required for large DMDs in the visual axis.

The management of DMD after glaucoma surgeries is challenging as achieving adequate tamponade of the Descemet's membrane may be difficult in the presence of a filtering bleb or tube. Multiple injections of air, gas, and OVD may be required for successful re-attachment of DMD post-trabeculectomy [21]. Drainage of interface fluid along with suture-fixation of the DM and viscoelastic tamponade has been reported [22]. Co-existent choroidal effusion and shallow AC may require transconjunctival suturing of the scleral flap to close the functional bleb in conjunction with choroidal tap and DM tamponade with 20% SF6 [20].

Long-standing DMD may induce significant corneal scarring and keratoplasty may be required for visual rehabilitation. Endothelial or penetrating keratoplasty is also required in cases with corneal decompensation following DMD.

18.3.1.4 Prevention

Post-surgical DMD may be minimized by avoiding the use of blunt surgical instruments and performing careful surgical manipulations. Excessive and forceful OVD injection during visco-dilation may be avoided.

18.3.2 Tube Migration with Tube-Corneal Touch

Glaucoma drainage devices typically consist of one or more plates to anchor the device to the globe, and a tube inserted in the anterior chamber to provide a conduit for aqueous outflow. The tube may migrate into the AC due to the anterior movement of the anchoring plate and has been reported in 35% cases, with up to 20% cases with an Ahmed glaucoma device developing a tube-corneal touch [23–26].

18.3.2.1 Predisposing Factors

Large buphthalmic eyes are predisposed to develop tube migration with tube-corneal touch [25]. Continued elongation of the globe in pediatric eyes combined with a low scleral rigidity lead to a relative anterior migration of the anchoring plate with increased likelihood of tube-corneal touch. Anterior migration of tube may also result from vigorous eye-rubbing.

18.3.2.2 Diagnosis

Diagnosis of tube migration and tube-corneal touch is usually established on a careful clinical examination using slit-lamp biomicroscopy (Fig. 18.4). Localized corneal decompensation may be present in cases of tube-corneal touch, and an ASOCT or UBM can help to visualize the lumen of the tube and establish its relation to the corneal endothelium in these cases.

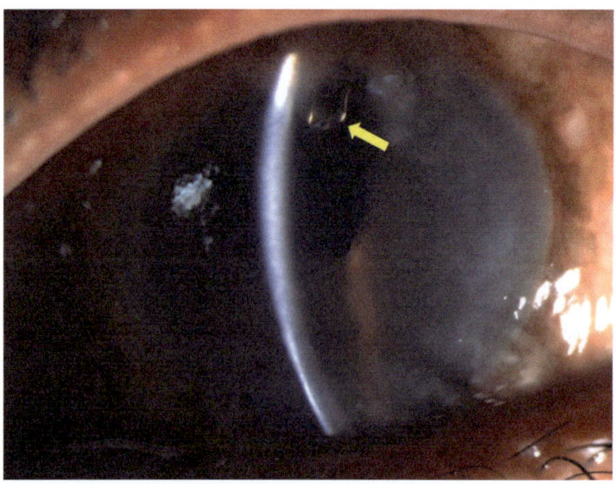

Fig. 18.4 Anterior migration of glaucoma drainage device with tube-corneal touch and endothelial decompensation

18.3.2.3 Management

Management of a tube-corneal touch is an emergency as it results in progressive endothelial cell loss and corneal decompensation. Surgical trimming of the tube is required in cases with a tube-corneal touch, and the plate may need to be anchored more posteriorly. Pars plana implantation of the tube into the vitreous cavity may be considered in cases with difficult anterior segment anatomy and persistent tube-corneal touch.

18.3.2.4 Prevention

The plate should be anchored securely to the sclera using sutures. The anchoring plate along with the external part of tube should be adequately covered by a patch graft if required. A long scleral tunnel should be made to insert the tube into the anterior chamber in a fashion that the tube is parallel to the iris plane. The tube should be positioned as posteriorly as possible in the anterior chamber to prevent an inadvertent tube-corneal touch [27]. Patients should be taught to avoid eye-rubbing. Postoperative regular follow-up is essential to monitor the position of the tube in the anterior chamber and detect any anterior migration of the tube at its earliest.

18.3.3 Blebitis and Keratitis

Bleb-related infections may be limited to the filtering bleb (blebitis), associated with adjacent keratitis or progress to fulminant bleb-related endophthalmitis [28]. They may occur after glaucoma-filtration surgeries including trabeculectomy and combined trabeculectomy + trabeculectomy with the formation of a bleb. Children are more frequently affected with an incidence ranging from 0% to 17% [29, 30].

18.3.3.1 Pathogens

The pathogenic micro-organisms associated with bleb-related infections are more virulent and include *Streptococcus* species, *Staphylococcus*, *Haemophilus influenzae*, and *Pseudomonas aeruginosa* [31].

18.3.3.2 Predisposing Factors

Bleb morphology is most commonly implicated in bleb-related infections, with avascular, thin-walled cystic blebs predisposing to an increased risk of developing blebitis and endophthalmitis. Excessive use of antimetabolites including mitomycin C (MMC) and 5-Fluorouracil (5-FU) is associated with thin avascular blebs postoperatively with an increased risk of developing bleb-related infections [32–34]. Chronic bleb leak, inferior location of filtering bleb after trabeculectomy, use of releasable sutures, ocular surface disorders, use of contact lens, and bacterial conjunctivitis also predispose to the development of bleb-related infections [32, 33]. Systemic co-morbidities such as diabetes mellitus and immunosuppression also increase the risk of infections. Past history of bleb-related infections is associated with a 12-fold increased risk of developing endophthalmitis.

18.3.3.3 Diagnosis

The diagnosis of bleb-related infections is usually established clinically due to the presence of classical signs and symptoms. The patient is usually symptomatic and presents with foreign body sensation, blurring of vision, redness, photophobia, and purulent discharge. Rapid progression of symptoms points towards a more fulminant course and is suggestive of endophthalmitis, with blebitis having a relatively insidious evolution of symptoms over a few days.

Blebitis is indicated by the presence of intense localized conjunctival inflammation surrounding a white thin cystic avascular bleb, resulting in a characteristic "white on red" appearance. Mucopurulent infiltration of the bleb with a purulent discharge is present in advanced blebitis and bleb leak may be observed. Adjacent keratitis may be observed in cases with corneal involvement. Associated vitritis is present in endophthalmitis which may be confirmed by B-scan ultrasonography.

18.3.3.4 Management

Frequent instillation of broad-spectrum topical antimicrobials should be commenced at initial presentation, which may be later tailored based on the culture reports and sensitivity pattern of the causative micro-organism. Systemic antibiotics are recommended in addition to topical medications especially in pediatric cases, and intravenous antibiotics may be required in concomitant endophthalmitis.

After resolution of active infection, bleb revision with excision of the bleb and advancement of the conjunctiva may be required to correct the underlying cause. Any scleral thinning or a full-thickness sclerostomy evident at the time of the revision should be addressed accordingly. Endophthalmitis, if present, should be adequately managed by a retina specialist with intravitreal injections and/or vitrectomy as required.

18.3.3.5 Prevention

Judicious intraoperative use of antimetabolites may help minimize the incidence of thin cystic blebs and prevent bleb-related infections. It is advisable to bury all releasable sutures and avoid making inferior blebs. Co-existent ocular and systemic co-morbidities should be adequately managed in the preoperative period.

18.4 Corneal Emergencies in Strabismus Surgeries

Complications after strabismus surgeries are uncommon, with corneal complications being extremely rare. Anterior segment ischemia is an extremely rare, sight-threatening complication that may be observed after strabismus surgeries. It involves the entire anterior segment including the cornea.

18.4.1 Anterior Segment Ischemia

The incidence of anterior segment ischemia is 1 in 13,000 cases [35]. It is most commonly associated with strabismus surgeries.

18.4.1.1 Predisposing Factors

The most significant factor associated with the development of anterior segment ischemia is surgery on 3–4 recti muscles in the same sitting compromising the anterior segment circulation. The interruption of anterior ciliary arteries may be accompanied by the interruption of deep episcleral collateral vessels, leading to hypoperfusion of the anterior segment, tissue hypoxia, and inflammation. Other predisposing factors for the development of anterior segment ischemia include advanced age, past history of rectus muscle surgery, and a history of vasculopathy such as diabetes or hypertension [35, 36].

18.4.1.2 Diagnosis

Diagnosis of mild cases of anterior segment ischemia may be established based on iris fluorescein angiography findings of reduced iris perfusion. Severe cases may be diagnosed clinically based on a spectrum of findings including changes in pupil shape and reactivity, postoperative uveitis, cataract, keratopathy, hypotony, loss of vision, and even phthisis bulbi [36].

18.4.1.3 Management

Intensive corticosteroids are the mainstay of management of anterior segment ischemia. Mild manifestations may be managed by topical steroids alone, whereas oral or intravenous corticosteroids are required for severe disease [36]. In addition, cycloplegics are prescribed to prevent synechiae, hypertonic saline to manage corneal edema and anti-glaucoma medications for IOP management, if required.

18.4.1.4 Prevention

The number of rectus muscles operated upon during strabismus surgeries should be limited, and three or four muscle surgeries involving the rectus muscles should be avoided. Techniques to preserve anterior ciliary arteries may be performed to minimize the risk of anterior segment ischemia [36, 37].

18.5 Corneal Emergencies in Ocular Surface, Lid and Orbital Surgeries

Ocular surface, lid and orbital surgeries often result in minor corneal epithelial abrasions and defects, which resolve spontaneously with conservative management. Rarely, corneal perforation may be observed which is an ocular emergency.

18.5.1 Corneal Perforation

Corneal perforation is an extremely rare complication that has been reported after laser blepharoplasty [38]. Excessive corneal thinning with inadvertent full-thickness dissection may be observed during lamellar dissection performed in various ocular surface surgeries, including pterygium surgeries, dermoid excision, or excision of ocular surface squamous neoplasms [39].

18.5.1.1 Predisposing Factors

Corneal perforation has been reported after laser blepharoplasty due to the elevation of cornea superior to the protective corneal shields during laser application [38]. The Bell's phenomenon leads to up-rolling of the eye on closure, which explained the exposure of cornea to the laser beam above the protective shields. Excessive use of laser power and prolonged exposure can lead to inadvertent perforation.

Excessive use of cautery and antimitotic agents and aggressive lamellar dissection can lead to inadvertent limbal perforation during pterygium excision, dermoid excision, or other ocular surface surgeries.

18.5.1.2 Management

The management of corneal perforations is based on the size of perforation. Tissue adhesives with bandage contact lens may be used to manage small perforations. Patch graft may be needed for larger perforations.

18.5.1.3 Prevention

Preoperative investigations including ASOCT and UBM can help to assess the depth of lesions and corneal thickness and aid in proper surgical planning. Intraoperative OCT provides a real-time assessment of the residual stromal bed and helps prevent inadvertent perforation. Laser power and corneal protection should be checked before application.

18.6 Corneal Emergencies in Vitreoretinal Surgeries

Corneal complications during vitreoretinal surgeries interfere with adequate visualization of the posterior segment and impede the surgical steps. Corneal clouding and epithelial damage are frequently observed during vitreoretinal surgeries. An urgent management is necessary to restore corneal clarity and successfully complete the vitreoretinal procedure. In addition, any corneal wound may dehisce or leak due to the intraocular pressure fluctuations that occur during these surgeries and need to be managed adequately. Anterior segment ischemia may rarely be observed after 360 degrees buckling surgeries, and has been described in detail in the earlier section.

18.6.1 Corneal Clouding

Corneal clouding may be observed during pneumatic retinopexy, buckling surgery or pars plana vitrectomy and impedes posterior segment visualization.

18.6.1.1 Predisposing Factors

Corneal edema may be observed in combined procedures with phacoemulsification and pars plana vitrectomy. Epithelial damage can result from trauma due to the irrigating lens/wire vectis, low quality irrigating fluids, or excessive scraping of the corneal epithelium during surgery. In addition, frequent IOP fluctuations during surgery with high IOP spikes can cause corneal clouding.

18.6.1.2 Diagnosis

Haziness of the cornea can be directly visualized under the operating microscope. Epithelial defects may be present.

18.6.1.3 Management

Rolling of the cornea with cotton tips or gently scraping off the epithelium can help improve visualization through cloudy corneas.

18.6.1.4 Prevention

Good surgical skills with gentle intraocular manipulations can help minimize corneal clouding. Staged phacoemulsification and pars plana vitrectomy procedures may be preferred rather than combined surgery, especially in complicated cases.

18.6.2 Wound Leak

Wound leak or gape of clear corneal incisions can be observed during retinal surgeries due to the increased pressure on the cornea. A leaky or gaping wound interferes with surgery and needs to be managed immediately.

18.6.2.1 Predisposing Factors

Clear corneal incisions made during combined procedures are more likely to dehisce, especially while inserting the pars plana ports. Excessive pressure exerted by the wide-angle or irrigating lens can lead to wound dehiscence.

18.6.2.2 Diagnosis

Corneal folds with a flat anterior chamber point towards wound leak and hypotony. Aqueous leak can be visualized from the site of dehiscence.

18.6.2.3 Management

Corneal hydration is ineffective in adequately sealing the incision during retinal surgeries, and all corneal incisions should be sutured. Multiple sutures may be required.

18.6.2.4 Prevention

Suture clear corneal incisions if phacoemulsification has been performed recently. Undue pressure on the cornea with the wide-angle lens/irrigating contact lens should be avoided.

18.7 Conclusion

Corneal emergencies may be observed after any intraocular surgery, including phacoemulsification, glaucoma surgeries, strabismus surgeries, oculoplasty procedures, and vitreoretinal surgeries. Emergent management of these complications is essential for two reasons—firstly, corneal involvement precludes adequate visualization of the intraocular structures and hampers the surgical procedure. Secondly, delay in timely diagnosis and management can lead to vision-threatening sequelae including corneal scarring, endothelial decompensation, corneal perforation, and even phthisis bulbi. It is essential for ophthalmic surgeons to be aware of the potential corneal complications that may occur during other intraocular surgeries, take preventive measures to minimize their incidence and adequately manage the corneal emergencies.

Key Points

- Corneal emergencies may be observed after any intraocular surgery, including phacoemulsification, glaucoma surgeries, strabismus surgeries, oculoplasty procedures, and vitreoretinal surgeries.
- Prompt diagnosis and appropriate management is essential to prevent long-term sequelae such as corneal decompensation or scarring.
- Descemet membrane detachment is a commonly encountered corneal emergency in patients undergoing phacoemulsification.
- Management of DMD is based on the size, location, and extent of DMD. Anterior segment optical coherence tomography is a useful adjunct for the timely diagnosis of DMD, classification and formulation of management algorithm.
- Post-surgical TASS often shows a dramatic response to steroid therapy and needs to be differentiated from endophthalmitis.
- Glaucoma drainage devices are associated with a high risk of corneal complications including Descemet membrane detachment, progressive endothelial cell loss, and endothelial decompensation.
- Managing DMD after glaucoma surgeries is more challenging as the presence of a filtering bleb/tube facilitates the escape of air/gas bubble from the anterior chamber.
- Corneal complications after strabismus, oculoplasty, and vitreoretinal surgeries are relatively uncommon and include anterior segment ischemia, accidental corneal perforation, corneal clouding, and wound leak.

Financial Disclosures and Conflicts of Interest No author has any financial interest in the study. There are no relevant conflicts of interest for any author.

References

1. Calladine D, Tanner V. Optical coherence tomography of the effects of stromal hydration on clear corneal incision architecture. J Cataract Refract Surg. 2009;35:1367–71.
2. Xia Y, Liu X, Luo L, et al. Early changes in clear cornea incision after phacoemulsification: an anterior segment optical coherence tomography study. Acta Ophthalmol. 2009;87:764–8.
3. Sharma N, Bandivadekar P, Agarwal T, et al. Incision-site Descemet membrane detachment during and after phacoemulsification: risk factors and management. Eye Contact Lens. 2015;41:273–6.
4. Titiyal JS, Kaur M, Ramesh P, et al. Impact of clear corneal incision morphology on incision-site Descemet membrane detachment in conventional and femtosecond laser-assisted phacoemulsification. Curr Eye Res. 2018;43:293–9.
5. Singhal D, Sahay P, Goel S, et al. Descemet membrane detachment. Surv Ophthalmol. 2020;65:279–93.
6. Mackool RJ, Holtz SJ. Descemet membrane detachment. Arch Ophthalmol. 1977;95:459–63.
7. Kumar DA, Agarwal A, Sivanganam S, Chandrasekar R. Height-, extent-, length-, and pupil-based (HELP) algorithm to manage post-phacoemulsification Descemet membrane detachment. J Cataract Refract Surg. 2015;41:1945–53.
8. Jhanji V, Agarwal T, Titiyal JS. Inadvertent corneal stromal staining by trypan blue during cataract surgery. J Cataract Refract Surg. 2008;34:161–2.
9. Nandini C, Matalia H, Zameer L, Matalia J. Corneal staining during cataract surgery: natural course, ASOCT features, and preventive measures. Indian J Ophthalmol. 2019;67:557.
10. Sengupta S, Chang DF, Gandhi R, et al. Incidence and long-term outcomes of toxic anterior segment syndrome at Aravind Eye Hospital. J Cataract Refract Surg. 2011;37:1673–8.
11. Mamalis N, Edelhauser HF, Dawson DG, et al. Toxic anterior segment syndrome. J Cataract Refract Surg. 2006;32:324–33.
12. Bodnar Z, Clouser S, Mamalis N. Toxic anterior segment syndrome: update on the most common causes. J Cataract Refract Surg. 2012;38:1902–10.
13. American Society of Cataract and Refractive Surgery, American Society of Ophthalmic Registered Nurses, Hellinger WC, et al. Recommended practices for cleaning and sterilizing intraocular surgical instruments. J Cataract Refract Surg. 2007;33:1095–100.
14. Cosar CB, Cohen EJ, Rapuano CJ, Laibson PR. Clear corneal wound infection after phacoemulsification. Arch Ophthalmol. 2001;119:1755–9.
15. Valenton M. Wound infection after cataract surgery. Jpn J Ophthalmol. 1996;40:447–55.
16. Sorensen T, Chan CC, Bradley M, et al. Ultrasound-induced corneal incision contracture survey in the United States and Canada. J Cataract Refract Surg. 2012;38:227–33.
17. Jaramillo A, Foreman J, Ayyala RS. Descemet membrane detachment after Canaloplasty: incidence and management. J Glaucoma. 2014;23:351–4.
18. Zhang B, Kang J, Chen X. A system review and meta-analysis of canaloplasty outcomes in glaucoma treatment in comparison with trabeculectomy. J Ophthalmol. 2017;2017:2723761.
19. Wimmersberger Y, Bergin C, Sharkawi E. Reattachment of Descemet's membrane using C3F8 gas in an eye with a Baerveldt aqueous shunt. Klin Monatsbl Augenheilkd. 2013;230:363–4.
20. Sharifipour F, Nassiri S, Idan A. Descemet's membrane detachment management following trabeculectomy. J Ophthalmic Vis Res. 2016;11:323–5.
21. Li Y-H, Shi J-M, Fan F, et al. Descemet membrane detachment after trabeculectomy. Int J Ophthalmol. 2012;5:527–9.
22. Rasouli M, Mather R, Tingey D. Descemet membrane detachment following viscoelastic injection for posttrabeculectomy hypotony. Can J Ophthalmol. 2008;43:254–5.

23. Al-Mobarak F, Khan AO. Two-year survival of Ahmed valve implantation in the first 2 years of life with and without intraoperative mitomycin-C. Ophthalmology. 2009;116:1862–5.
24. Mullaney PB, Selleck C, Al-Awad A, et al. Combined trabeculotomy and trabeculectomy as an initial procedure in uncomplicated congenital glaucoma. Arch Ophthalmol. 1999;117:457–60.
25. Nassiri N, Nouri-Mahdavi K, Coleman AL. Ahmed glaucoma valve in children: a review. Saudi J Ophthalmol. 2011;25:317–27.
26. Hill RA, Heuer DK, Baerveldt G, et al. Molteno implantation for glaucoma in young patients. Ophthalmology. 1991;98:1042–6.
27. Englert JA, Freedman SF, Cox TA. The Ahmed valve in refractory pediatric glaucoma. Am J Ophthalmol. 1999;127:34–42.
28. Parker JS, Dockery PW, Parker JS, et al. Bacteroides Spp. blebitis, keratitis, and endophthalmitis following uncomplicated trabeculectomy. J Glaucoma. 2019;28:e118.
29. Sidoti PA, Belmonte SJ, Liebmann JM, Ritch R. Trabeculectomy with mitomycin-C in the treatment of pediatric glaucomas. Ophthalmology. 2000;107:422–9.
30. Beck AD, Wilson WR, Lynch MG, et al. Trabeculectomy with adjunctive mitomycin C in pediatric glaucoma. Am J Ophthalmol. 1998;126:648–57.
31. Yassin SA. Bleb-related infection revisited: a literature review. Acta Ophthalmol. 2016;94:122–34.
32. Ramakrishnan R, Bharathi MJ, Maheshwari D, et al. Etiology and epidemiological analysis of glaucoma-filtering bleb infections in a tertiary eye care hospital in South India. Indian J Ophthalmol. 2011;59:445.
33. Soltau JB, Rothman RF, Budenz DL, et al. Risk factors for glaucoma filtering bleb infections. Arch Ophthalmol. 2000;118:338–42.
34. Yap ZL, Chin YC, Ku JY-F, et al. Bleb related infections: clinical characteristics, risk factors, and outcomes in an Asian population. Clin Ophthalmol. 2016;10:2303–9.
35. France TD, Simon JW. Anterior segment ischemia syndrome following muscle surgery: the AAPO&S experience. J Pediatr Ophthalmol Strabismus. 1986;23:87–91.
36. Olver JM, Lee JP. Recovery of anterior segment circulation after strabismus surgery in adult patients. Ophthalmology. 1992;99:305–15.
37. Pineles SL, Chang MY, Oltra EL, et al. Anterior segment ischemia: etiology, assessment, and management. Eye (Lond). 2018;32:173–8.
38. Lee S, Moon D, Kang H. Corneal perforation during laser assisted blepharoplasty. Acta Ophthalmol. 2016;94 https://doi.org/10.1111/j.1755-3768.2016.0268.
39. Pirouzian A. Management of pediatric corneal limbal dermoids. Clin Ophthalmol. 2013;7:607–14.

Keratomalacia 19

Deepak Soni, Bhavana Sharma, Priti Singh, and Suraj Kubrey

19.1 Introduction

Keratomalacia constitutes an important corneal emergency in vitamin A deficiency disease, which requires prompt intervention to salvage visual and structural integrity. It is an important cause of preventable corneal blindness with a reported incidence varying between 8% and 27.3% [1, 2]. Retinol is essential for the production of visual pigment Rhodopsin by the rod photoreceptors [3]. Mild cases of xerophthalmia present with nyctalopia or night blindness as opposed to those with advanced disease who present with severe grades of ocular surface xerosis and corneal melting. Timely institution of vitamin A therapy in the early stages of the disease leads to rapid response usually within 2 days of initiating treatment [4]. Therefore, early detection and adequate management is critical in preventing progression of disease.

19.2 Clinical Features

The earliest symptom of vitamin A deficiency is impaired dark adaptation. It is characterised by diminished adjustment to vision in the dim light conditions or darker ambience. Impaired dark adaptation is the result of dysfunctional rods and is closely correlated with the serum retinol concentrations. A serum retinol concentration of <1.0 μmol/L is observed to be associated with the initiation of impaired dark adaptation, while its level below 0.35 μmol/L is associated with manifest

D. Soni · B. Sharma (✉) · P. Singh
All India Institute of Medical Sciences, Bhopal, Madhya Pradesh, India
e-mail: head.ophtho@aiimsbhopal.edu.in

S. Kubrey
Gandhi Medical College, Bhopal, Madhya Pradesh, India

B. Sharma, J. S. Titiyal (eds.), *Corneal Emergencies*,
https://doi.org/10.1007/978-981-16-5876-1_19

Table 19.1 World Health Organization (WHO) classification of the clinical signs of xerophthalmia[a]

Classification	Signs
XN	Night blindness
X1A	Conjunctival xerosis
X1B	Bitot's spot
X2	Corneal xerosis
X3A	Corneal ulceration—keratomalacia involving one-third or less of the cornea
X3B	Corneal ulceration—keratomalacia involving equals to or more than one-third of the cornea
XS	Corneal scars
XF	Xerophthalmic fundus

[a]Reprinted with permission. Adapted from Control of vitamin A deficiency and xerophthalmia. Report of a joint WHO/USAID/UNICEF/HKI/IVACG meeting (WHO Technical Report Series, No. 672), Geneva, 1982, World Health Organization

xerophthalmia [5, 6]. Night blindness usually has a very good response to early institution of vitamin A therapy. Prompt and adequate treatment of xerophthalmia may restore almost complete preservation of eyesight and halts further progression of the diseases to advanced stages [4, 7]. Most referred staging system of xerophthalmia as formulated by WHO [4] is described in Table 19.1.

19.2.1 Conjunctival Xerosis (X1A) and Bitot's Spots (X1B)

19.2.1.1 Conjunctival Xerosis

Conjunctival xerosis is a result of squamous metaplasia (columnar to stratified squamous epithelium) of the conjunctival epithelium along with decrease in the number of goblet cells, and the consequent keratinisation of ocular surface.

Clinical features: On slit lamp examination conjunctiva shows one or more patches of dry non-wettable conjunctiva. The typical appearance which is described as 'emerging like sand banks at receding tide' when the child ceases to cry is usually seen in the temporal interpalpebral areas of the conjunctiva [4]. As the disease progresses a complete involvement of the bulbar conjunctiva may be seen with variable degree of conjunctival wrinkling, thickening, and pigmentation.

19.2.1.2 Bitot's Spot

Bitot's spot is an extension of the same xerotic process as in X1A and represents persistent areas of squamous metaplasia.

Clinical Features

Triangular foamy white patches at 3/9 o'clock position of bulbar conjunctiva, more frequently over temporal side (Fig. 19.1). Clinically there are no definitive clinical features to differentiate between active and the inactive lesions. However, active lesions do respond to vitamin A therapy and this is the only way one can differentiate between both.

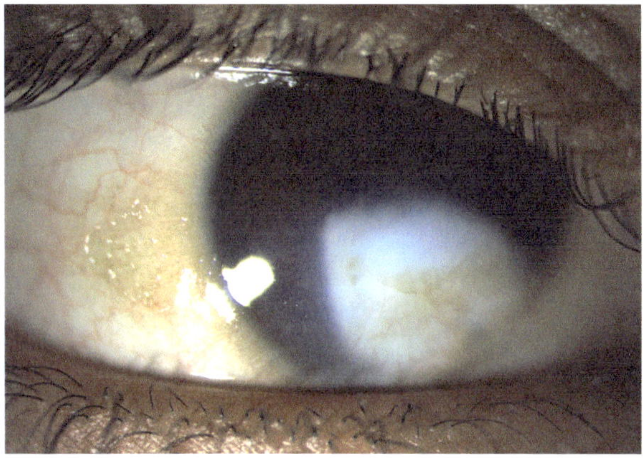

Fig. 19.1 Slit lamp picture showing leucomatous corneal opacity with surface degeneration involving inferior one-third of cornea, extending up to centre, status post keratomalacia. Also seen is the presence of Bitot's spot at 9 o'clock position

Response to Therapy

After the initiation of vitamin A therapy, active conjunctival xerosis begin to resolve within a duration of 2–5 days. With continued vitamin A therapy majority of the signs show complete resolution within a period of 2 weeks. However, a significant proportion of temporal lesions particularly Bitot's spots may persist in shrunken form even after receiving adequate treatment [4, 7].

19.2.2 Corneal Xerosis (X2)

Corneal manifestations begin early in the course of vitamin A deficiency. The earliest change begins usually in the lower nasal quadrant in the form of punctate keratopathy, which can be easily appreciated on slit lamp examination in a fluorescein-stained eye [8]. Corneal xerosis too begins in the inferior sector along with punctate keratopathy and accompanying stromal edema.

Clinical Features

Corneal xerosis presents with a typical dry, lustreless appearance of cornea along with superficial punctuate erosions which later progress to involve the whole cornea. In advanced stages, the corneal surface attains epithelial keratinisation (Fig. 19.2).

Response to Therapy

With the start of vitamin A therapy, the corneal plaques start to peel off, at times leaving a superficial corneal erosion that heals quickly. Treatment to response time usually varies from 2 to 5 days and most of the xerotic changes completely disappear within 1–2 weeks [4, 7].

19.2.3 Corneal Ulceration/Keratomalacia (X3A, X3B)

Keratomalacia, also known as corneal ulceration, is a condition in which a part or all of the corneal stroma shows melting resulting in permanent structural changes.

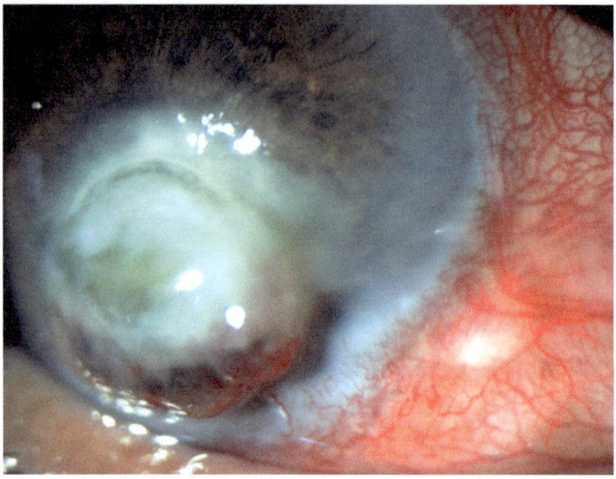

Fig. 19.2 Slit lamp image of keratomalacia stage X3A, showing liquefactive necrosis of inferior one-third of the cornea

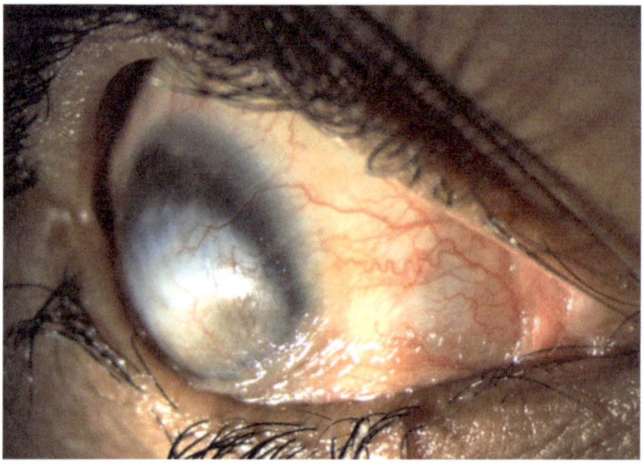

Fig. 19.3 Slit lamp photograph showing vascularised leucomatous corneal opacity with partial anterior staphyloma status post keratomalacia. Also note the wrinkling of inferior bulbar conjunctiva

It involves liquefactive necrosis of corneal layers which result in formation of corneal ulcers involving deep stroma leading to corneal melts; categorised as X3A—keratomalacia involving less than one-third of the corneal surface (Fig. 19.3) and X3B—keratomalacia involving more than one-third of the corneal surface.

Response to Therapy

Role of early vitamin A therapy in treatment of keratomalacia remains limited and varies as per stage. Stage X3A generally spares the pupillary zone, and timely vitamin A therapy usually preserves the functional vision. While a more advanced stage with extensive involvement as seen with stage X3B, especially generalised liquefactive necrosis, remains unresponsive to vitamin A therapy. The further course in such scenario usually results in corneal perforation, extrusion of intraocular contents, and loss of the ocular integrity. However, emergency management and prompt therapy

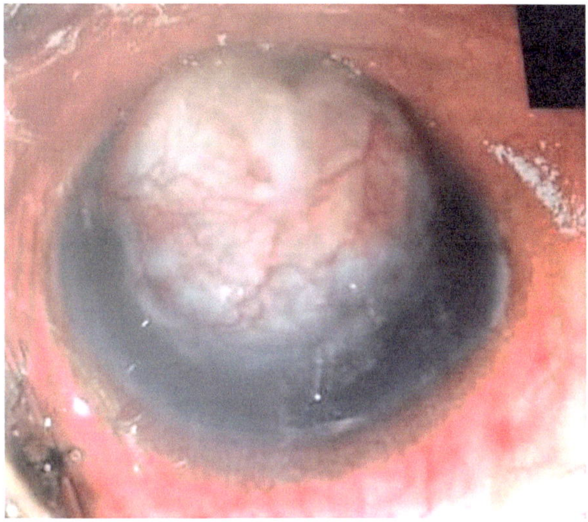

Fig. 19.4 Anterior staphyloma status post vitamin A deficiency induced keratomalacia

may still be able to preserve ocular integrity in preparation for future surgical procedures.

19.2.4 Corneal Scars (XS)

Opacities or scars of different density (nebula, macula, leukoma) and weakening and outpouching of the remaining corneal layers in the form of staphyloma are healed sequelae of past corneal disease associated with vitamin A deficiency (Fig. 19.4).

19.3 Keratomalacia

19.3.1 Pathogenesis

Keratomalacia is a condition marked by specific ocular abnormalities caused by severe vitamin A deficiency, the severity of which is inversely proportional to age. Vitamin A is an integral part of corneal metabolism owing to specific retinol-binding phenomenon seen in the cells of epithelium, keratocytes, and endothelium [9]. Without adequate treatment, increased softening of all or a part of the cornea (keratomalacia) may lead to sight threatening complications and/or sequelae:

- Corneal ulceration,
- Chronic perforation,
- Degenerative tissue changes, e.g., ectasia, staphyloma, and phthisis bulbi (Fig. 19.4).

19.3.2 Associated Corneal Emergencies

19.3.2.1 Corneal Ulceration

Keratomalacia is associated with stromal defects that can take several forms from small to large ulcers. Ulcers are classically round or oval 'punched-out' defects, as if a trephine or cork-borer had been applied to the eye [4]. The surrounding cornea is usually xerotic, but transparent, and does not have the grey, infiltrated appearance of bacterial ulcers. Small ulcers (1–3 mm) are circular in shape with well-marked boundaries and are almost always restricted to the periphery, particularly the inferior and nasal sides. Ulcers can range in depth from shallow to deep. Large ulcers and necrotic zones have a centripetal extension and might affect the entire cornea. In most cases, surface ulcers heal with little scarring, whereas deeper lesions, particularly perforations result in adherent leukomas.

19.3.2.2 Corneal Perforation

Localised keratomalacia may progress rapidly and affect the entire thickness of the cornea. It first shows as a mound or outpouching of the corneal surface that is opaque and grey to yellow. The necrotic stroma sloughs off in advanced cases, forming a large sized ulcer or descemetocele that eventually perforates. Subsequently, iris plugs the perforation with ensuing healing.

19.3.2.3 Secondary Keratitis

Corneal lesions can acquire superimposed secondary microbial infections. In such cases it becomes difficult to differentiate ulceration/necrosis caused by vitamin A deficiency from those caused by microbial infections. Secondary infection can occur because of inflamed conjunctiva and consequent decreased ocular surface barrier function. The generalised depressed immune status of the vitamin deficient child further increases the chance of secondary corneal infections. A thorough slit lamp examination is required to elicit features of secondary keratitis.

19.3.2.4 Phthisis Bulbi

Chronically inflamed and untreated advanced cases progress to perforation with loss of intraocular contents, subsequently to shrinkage of globe and development of phthisis bulbi.

19.3.3 Treatment

Treatment of Xerophthalmic manifestations at an early stage is pivotal to stop transition to advanced stage of the disease and avoidance of severe complications [4]. Stage III A with pupil sparing carries a relatively good prognosis with recovery of visual function as opposed to more advanced stages. Even if vitamin A deficiency has led to the stage of keratomalacia and irreversible loss of sight, it is imperative to administer treatment in order to save the other eye and the life of the patient [4, 10]. Vitamin A accelerates the development of epithelium, prevents keratinisation of

Table 19.2 Treatment schedule for xerophthalmia or keratomalacia[a]

WHO recommendations for Vitamin A dosage	
Immediately on diagnosis (Day 1)	110 mg Retinol palmitate, or 66 mg Retinol acetate (200,000 IU) orally, or 55 mg Retinol palmitate (100,000 IU) by intramuscular injection
Next day (day 2)	110 mg Retinol palmitate, or 66 mg Retinol acetate (200,000 IU) orally
Prior to discharge/clinical deterioration occurs/2–4 weeks later	110 mg Retinol palmitate, or 66 mg Retinol acetate (200,000 IU) orally
For children <1 year old these doses should be halved	

Recommended preparations of Vitamin A		
Formulation	Route	Dose
Oil-based solution of retinol palmitate or acetate, as capsule or liquid (with or without added Vitamin E)	Oral	110 mg Retinol palmitate or 66 mg Retinol acetate (200,000 IU)
Water miscible retinol palmitate	Intramuscular	55 mg (100,000 IU)

[a]Reprinted with permission. Adopted from: Control of vitamin A deficiency and xerophthalmia Report of a joint WHO/UNICEF/USAID/Helen Keller International/IVACG meeting, World Health Organization

epithelium and provides fatty acids that combines with vitamin A. Treatment protocol has been described in Table 19.2 [4].

19.3.3.1 Adjunctive Modalities

Corneal lesions in Xerophthalmia are considered an emergency. In addition to the immediate administration of retinol, prevention and treatment of secondary bacterial infections with broad spectrum antibiotic ointment (1% tetracycline eye ointment, every 8 h) with protection of eye with an eye-pad after each application especially in stage X3 is required. Topical tear substitutes should be initiated and exposure of corneal surface should be avoided.

Every effort should be made to preserve the structural integrity of the eye due to active keratomalacia, ulceration, or thinning. The eye must be protected from undue pressure examinations, applications of drugs, and dressing changes should be performed with utmost care. Eye should be covered, at all other times, by a plastic shield. If necessary, child's hands can be restrained to avoid undue rubbing.

19.3.3.2 Medical Status and Diet

Children with xerophthalmia, particularly in blinding and advanced stages, are often severely ill, malnourished, and dehydrated [7]. General supportive care, rehydration, and frequent feeding (by nasogastric tube if necessary) with easily digestible energy- and protein-rich foods is to be considered. Concurrent illnesses, such as respiratory and gastrointestinal infections, tuberculosis, worm infestations, and amoebiasis, should be treated with appropriate agents (antibiotics, antihelminthic, etc.).

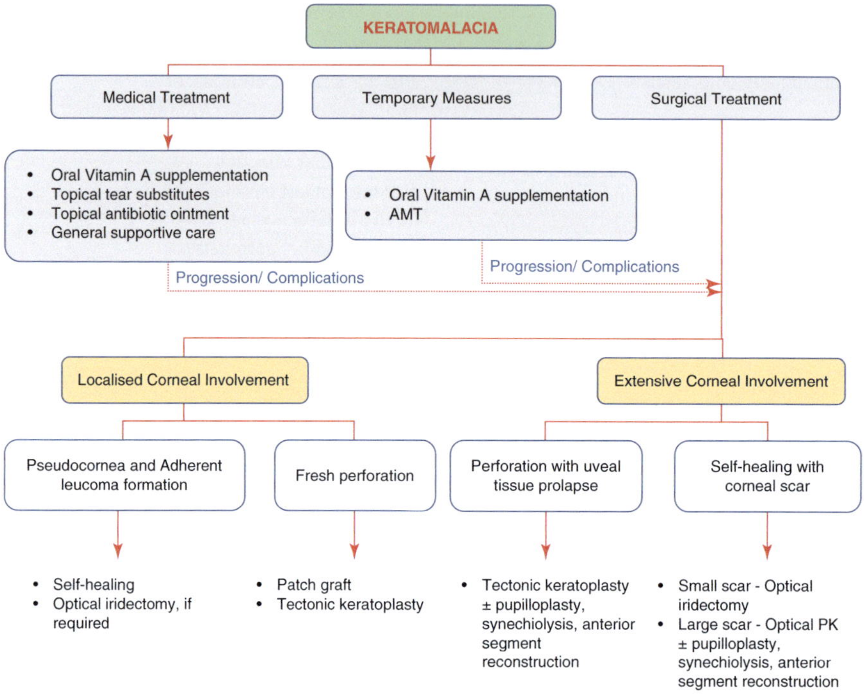

Fig. 19.5 Management options for keratomalacia. AMT: Amniotic membrane transplantation, PK: Penetrating keratoplasty

19.3.3.3 Surgical Management

Small perforated corneal ulcers are plugged by iris tissue and heal with adherent leukoma formation. Advanced necrosis of the cornea with or without perforation requires surgical intervention in the form of patch grafts and tectonic keratoplasty. Keratoplasty in paediatric eyes calls for careful planning and execution owing to the small anatomical configuration and decreased ocular rigidity [11]. Emergency tectonic/optical penetrating keratoplasty performed under GA with an oversized graft of 0.5–1 mm is the treatment of choice in such cases; procedure can be supplemented with pupilloplasty, synechiolysis, anterior segment reconstruction, and cataract extraction when necessary [11]. Amniotic membrane transplantation (AMT) in conjunction with oral vitamin A supplementation can be a useful temporary measure. Large grafts are invariably required because of the total corneal involvement by the melting process (Fig. 19.5).

19.4 Prevention

The ultimate aim for preventing corneal emergencies encountered in xerophthalmia should be directed towards early detection of vitamin A deficiency along with provision of regular, adequate dietary intake of vitamin A to vulnerable children especially in endemic regions. Early detection and stage-based intervention is critical to stop progression to sight threatening complications [7] (Box 19.1).

In few conditions, routine prophylactic vitamin A supplementation may also be required, such as for cases with impaired vitamin A absorption, storage, or transport. In developing countries where keratomalacia is a major cause of blindness, regular prophylactic vitamin A supplementation is recommended for children in appropriate doses as determined by age and other factors [2] (Table 19.3).

Box 19.1

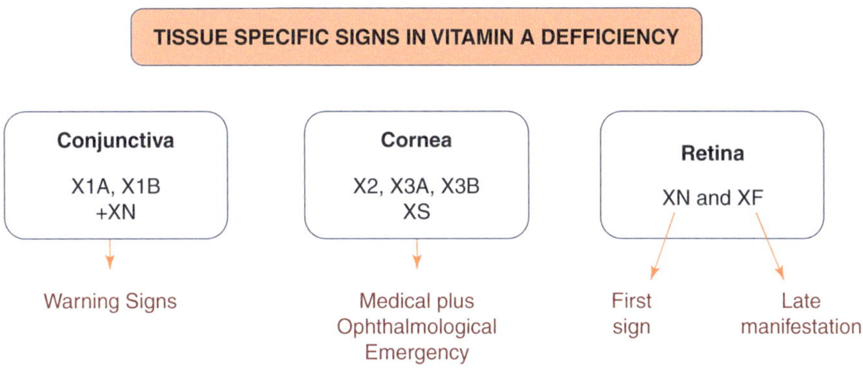

Table 19.3 WHO recommendation for prophylactic Vitamin A supplementation[a]

Suggested vitamin A supplementation scheme for infants and children 6–59 months of age		
Target group	Infants 6–11 months of age (including HIV+)	Children 12–59 months of age (including HIV+)
Dose	100,000 IU (30 mg Retinol equivalent) vitamin A	200,000 IU (60 mg Retinol Equivalent) vitamin A
Frequency	Once	Every 4–6 months
Route of administration	Oral liquid, oil-based preparation of retinyl palmitate or retinyl acetate	
Settings	Populations where the prevalence of night blindness is 1% or higher in children 24–59 months of age or where the prevalence of vitamin A deficiency (serum retinol 0.70 μmol/L or lower) is 20% or higher in infants and children 6–59 months of age	

In settings where vitamin A deficiency is a public health problem [prevalence of night blindness is 1% or higher in children 24–59 months of age or where the prevalence of vitamin A deficiency (serum retinol 0.70 μmol/L or lower) is 20% or higher in infants and children 6–59 months of age], high-dose vitamin A supplementation is recommended in infants and children 6–59 months of age

[a]Reprinted with permission. Adapted from: WHO Guideline: Vitamin A supplementation in infants and children 6–59 months of age. (https://www.who.int/publications/i/item/9789241501767)

19.5 Conclusion

Keratomalacia presents as a medical and ophthalmological emergency, usually with bilateral presentation, in vitamin A deficiency disease. Despite aggressive and timely intervention, keratomalacia remains a bilaterally blinding although a preventable disorder in young children with poor visual recovery and suboptimal functional results. Prompt diagnosis and appropriate treatment of xerophthalmia with vitamin A supplementation can stop the progression from benign stage to a stage of emergency.

Key Points

1. Xerophthalmia is a significant cause of corneal emergency in clinical practice.
2. To prevent the burden of xerophthalmia, a prompt diagnosis based on the detection of early signs is pivotal for management.
3. Prompt treatment of xerophthalmia with vitamin A supplementation can stop the progression to advanced stage manifesting as emergency.
4. Patients with advanced disease benefit with careful selection of surgical intervention.

References

1. Sommer A, Quesada J, Doty M, et al. Xerophthamia and anterior segment blindness among preschool-age children in El Salvador. Am J Ophthalmol. 1975;80:1066–72.
2. Dada T, Sharma N, Vajpayee RB. Indications for pediatric keratoplasty in India. Cornea. 1999;18:296–8.
3. McLaren DS. Vitamin A deficiency disorders. J Indian Med Assoc. 1999;97(8):320–3.
4. Sommer A. Vitamin A deficiency and its consequences: a field guide to detection and control. World Health Organization; 1995. http://whqlibdoc.who.int/publications/1995/92415447783_eng.pdf. Accessed 25 Aug 2020
5. Natadisastra G, Wittpenn JR, West KP, Sommer A. Impression cytology for detection of vitamin A deficiency. Arch Ophthalmol. 1987;105(9):1224–8.
6. Sommer A. Nutritional blindness. Xerophthalmia and keratomalacia. New York: Oxford University Press; 1982.
7. WHO/UNICEF/IVACG Task Force. Vitamin A supplements. A guide to their use in the treatment and prevention of vitamin A deficiency and xerophthalmia. 2nd ed. Geneva: World Health Organization; 1997. http://whqlibdoc.who.int/publications/1997/9241545062.pdf. Accessed 25 Aug 2020
8. Sommer A, Emran N, Tamba T. Vitamin A-responsive punctate keratopathy in xerophthalmia. Am J Ophthalmol. 1979;87(3):330–3.
9. Anderson JA, Richard NR, Rock ME, Binder PS. Requirement for vitamin A in long-term culture of human cornea. Invest Ophthalmol Vis Sci. 1993;34(12):3442–9.
10. Feroze KB, Kaufman EJ. Xerophthalmia. [updated 2020 Jun 22]. In: StatPearls [internet]. Treasure Island (FL): StatPearls Publishing; 2020. Available from: https://www.ncbi.nlm.nih.gov/books/NBK431094/. Accessed 25 Aug 2020.
11. Vajpayee RB, Vanathi M, Tandon R, Sharma N, Titiyal JS. Keratoplasty for keratomalacia in preschool children. Br J Ophthalmol. 2003;87(5):538–42.

20 Public Awareness, Preventive and Medicolegal Aspects in Corneal Emergencies

Deepak Soni, Aditi Dubey, Vidhya Verma, and Bhavana Sharma

20.1 Introduction

Ocular emergencies are an important cause of visual morbidity worldwide. Corneal emergencies add to a significant subtype of such visual crises. Studying their spectrum and presentation is vital for formulating preventive strategies. Corneal trauma, ulcers, and surgical procedures are the main entities which are associated with corneal emergencies. Amongst them, traumatic corneal injuries constitute a major segment. Public awareness and preventive measures are the mainstem of reducing corneal blindness secondary to lack of knowledge among the general population and inadequately managed corneal emergencies at the primary care level. Medicolegal aspects call for special attention as the majority of corneal emergencies carry a guarded prognosis and necessitate well-timed appropriate interventions to salvage achievable visual and structural integrity. This chapter intends to provide a comprehensive knowledge on prevention awareness and medicolegal aspects of corneal emergencies.

20.2 Awareness

Awareness and information regarding corneal emergencies are largely deficient amongst the general population, especially in developing countries with lower literacy rates. Community ophthalmologists and fieldworkers have consistently emphasized the need for increasing public awareness regarding the prevention and

D. Soni · V. Verma · B. Sharma (✉)
All India Institute of Medical Sciences, Bhopal, Madhya Pradesh, India
e-mail: head.ophtho@aiimsbhopal.edu.in

A. Dubey
Gandhi Medical College, Bhopal, Madhya Pradesh, India

B. Sharma, J. S. Titiyal (eds.), *Corneal Emergencies*,
https://doi.org/10.1007/978-981-16-5876-1_20

management of corneal emergencies. Awareness and knowledge are important for early consultation and maximization of visual prognosis in the majority of cases, so as to preserve the quality of life.

Preventable blindness is that which can be restricted/prevented by awareness at the community level and targeting the causative factor at an appropriate time. Blindness from corneal opacity is a significant public health burden that accounts for about 4.5% of cases of blindness worldwide [1]. Reduction in the prevalence of preventable and curable corneal blindness is one of the important objectives of the National Program For Control Of Blindness (NPCB) to bring down the overall incidence of blindness [2].

Conscious efforts directed to facilitate awareness supplemented with adequate protective measures can lessen the severity or even prevent many blinding corneal conditions. Such avoidable corneal emergencies comprise corneal ulcer, trachoma, keratomalacia, corneal trauma, i.e., mechanical (penetrating and blunt), chemical (acid, alkali, splashes, and fumes), radiational/thermal (ultraviolet, heat, or infrared radiation), foreign objects (projectile, dust, concrete, metal, wood, and other particles), fireworks and occupational/workplace-related injuries. Voon et al. reported that corneal trauma constitutes more than 75% of cases of corneal emergencies [3].

Strategies to control corneal blindness include prevention of eye infection, eye injuries, trachoma, and Xerophthalmia. The need for protective eyewear should be emphasized for industrial workers and agriculturists. Furthermore, promoting eye donation and keratoplasty through mass awareness remains an important goal to curb corneal blindness. Information, education, and communication (IEC) plays a vital role in achieving awareness among the general population, high-risk individuals and school-going children to reduce the burden of preventable corneal blindness secondary to corneal emergencies. Specific preventive measures (Fig. 20.1), targeted towards avoidance of sight-threatening corneal emergencies are described as follows:

20.2.1 Traumatic Corneal Emergencies

Corneal injuries contribute significantly to the burden of ocular injuries encountered in day-to-day practice. Owens et al. reported an annual incidence of more than 2.5 million eye injuries, out of which 2% of patients suffer permanent visual impairment [4]. They can occur in a wide variety of settings, including household, sports as well as work-related events. The probability of a particular type of injury is predominantly specific for a particular group of individuals, and accordingly, if a unique set of precautionary measures are undertaken, the risk of sustaining such injuries can be minimized. Corneal injuries are particularly frequent in developing countries owing to illiteracy, lack of knowledge about their devastating outcomes and hazards of the workplace not appreciated either by employers or employees. Approximately 44% of these injuries occur with household activities [5], as opposed to nearly 1 lac workplace-related eye injuries every year [6, 7]. Sports-related injuries have been seen to be commoner amongst children aged 5–14 years, and the

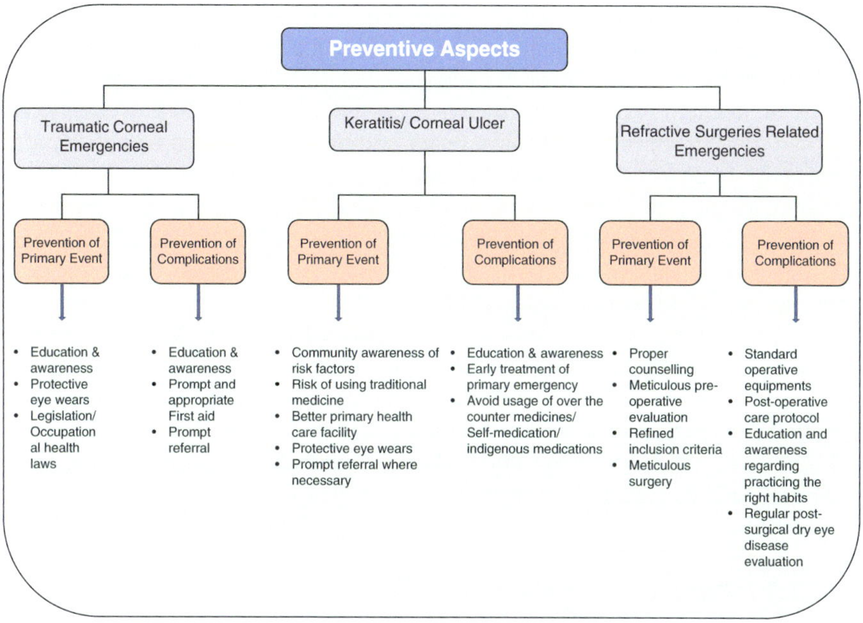

Fig. 20.1 Preventive aspects in different corneal emergencies

majority of them involve cornea [5]. The commonest cause of trauma in such cases has been reported to be wooden and sharp objects, broken toys and playtime activities [8]. Chemical injuries in pediatric patients are more commonly encountered in the pre-school age group [9], while in adults, it is more commonly correlated with occupation. The reported incidence of ocular chemical injuries in developing countries is approximately 1.25–4.4% [10].

Vajpayee et al. reported chemical injury from bursting of chuna packets as the most common mode of chemical injury in pediatric patients, especially in pre-school age group with an overall incidence of about 65% [9]. Management of severe chuna alkaline injuries typically requires a long period of treatment for restoration of visual acuity. Therefore, prevention becomes more significant in the pediatric age group, as there is an additional risk of the development of amblyopia. These pouches are malleable, and pre-school children view them as toys; when squeezed hard, the packet bursts, injuring the eye with calcium hydroxide. Increasing awareness towards the danger of chuna injury caused by these easily available and cheap pouches, keeping packets beyond the reach of children, ban on the use of these malleable pouches and replacement of packing with sturdy alternative material with a written warning on the possibility of eye damage can be done for decreasing their incidence. Awareness about first aid with copious irrigation and washing of eyes immediately after injury are important measures that can be utilized for the prevention of such injuries. Additionally, farmers, factory workers and persons involved in pharmaceutical manufacturing are predisposed for corneal chemical injuries, which require emergency management.

Firecracker injuries is one of the commonly seen causes of childhood corneal trauma, particularly during religious festivals [11]. In a retrospective study to document the profile of ocular firework injuries in children during the festive season of Diwali in Southern India, corneal trauma constituted more than 50% of cases [11].

Road traffic accidents constitute a major portion of mechanical corneal injuries irrespective of age group. Despite the different causes of corneal injuries, prevention remains the prime focus, and it includes awareness, required use of protective eye gears and legislative changes. However, more than 90% of ocular trauma, which includes corneal injuries in around 50% of cases, is preventable with the use of abovementioned preventive strategies [5–7].

The outcome can be devastating due to primary wound, secondary infection and sympathetic ophthalmia. The exacerbation of both injury and infection is often due to delay in proper management, delayed referral and inappropriate indigenous medication. Valuable time is hence lost for salvaging the visual and structural integrity. Primary care providers must be able to diagnose, initiate first aid and refer to identifiable corneal emergencies as any delay in treatment can result in permanent loss of vision.

20.2.1.1 Preventive Measures

Well planned and executed preventive measures can play a vital role in bringing down the incidence of visual impairment caused due to of corneal injuries. Training sessions can be used for educating employees on eye injury, their statistics and demonstrating the right ways to use eye safety gear. Acute chemical corneal injury treated immediately with copious irrigation and removal of trapped debris is associated with a significantly better visual outcome [9]. Early management aims to preserve the globe integrity, whereas subsequent treatment is targeted at promoting ocular surface epithelial recovery, augmenting corneal repair, minimizing ulceration, and controlling the inflammatory response [9, 12].

20.2.1.2 Information, Education, and Communication (IEC)

IEC is a method to educate and empower people to take decisions and adapt changes for positive outcomes. IEC in the prevention of corneal emergencies aims to increase awareness and change the pre-adapted practices in a targeted subset of people. A detailed knowledge of common modes of corneal trauma and the role of using protective gears in preventing sight-threatening corneal injuries can be effectively executed to educate susceptible groups through IEC.

IEC along with school curriculum can be used to inform and educate children about ocular and corneal injuries and their preventive measures. IEC activities can also be used to emphasize first aid management for corneal injuries that can improve the visual prognosis dramatically. The general population should be made aware of immediate referral of ocular trauma cases to eye specialists or tertiary care facilities for effective management. Likewise, the prevention of serious visual morbidity post chemical injury can also be achieved by raising awareness through IEC about the importance of immediate and copious irrigation after corneal exposure to chemicals.

20.2.1.3 Legislation

Legislative changes are important measures of prevention from corneal injuries, especially in underdeveloped countries. It becomes more reasonable in context to occupational, and sports-related corneal injuries. Prevention of sports-related corneal trauma involves the mandated use of protective gears in high-risk sports. Legislative enforcement in the USA lead to the dramatic decrease in the incidence of corneal ocular injuries related to hockey after protective eyewear was mandated [13]. Goggles that are closely fitted to the face of a soldier are superior to protective spectacles because they prevent the negative pressure associated with a blast from communicating with the space around the eye. Regulations and or prohibition towards the purchase and use of fireworks, especially for minors, and their restricted usage to unsupervised minors can be important in decreasing firework-related corneal trauma.

Preventive measures play the most important role in chemical injury-related trauma. Cases of vitreolage can be prevented through strict regulations pertaining to the sale and legitimate usage of chemicals in addition to the penalization of acid offenders. Legislative endeavors which can be adopted for the prevention of corneal injuries have been summarized in Box 20.1.

Box 20.1: Legislative Endeavor's Which Can Be Adopted for Prevention of Corneal Injuries

- Enforcement of safety standards with regard to workplace like proper illumination for industrial setups.
- Regulations on the sale and use of fireworks to minors.
- Mandatory usage and provision of protective devices in high-risk areas.
- Mandatory provision of first aid measures, in high-risk industries, particularly in chemicals-related work.
- Mandatory usage of seatbelts in cars.
- Mandating the distribution and documentation of dangerous chemicals to authorized persons.
- Improved primary health care service: primary health care workers should plan and execute preventive measures, facilitate the initial management and optimize referrals.

Key Points in Prevention of Corneal Injuries

- Health education can reduce incidences of corneal trauma by sharp toys and wooden objects, agricultural and industrial practices and household injuries.
- The provision of facilities for first aid can help reduce the magnitude of corneal trauma.
- Education for ocular protection should be integrated into the school curriculum at all levels. Safe playgrounds and parks that do not pose eye hazards should be provided in schools and residential areas.

- Mass media services should be utilized to create awareness regarding modes of corneal trauma, the need to prevent such accidents and protective measures.
- In addition to health personnel, school teachers and staff, senior grade students and social workers can be trained to disseminate information on the prevention of ocular injuries.
- Industrial injuries can be prevented by improving the safety features of machines, adequate illumination of work areas, ocular examination and visual fitness of workers, benchmark visual standards before deployment and usage of protective devices.

Preventive strategies in various types of corneal traumatic injuries are summarized in Table 20.1.

20.2.2 Infectious Keratitis

Infectious keratitis, as discussed in Chap. 5, has multiple etiologies, which varies with geographical areas, climatic conditions and socioeconomic status. Bacterial keratitis is more common among people who wear contact lenses in the developed world, while in developing countries, it is more commonly caused by occupation-related ocular trauma [14]. HSV keratitis is one of the emerging causes of unilateral infectious blindness and significantly impacts the quality of life even when patients are not experiencing an active infection. Fungal keratitis warrants targeted preventive efforts due to its higher prevalence among the lower socioeconomic and illiterate group. Education about right practices and information about first aid is the best preventative measures irrespective of the causative agent. Contact lens-related keratitis, being a rapidly emerging cause of recurrent and painful keratitis, needs more attention through preventive measures.

20.2.2.1 Preventive Measures

Health education and improvement in personal hygiene can reduce the incidence of corneal and other eye infections. Early treatment of corneal infections will prevent the conversion of less severe conditions into vision-threatening corneal blindness. In underdeveloped countries, eye care facilities are not easily approachable and accessible. Over-the-counter self-medication, particularly with topical steroids, remains one of the most important predisposing factors of mycotic keratitis, in addition to the progression of mild keratitis into severe corneal ulcers. Educating masses regarding avoidance of use of over-the-counter drugs for their potential consequences and to seek immediate medical assistance in case of acute eye symptoms instead of using self-medication, can significantly reduce the burden of infectious keratitis-related blindness. Prevention of viral keratitis is achievable by way of hand hygiene and spreading awareness to avoid touching the eyes, eyelids, and skin around eyes with unclean hands. Farmers and people employed in agriculture-related work should be informed about the potential risks of ocular contamination with organic matter, particularly livestock related and to avoid them through

Table 20.1 Prevention measures in different types of corneal traumatic emergencies

S No	Type of corneal trauma	Mode of injury	Preventive measures		
			Education	Protective eye gears	Legislation
1	Mechanical (corneal epithelial defects, laceration, perforation)	RTA	Awareness about precautionary measures such as seat belts, helmets Avoid driving under the influence of alcohol Eye should not be pressed and a protective eye shield should be applied as early as available	Use of polarized glasses for enhanced contrast and depth perception	To follow traffic rules Strict adherence with the use of protective safety gears
		Sport-related	Information about the potential hazards Avoid the use of spectacles during play, Players and staff should have adequate knowledge of first aid to be provided	Protective eye wear in high-risk sports, as the use of helmet-visors in American football or goggles in hockey. Protective eyewear—strong enough to withstand contact with high-speed implements without breaking. Protective goggles must be transparent providing distortion and fog free vision and allowing for peripheral vision	Mandatory use protective eye wears in high-risk sports
		Occupational	Training of employees to use personal protective equipment's at work. Employees should be provided comprehensive guidelines on preventing eye injuries and training on basic first aid treatment for eye injury	Wearing appropriate eyewear like safety goggles, face shields, full-facepiece respirators and helmets as needed	Well equipped first aid rooms
		Firecracker	Awareness programs should be directed towards explaining the hazards of firework-related ocular injuries to high-risk groups Parental education	Maintaining a safe distance and supervised firework remains the only protective gear available to avoid severe corneal injuries	Strict legislative rules on the prohibition of sell of firecrackers to unsupervised minors Implementation of firework laws

(continued)

Table 20.1 (continued)

S No	Type of corneal trauma	Mode of injury	Preventive measures		
			Education	Protective eye gears	Legislation
2	Chemical	Occupational	Written drafts of eye safety measures and their display Avoiding contact of chemicals with eye Avoid rubbing eyes with dirty hands or clothes. Clean eyewear before and after use. Awareness about initial first aid that involves passive opening of the eyelids and effective copious irrigation of the eye	Safety goggles, face shields	Mandatory establishment of easily accessible eyewash stations in areas where chemicals are used will help workers wash their eyes immediately. Regular inspection of safety gears
		Assault	Awareness of general population regarding prevention and first aid of chemical injuries		Legislation on the sale and distribution of strong acids and alkalis
3	Radiational and thermal	Occupational	Awareness about proper safety measures and first aid	Welding helmets, face shields, goggles, and full-face respirator	Laws to provide the right safety training and incorporate different safety elements to keep protection against thermal and radiational ocular trauma

personal measures. Primary care providers must be able to diagnose, initiate first aid and refer to identifiable corneal emergencies as any delay in treatment can result in permanent loss of vision.

20.2.2.2 IEC

Disseminating pertinent information to the general public on predispositions and pathogenesis of corneal ulcers, particularly to the illiterate and lower socioeconomic strata, is an effective measure for bringing down the incidence. Risk of developing a corneal ulcer in predispositions like trauma, lid infections, ocular allergies, contact lens wear, contact with contaminated water bodies, touching the eyes with contaminated fingers, systemic immune-compromised states like diabetes mellitus should be informed to masses through mass media. Vision-threatening outcomes of self-medication, indigenous medications, topical, and systemic steroids should be highlighted. Symptoms pertaining to corneal ulcer in patients with predispositions should be informed so that a prompt consultation and treatment by health care provider can be initiated. Important considerations while designing IEC module for prevention of corneal ulcer is described in Box 20.2.

Box 20.2: Important Considerations While Designing IEC Module for Prevention of Corneal Ulcer

- Wear protective glasses
- Avoid ocular contamination with organic matter
- Irrigate the eyes with clean water in the event of accidental entry of foreign body including organic matter.
- Avoid rubbing of eyes
- Avoid eye makeup
- Maintain hand hygiene
- Avoid sharing makeup, linen, or eye drops with others
- Follow contact lens hygiene.
- Discontinue wearing contact lenses while sleeping
- Take prescribed medications on time
- Avoid self-medication/over-the-counter medication
- Avoid using topical and systemic steroids without prescription
- Take proper treatment of systemic predispositions
- Wear an eye patch to avoid symptoms such as sensitivity to light
- If an eye surgery has been performed, do not allow water to enter your eye

Contact Lens-Related Keratitis

Contact lens wearers have an increased risk of corneal ulcers, especially when using extended-wear soft contact lenses. Failing to keep contact lenses or a contact lens case clean is an important predisposing factor. It is important to educate the contact lens user to follow cleaning and hygiene guidelines for contact lenses: Box 20.3.

Box 20.3: Cleaning and Hygiene Guidelines for Contact Lens Use

- Wash your hands thoroughly before handling your contact lenses or touching your eyes.
- Do not use tap water, bottled water, saline solution or rewetting drops to disinfect or store contact lens.
- Be sure to clean, rub, and rinse your lens each time you remove your lens before soaking it for disinfection. Rubbing and rinsing your contact lens will aid in removing harmful microbes and residues.
- Replace your contact lenses as recommended.
- Do not sleep in lenses you are supposed to remove every day.
- Do not wear contact lenses when you go swimming or for a shower.
- If there is any eye irritation, remove contact lenses, do not rub your eyes and seek medical attention.
- Close all bottles of contact lens solution properly after use.
- Discard contact lens solutions 1 month after opening.
- Replace your lenses and storage cases as recommended.

20.2.3 Keratomalacia

Non-infective keratitis particularly related to malnutrition can be effectively addressed through proper preventive measures. The World Health Organization (WHO) estimated that about 254 million children have Vitamin A deficiency and 2.8 million children have Xerophthalmia [15]. Corneal xerosis, corneal ulceration/keratomalacia and corneal scarring are major corneal manifestations of xerophthalmia. It is the most common cause of childhood blindness, with 3,50,000 new cases every year [16]. A one-year follow-up of corneal xerophthalmia cases shows that only 40% survive, and of the survivors, 25% are blind and 50% to 60% partially blind [16]. Looking at the large contribution of the disease to blindness, preventive measures play a major role. For the prevention and control of vitamin A deficiency, WHO recommended periodic administration of vitamin A supplements in areas where vitamin A deficiency is endemic, as summarized in Fig. 20.2 [17].

20.2.4 Corneal Refractive Surgeries

Meticulous pre-operative evaluation is the best preventive measure to avoid complications like corneal ectasia, flap complications, visual aberrations and DED. Furthermore, prophylactic topical antibiotics and pre-operative ocular and systemic examination is the best preventive measure for reducing the incidence of microbial keratitis in the immediate post-operative period. Meticulous attention to microkeratome assembly, cleaning, handling, storage, and intraoperative care for

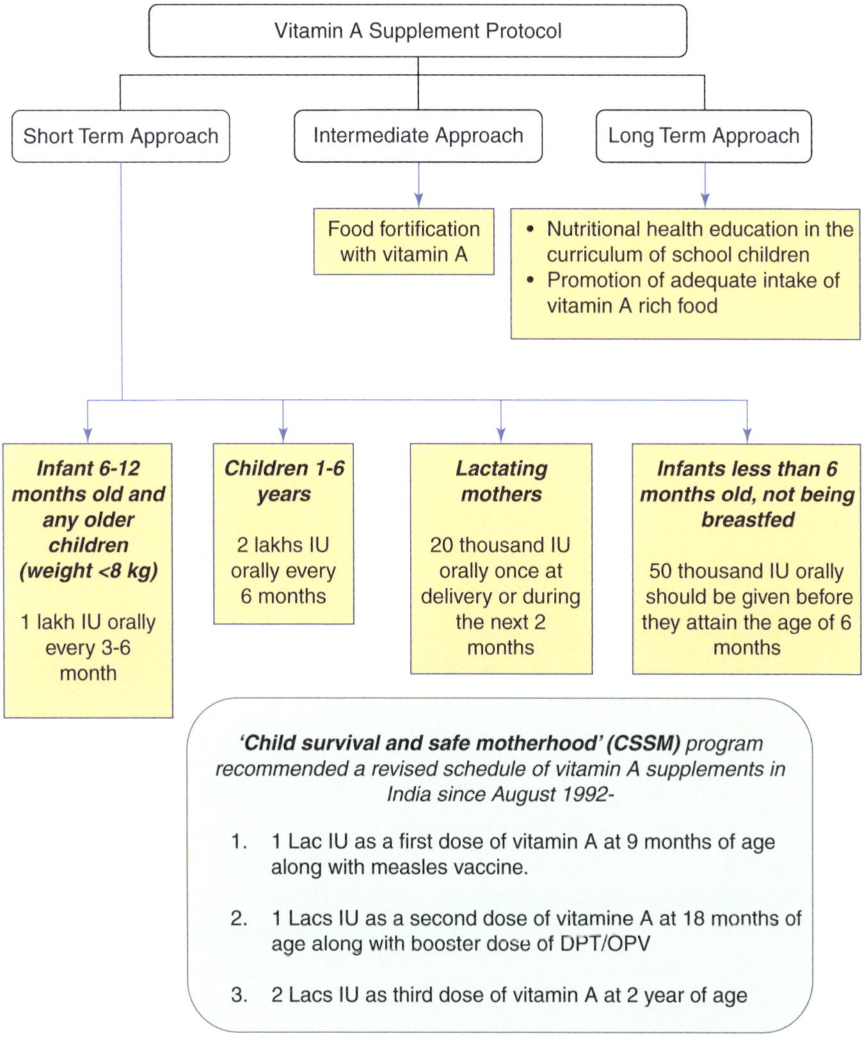

Fig. 20.2 WHO recommended guidelines for Vitamin A supplementation

the smooth translation of the keratome head may prevent various intraoperative complications.

Thin flaps and buttonholing are serious intraoperative complications that can be prevented by proper maintenance and handling of microkeratome. Eyes with previous scleral buckling and conjunctival scarring should be properly evaluated preoperatively to prevent any such intraoperative complications. A careful keratometry and topography prevent free cap formation in susceptible eyes, especially those with flat corneal curvature.

Precautions should be taken in the first 24 h after LASIK, as flap dislodgement occurs as a result of mechanical disruption due to blinking, lid squeezing and eye rubbing, and the same can be prevented with well-explained procedure, precautions, and consequences. The corneal ectatic disorder may increase the risk of drastic complications of corneal perforation, which requires emergency management. Due to improper adjustment of the thickness plate, the microkeratome blade can perforate the cornea during the pass. With newer microkeratomes that have pre-assembled fixed thickness plates inadvertent corneal perforation is not usually seen.

During laser ablation, corneal perforation can be an outcome of either improper calculation of stromal bed or excessive dehydration of the bed, which can be prevented by a meticulous pre-operative pachymetry. While intraoperative pachymetry before raising the corneal flap, after raising the corneal flap and after stromal ablation seems helpful in the prevention of corneal ectasia [18]. Patient cooperation during the procedure is essential for well-centered ablation, which requires good pre-operative counseling. Active eye-tracking systems can overcome the effects of Patient's involuntary eye movement to prevent decentered ablation. To prevent post-LASIK complications like keratitis, flap dislodgement and dry eyes, "care plan" will often include measures as described in Box 20.4.

Box 20.4: Care Plan to Prevent Post-LASIK Complications

- Topical tear substitutes
- During the healing process, it is important to avoid rubbing of eyes and use of protective eye shield for as long as recommended. Wear sunglasses when out in the sun for at least a month.
- Regular follow-ups should be continued for at least 6 months after surgery
- Prevent contact of shampoo, shower water, and soap from eyes
- Do not participate in any strenuous activities for the first 2 or 3 days.
- Avoid dry dusty or polluted environment for at least a week.

20.3 Medicolegal Implications

Ocular trauma cases account for 6–9% of all ophthalmology-related litigations [19]. Partial or complete loss of vision is an emotionally challenging event likely to decrease patient's quality of life and in turn persuade him or her to seek litigation. The following steps will minimize the medicolegal risk of the ophthalmologists when dealing with such corneal emergency cases, Box 20.5.

Box 20.5: Recommendations in Corneal Trauma

- Immediate primary care which is available should be provided to all emergency cases presenting with corneal trauma
- Detailed and meticulous documentation, best to document precise values and evident findings
- Explain potential risks and long-term squeal while taking informed consent
- Rule out intraocular foreign body associated with corneal trauma
- Use Steroids only where indicated and recommended
- Maintain good patient rapport
- Timely referral in cases requiring emergency management, not available at primary setup, to higher centers after providing primary care

20.3.1 Approach to Deal with Emergency Cases

The rule of thumb while dealing with corneal emergencies is "all emergency cases must be attended without delay and at least first aid should be provided before referring." In the event of non-adherence to this or denial to attend the same, especially while dealing with sight-threatening corneal emergencies, can invite legal proceedings. As per the supreme court of India "The priority of doctor should be saving lives of injured and not to make entries."

As per ICMR 2002 regulation no 2.1.1—"A physician advising a patient to seek service of another physician is acceptable, however, in case of emergency a physician must treat the patient. No physician shall arbitrarily refuse treatment to a patient. However, for good reason, when a patient is suffering from an ailment which is not within the range of experience of the treating physician, the physician may refuse treatment and refer the patient to another physician." [20] For instance, if any case of traumatic corneal perforation comes, then patient must be given primary care followed by primary repair of the wound, and once the emergent situation is satisfactorily dealt with the patient may be given an option to visit a concerned specialist for other ocular injuries if the trained person is not available at the site of primary care or if the patient wants the second opinion.

As per ICMR 2002 regulation no 2.4—"A physician is free to choose whom he will serve. He should, however, respond to any request for his assistance in an emergency. Once having undertaken a case, the physician should not neglect the patient, nor should he withdraw from the case without giving adequate notice to the patient and his family." [20] However, the treating doctor should exercise conscious efforts to administer specifically that treatment that falls within his expertise even though it may be an emergency. It is always prudent to address the corneal emergency in patients with the stable general condition. In case of unstable general condition, the patient should first be referred for management of systemic status and later for ocular intervention.

In a case where a patient of ocular trauma seeks treatment from practicing general ophthalmologist and if the ocular condition is beyond his expertise, it is advisable to refer the case after administering primary treatment. A referral letter to the patient with a receiving signature of patient or guardian with the date and time should be kept as a record. The Doctor should record the corneal injuries in detail with figures or photographs, all necessary investigations, consents, and prognosis must be documented. The patient should be treated as per the standard recommended norms.

As per ICMR 2002 regulation no 2.3—"The physician should neither exaggerate nor minimize the gravity of a patient's condition. He should ensure that the patient, his relatives or his responsible friends have such knowledge of the patient's condition as will serve the best interests of the patient and the family." [20] Cases presenting with corneal emergencies carry a wide variation in potential prognosis from very good to vision threatening. Patient and relatives must be explained clearly about the expected visual prognosis based on presenting clinical scenario. Counseling for prognosis becomes more important when a surgical intervention is planned.

20.3.2 Clinical Examination

A careful and detailed clinical examination to elucidate, quantify, and record the extent of damage is the most vital aspect in the management of a case of corneal emergency. Take photographs or draw simple sketches of the ocular condition wherever possible. This is particularly important while informing the status of damage and also its prognosis to the patient and their relatives. Clinical features which should be examined are as follows:

Corneal laceration—The type, location, grade, direction, dimensions, coexistent damage to other tissues and presence or absence of foreign bodies in the wound should be carefully noted. All descriptions relating to measurement should be accurate while avoiding terms like "about" "approximately" "likely."

Infectious keratitis—Meticulous clinical examination based on history and presentation is pre-requisite for preventing the progression of infectious keratitis to the visual threatening corneal emergency. Morphological features like size, location and depth of ulcer and infiltration, condition of uninvolved cornea and limbus, presence of hypopyon/anterior chamber reaction, satellite lesions, involvement of contiguous tissues and descemetocele/perforation should be noted.

Keratomalacia—Slit-lamp evaluation to look for dryness with loss of luster and melting/ulceration and perforation of the cornea, with the typical absence of inflammatory reactions, particularly in malnourished children.

Contact lens wear—Clinical features which should be looked for comprising of mucopurulent discharge, conjunctival injection, stromal edema and epithelial defect with underlying stromal infiltration in the midperiphery with or without anterior chamber reaction.

Chemical Injuries—Extent and depth of injury using a standard classification system should be documented to quantify the degree of corneal, conjunctival, and limbal involvement. Both the palpebral and bulbar conjunctiva need to be examined with fluorescein under a cobalt blue light. IOP documentation especially in cases with alkaline chemical injuries.

Post-surgical—Slit-lamp evaluation on the first post-operative day is crucial in timely management of early complications associated with corneal surgical procedures and consequent emergencies. Post corneal refractive surgery cases should be looked for position of flaps, corneal edema and infiltration. Post-keratoplasty cases require evaluation of sutures, anterior chamber integrity and signs of anterior chamber inflammation. Features suggestive of infection and raised IOP needs immediate attention in both situations.

20.3.3 Record Keeping

Document is the best evidence as law adheres to evidence; hence all records should be meticulously maintained in the form of prescription, intervention, referral notes, etc. In corneal emergencies, documenting the clinical findings in the form of corneal drawings should be mandatorily performed. The basic scheme for corneal drawings is illustrated in Fig. 20.3 [21]. It is always advisable to follow the standard protocol for corneal drawings rather than developing one's own as these can be uniformly followed and easily interpreted by other ophthalmologists. It is a good practice to avoid writing codes and unfamiliar short forms.

The Medical Council of India has mandated to preserve the records for a period of 3 years [20, 22]. Proper documentation and recording of minute details of the ocular treatment is pre-requisite for avoiding the charge of negligence. The prescription should be in own letterhead with details of patient and date which should be legible and signed. Computer records may not serve as authentic documents; hence a hard copy should be kept as a record [20, 23].

Medico Legal Case Register should record all MLC cases with date, time, finding, and description of injury—simple or grievous [24]. Record of all investigations should be mandatorily preserved data. It should be clear, detailed, accurate, and objective [24]. It is imperative for a medical establishment to inform the police whenever such cases come for treatment. Certificates pertaining to the type of injury and extent of damage should be issued to police or court on request. Medical Information of a patient is protected by the code of Professional Conduct framed under Section 33(m) read with Section 20-A of the Indian Medical Council Act. 1956 [20]. There is an exception to the general rule of maintaining the confidentiality of information of the patient, in as much as such information can be disclosed in public interest or disclosure is solicited by the court of law [20].

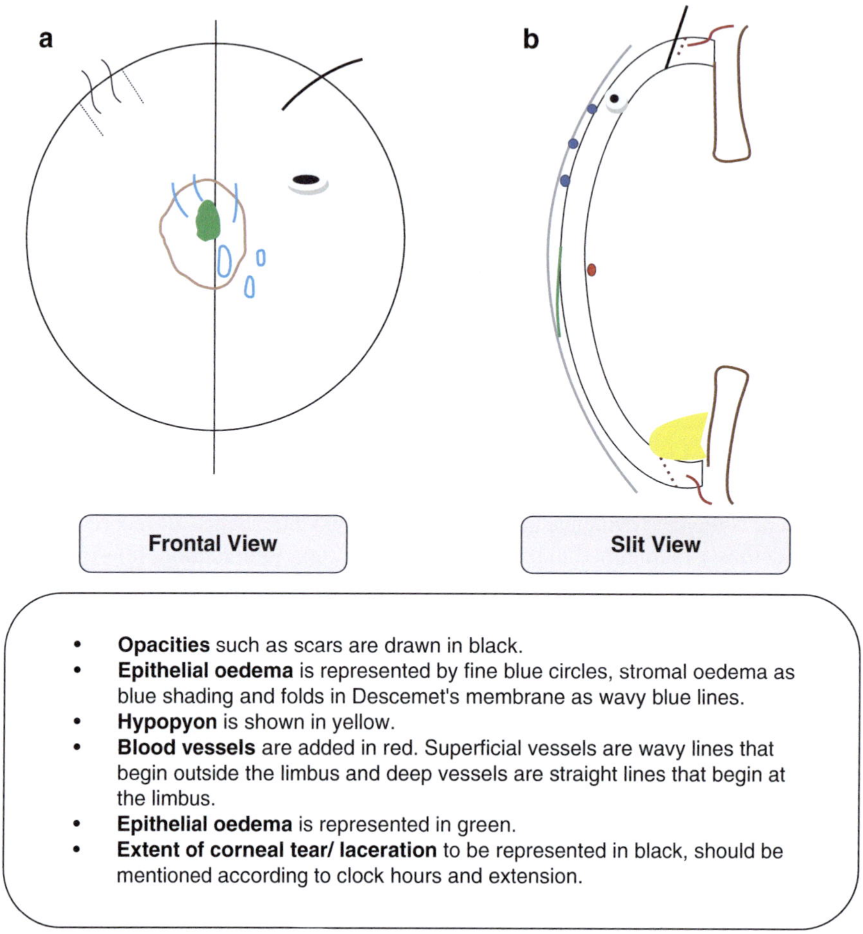

Fig. 20.3 Corneal draw chart

20.3.4 Informed and Documented Consent

Medical or Surgical intervention in each case should be cautiously planned with informed consent in patient's language. It is defined as "Voluntary agreement, compliance, or permission for specified act or purpose" [25]. The Indian contract Act Section 13, states "two or more persons are said to consent when they agree up on the same thing in the same sense" [25]. Any intervention medical or surgical without consent will be considered as an internal interference with the patient's body without legal sanction and liable for damage claim. Consent is to be obtained from conscious, mentally sound adults or from the parent of a child who is <12 years of age [26]. Cataract and corneal surgeries account for the majority of the claims filed in courts [27]. Permanent privation of the sight of either eye has been termed as grievous injury, which makes it a punishable offense under IPC Section 320 [28].

The valid consent—not only protects the ophthalmologist from civil liability but also from criminal liability—Sec 87 of IPC Act [25]. Informed consent is the process in which a health care provider educates a patient about the risks, benefits, and alternatives of a given procedure or intervention in a language understandable by the patient/legal guardian and documenting the same with a witness signature. Various essential components of the consent have been recommended by different ophthalmologic organizations [25, 29–32]. Parts of valid consent includes:

1. The nature of the procedure including type of anesthesia to be administered.
2. The risks and benefits of the procedure.
3. Reasonable alternatives.
4. Risks and benefits of alternatives.
5. Assessment of the patient's understanding of above.

However, consent does not give complete immunity from being negligent. Consent is de facto given for the risk associated with the procedure for which the consent is obtained. If complication happens or risk materializes due to negligence—the consent will not be considered in court [25]. Exceptions to informed consent: (1) the patient is incapacitated, (2) life-threatening emergencies with inadequate time to obtain consent, and (3) voluntary waived consent [33]. In a recent judgment, the National Consumer Disputes Redressal Commission has held that "consent is implicit" in emergency cases where the patient was brought in seriously injured condition and waiting for the consent of patient or passer-by who brought the patient in the hospital is "deficiency in services."

Precautions to be taken prior to ophthalmic emergency surgery to make the surgeon safe:

(a) Take physical fitness from a Physician.
(b) Always have a qualified stand-by Anesthetist.
(c) O.T. should have an oxygen cylinder, suction machine, emergency drugs as per standard list.
(d) Written informed consent in patient's language.

While dealing with corneal injuries in emergency, police should be informed within 24 h from the admission in the hospital in cases of [25]:

1. Grievous injury with a history of assault (perforating corneal injuries and chemical injuries).
2. In cases of patient's death.
3. Where cause of death cannot be certified.
4. During surgical or interventional ophthalmological procedure, death occurs (death on table).

20.4 Conclusion

A major proportion of corneal blindness due to causes related to corneal emergencies are amenable to prevention or cure in the majority of cases, by the reasonable deployment of preventive measures and timely interventions. Blindness due to infectious and traumatic causes and nutritional deficiencies can be effectively prevented by concerted preventive measures adopted by authorities and masses. Similarly, predisposing factors relating to corneal surgeries, contact lens use, Stevens-Johnson syndrome and other corneal pathologies are largely avoidable and treatable with appropriate and timely interventions.

Areas with a high prevalence of corneal morbidity and where preventive strategies are not in place should be identified to initiate committed efforts for the prevention and management of such cases. Emphasis should be placed on developing primary eye care facilities and a rapid referral system. However, secondary and tertiary facilities should also be developed to provide therapeutic interventions, facilitate training and overall sensitization of the complete ocular health care network. Education for eye safety should be integrated into the school syllabus at all levels. The key to the prevention of corneal emergencies lies in the coordinated approach of health care providers, administrative authorities and the general population themselves towards whom the integrated efforts are targeted. Strengthening community cooperation in behavior, rituals, and environment can go a long way in the reduction/elimination of factors contributing to corneal emergencies and subsequent corneal blindness.

Guidelines for primary health care workers while dealing with ocular diseases with corneal involvement at primary set up as summarized in Box 20.6.

Box 20.6: Guidelines for Primary Health Care Worker While Dealing with Ocular Diseases with Corneal Involvement at Primary Set up

Conditions recognized and treated by the primary health care worker

- Conjunctivitis and lid infections
- Sub-conjunctival hemorrhage
- Conjunctival and corneal foreign bodies
- Corneal abrasion
- Xerophthalmia—conjunctival and corneal xerosis, Bitot's spots
- Chemical injuries—first aid

Conditions recognized and referred after treatment has been initiated

- Corneal ulcers
- Corneal lacerations
- Keratomalacia
- Chemical injuries

Conditions recognized and referred for further treatment to higher Center

- Any cause which has led to visual loss/visual deprivation
- Steven Johnson syndrome
- One-eyed patient

Key Points

- Prevention and awareness are major weapons to fight preventable blindness arising from corneal emergencies.
- Role of community ophthalmologists and field workers needs to be strengthened to create awareness and deal appropriately with corneal emergencies.
- Information, education, and communication (IEC) plays a vital role in achieving awareness among the most susceptible sections of society.
- Corneal trauma, ulcers, and refractive surgeries are the most common entities seen to be associated with corneal emergencies.
- Proper use of protective eye wears, provision of strict guidelines and adequacy of first aid is pivotal to the prevention and prognosis of occupational corneal traumatic emergencies.
- School-based awareness and strict legislation are pre-requisite to reduce the burden of childhood traumatic corneal emergencies.
- Education and awareness regarding healthy contact lens habits and stay away from the use of over-the-counter and traditional medications prevent the keratitis-related emergencies.
- Approach to deal with a case of corneal emergency and strict adherence to the rules of documentation and consent are a crucial part of medicolegal aspects.

References

1. Burton MJ. Corneal blindness: prevention, treatment and rehabilitation. Community Eye Health. 2009;22(71):33.
2. Verma R, Khanna P, Prinja S, Rajput M, Arora V. The national programme for control of blindness in India. Australas Med J. 2011;4(1):1–3.
3. Voon LW, See J, Wong TY. The epidemiology of ocular trauma in Singapore: perspective from the emergency service of a large tertiary hospital. Eye (Lond). 2001;15(Pt 1):75–81.
4. Owens PL, Mutter R. Emergency department visits related to eye injuries, 2008: statistical brief #112. 2011 may. In: Healthcare cost and utilization project (HCUP) statistical briefs [internet]. Rockville (MD): Agency for Healthcare Research and Quality (US); 2006. Available from: https://www.ncbi.nlm.nih.gov/books/NBK56035/.
5. American Academy of Ophthalmology and American Society of Ocular Trauma. United States eye injury registry summary report, 1998–2002. http://www.aao.org/newsroom/guide/upload/Eye-Injuries-BkgrnderLongVersFinal-l.pdf

6. National Institute for Occupational Safety and Health (NIOSH). Healthy people 2010. Vision. Fact sheet: eye safety at work is everyone's business. www.cdc.gov/Features/dsworkPlaceEye/
7. Harrison A, Telander DG. Eye injuries in the youth athlete: a case-based approach. Sports Med. 2002;31(1):33–40.
8. Singh S, Sharma B, Kumar K, Dubey A, Ahirwar K. Epidemiology, clinical profile and factors, predicting final visual outcome of pediatric ocular trauma in a tertiary eye care center of Central India. Indian J Ophthalmol. 2017;65(11):1192.
9. Vajpayee RB, Shekhar H, Sharma N, Jhanji V. Demographic and clinical profile of ocular chemical injuries in the pediatric age group. Ophthalmology. 2014;121(1):377–80.
10. Xie Y, Tan Y, Tang S. Epidemiology of 377 patients with chemical burns in Guangdong province. Burns. 2004;30:569–72.
11. John D, Philip SS, Mittal R, John SS, Paul P. Spectrum of ocular firework injuries in children: a 5-year retrospective study during a festive season in southern India. Indian J Ophthalmol. 2015;63(11):843–6.
12. Wagoner MD. Chemical injuries of the eye: current concepts in pathophysiology and therapy. Surv Ophthalmol. 1997;41(4):275–313.
13. Dain SJ. Sports eyewear protective standards. Clin Exp Optom. 2016;99(1):4–23.
14. Gopinathan U, Sharma S, Garg P, Rao GN. Review of epidemiological features, microbiological diagnosis and treatment outcome of microbial keratitis: experience of over a decade. Indian J Ophthalmol. 2009;57(4):273.
15. West KP Jr. Extent of vitamin A deficiency among preschool children and women of reproductive age. J Nutr. 2002;132(9 Suppl):2857S–66S.
16. Feroze KB, Kaufman EJ. Xerophthalmia [updated 2020 Jun 22]. In: StatPearls [internet]. Treasure Island (FL): StatPearls Publishing; 2020. Available from: https://www.ncbi.nlm.nih.gov/books/NBK431094/.
17. Underwood BA. Prevention of vitamin A deficiency. In: Prevention of micronutrient deficiencies: tools for policymakers and public health workers. Institute of Medicine; 1998. p. 103–66.
18. Sridhar MS, Rao SK, Vajpayee RB, Aasuri MK, Hannush S, Sinha R. Complications of laser-in-situ-keratomileusis. Indian J Ophthalmol. 2002;50(4):265.
19. Bettman JM. Seven hundred medicolegal cases in ophthalmology. Ophthalmology. 1990;97:1379–84.
20. Code of medical ethics regulation. ICMR guidelines 2002. https://www.mciindia.org/CMS/rules-regulations/code-of-medical-ethics-regulations-2002
21. Bowling B. Kanski's clinical ophthalmology: a systematic approach. 8th ed. Saunders; 2016. p. 172.
22. Aggarwal KK, Gupta I. Maintenance and preservation of medical records. Indian J Clin Pract. 2019;29(12):1184. https://ijcp.in/Admin/CMS/PDF/21.%20Medicolegal_IJCP_May2019.pdf
23. Thomas J. Medical records and issues in negligence. Indian J Urol. 2009;25(3):384–8.
24. Meera T. Medicolegal cases: what every doctor should know. J Med Soc. 2016;30(3):133.
25. Verma L. Legal aspects in ophthalmology. All India Ophthalmological Society. https://www.aios.org/cme/cmeseries27.pdf
26. Chaturvedi A. Consent-its medico-legal aspects. Medicine update; 2000. pp. 883–7. http://apiindia.org/wp-content/uploads/pdf/medicine_update_2007/153.pdf.
27. Agarwal D, Kumar A, Sundar D. Commentary: medico legal aspects in ophthalmology in India. Indian J Ophthalmol. 2019;67(10):1526.
28. Yadav M, Bansal MK. Critical analysis of grievous hurt section 320, 326, IPC: a case law. Indian Internet J Forensic Med Toxicol. 2019;17(4):93–7.
29. Pandey SK, Sharma V. Commentary: increasing cases of litigations against ophthalmologists: how can we minimize litigations during ophthalmic practice? Indian J Ophthalmol. 2019;67(10):1527.
30. Anderson OA, Wearne IM. Informed consent for elective surgery—what is best practice? J R Soc Med. 2007;100(2):97–100.

31. Skene L, Smallwood R. Informed consent: lessons from Australia. BMJ. 2002;324(7328):39–41.
32. Scanlan D, Siddiqui F, Perry G, Hutnik CM. Informed consent for cataract surgery: what patients do and do not understand. J Cataract Refract Surg. 2003;29(10):1904–12.
33. Shah P, Thornton I, Turrin D, et al. Informed consent. [updated 2020 Jun 1]. In: StatPearls [internet]. Treasure Island (FL): StatPearls Publishing; 2020. https://www.ncbi.nlm.nih.gov/books/NBK430827/.

Index

B. Sharma, J. S. Titiyal (eds.), *Corneal Emergencies*,
https://doi.org/10.1007/978-981-16-5876-1

S

MIX
Papier aus verantwortungsvollen Quellen
Paper from responsible sources
FSC® C105338

FSC
www.fsc.org

If you have any concerns about our products,
you can contact us on
ProductSafety@springernature.com

In case Publisher is established outside the EU,
the EU authorized representative is:
Springer Nature Customer Service Center GmbH
Europaplatz 3, 69115 Heidelberg, Germany

Printed by Libri Plureos GmbH
in Hamburg, Germany